"I am most delighted to welcome David Twicken's new book, *I Ching Acupuncture—The Balance Method*. This book lays a solid foundation for understanding the background theories of acupuncture. The simplicity and clarity of presenting a profound subject is truly fantastic."

—*Joseph Yu, founder of Feng Shui Research Center, Toronto, Canada*

"There have been many books on the *I Ching* and acupuncture, but rarely with such clear integration of a deeper and thorough understanding of this ancient philosophy and wisdom. David Twicken's book has given the readers what we need to know, 'The Balance Method,' in learning and partaking in these treasures from the sages of the old China."

—*Master Chungliang Al Huang, founder of Living Tao Foundation and author of* Embrace Tiger, Return to Mountain, Essential Tai Ji, Quantum Soup *and* The Chinese Book of Animal Powers

"I have followed David Twicken's work since 1998. He has authority of lineage and direct knowledge, which brings clarity and accuracy. This work is mature and it is my number one recommendation when learners ask me what resources there are for *Yijing* theory as it pertains to acupuncture."

—*William R. Morris, PhD, President, AOMA Graduate School of Integrative Medicine, Austin, Texas*

C000165328

"In classical Chinese medicine, the highest level doctors utilize the *Yijing* to deepen their understanding of the medicine itself, and to enhance their clinical results. In his book, *I Ching Acupuncture—The Balance Method*, David Twicken provides the serious practitioner with a method for far-reaching healing through the guidance of the *Yijing*."

—*Master Zhongxian Wu, lineage holder of four schools of Qi Gong and martial arts, and author of* Vital Breath of the Dao, Seeking the Spirit of the Book of Change *and* Chinese Shamanic Cosmic Orbit Qigong

"The most brilliant, concise, penetrating synthesis of Taoist cycles ever done. Suddenly, the *I Ching* trigrams, Ten Stem/ Twelve Branch Chinese calendar, Yin–Yang, Five Phase, twelve hour body clock and Six Channel medical theories all leap into sharp, unified focus. More amazingly, Twicken turns theory into easily grasped 'how-to' practice. Finally we have a clear map of Taoist body channels, natural models of healing and life-balance that acupuncturists, Taiji and Qi Gong players, energy healers, and feng shui and astrology adepts cannot do without."

—*Michael Winn, founder of HealingTaoUSA.com and co-author of seven Tao books with Mantak Chia*

I Ching Acupuncture

The Balance Method

of related interest

Seeking the Spirit of The Book of Change
Eight Days to Mastering a Shamanic Yijing (I Ching) Prediction System
Master Zhongxian Wu
Foreword by Daniel Reid
ISBN 978 1 84819 020 7

Yijing, Shamanic Oracle of China
A New Book of Change
Richard Bertschinger
ISBN 978 1 84819 083 2

Wan's Clinical Application of Chinese Medicine
Scientific Practice of Diagnosis, Treatment and Therapeutic Monitoring
Giorgio Repeti, LAc
With Marc S. Micozzi, MD, PhD
ISBN 978 1 84819 047 4

I CHING ACUPUNCTURE

THE BALANCE METHOD

CLINICAL APPLICATIONS OF THE BA GUA AND I CHING

DR. DAVID TWICKEN, DOM, LAc

To Joanne,

Happy birthday — and
happy needling!

Love,
Charlie & Clio xxx

16/12/21

SINGING
DRAGON

LONDON AND PHILADELPHIA

First published in 2012
by Singing Dragon
an imprint of Jessica Kingsley Publishers
116 Pentonville Road
London N1 9JB, UK
and
400 Market Street, Suite 400
Philadelphia, PA 19106, USA

www.singingdragon.com

Library of Congress Cataloging in Publication Data
A CIP catalog record for this book is available from the Library of Congress

British Library Cataloguing in Publication Data
A CIP catalogue record for this book is available from the British Library

ISBN 978 1 84819 074 0
eISBN 978 0 85701 064 3

Printed and bound in the United States

CONTENTS

DISCLAIMER 12

ACKNOWLEDGEMENTS .13

AUTHOR NOTE 14

INTRODUCTION 15
    Chinese Metaphysics Models   *16*

PART 1 ORIGINS, PRINCIPLES AND THEORY

CHAPTER 1 QI 21
    Life Cycles   *21*
    Qi   *23*

CHAPTER 2 YIN–YANG 27
    Opposition   *30*
    Interdependence   *30*
    Mutual Consumption   *30*
    Inner Transformation   *30*
    Tai Chi Theory   *31*

CHAPTER 3 EIGHT TRIGRAMS AND THE EARLY HEAVEN BA GUA 33
    Three Forces   *33*
    Yin and Yang Lines   *34*
    Eight Trigrams   *34*
    I Ching Numerology   *36*
    Formation of the Eight Trigrams and the Early Heaven Ba Gua   *38*
    Structure of the Eight Trigrams   *42*
    Structure of the Early Heaven Ba Gua   *46*
    Application of the Early Heaven Ba Gua in Acupuncture   *47*

CHAPTER 4 FIVE PHASES 49
    Five Phases Cycles   *51*
    Five Phases Correspondences   *55*
    Five Phases Shapes   *57*
    Integrating Eight Trigrams and Five Phases   *59*

CHAPTER 5 THE HE TU DIAGRAM. 65

The He Tu Diagram   *65*

Structure of the He Tu   *67*

CHAPTER 6 NINE PALACES. 71

The Nine Palaces Diagram   *71*

Structure of the Nine Palaces   *72*

CHAPTER 7 THE LATER HEAVEN BA GUA 75

The He Tu Diagram and the Nine Palaces as the Origins of the Later Heaven Ba Gua   *77*

Comparing the Later Heaven Ba Gua with the Early Heaven Ba Gua   *81*

CHAPTER 8 THE CHINESE CALENDAR. 91

The Ten Heavenly Stems   *91*

The Twelve Earthly Branches   *92*

The Stem and Branch Cycle of 60   *95*

The Twelve Earthly Branches and the Chinese Zodiac Animals   *97*

The Twelve-Stage Growth Cycle   *102*

The Chinese Calendar   *104*

The Origin of the Daily Meridian Clock   *108*

The Nine Palaces   *108*

The Cosmological Daily Meridian Clock   *120*

The Daily Meridian Clock, Channels and Internal Organs   *127*

PART II CLINICAL APPLICATIONS

INTRODUCTION TO PART II 137

The Acupuncture Layering System   *137*

CHAPTER 9 BALANCE METHOD 1: BALANCING SIX CHANNEL PAIRS 141

Theory and Applications   *142*

Chinese Metaphysics and Six Channel Pairings   *143*

CHAPTER 10 BALANCE METHOD 2: BALANCING YIN–YANG PAIRED CHANNELS 153

The Ba Gua and Yin–Yang Acupuncture Channel Pairs   *154*

The Ba Gua and Opposite Channel Pairs   *160*

Applying Balance Method 2   *162*

CHAPTER 11 BALANCE METHOD 3: BALANCING
WITH STREAM AND SEA ACUPOINTS—THE 3–6
BALANCE METHOD 163
   Assigning Acupuncture Points to Hexagrams   *164*
   Applying Balance Method 3   *165*
   Balance Method 3 Guidance   *170*

CHAPTER 12 BALANCE METHOD 4: BALANCING THE
DAILY MERIDIAN CLOCK. 171
   Applying Balance Method 4   *171*

CHAPTER 13 BALANCE METHOD 5: BALANCING
CHANNEL CORRESPONDING NAMES AND
POSITIONS 175
   Applying Balance Method 5   *177*

CHAPTER 14 BALANCE METHOD 6: BALANCING
HEXAGRAMS 181
   Hexagram 61   *185*
   Selecting Favorable Hexagrams   *187*
   A Step-by-Step Explanation for Balancing Hexagrams   *191*
   A Synopsis of the Favorable Hexagrams   *191*
   Guidance for Acupuncture Needling   *254*

  APPENDIX I SIX CLINICAL CASES FOR BALANCE METHOD 6 255
   Case 1   *255*
   Case 2   *256*
   Case 3   *257*
   Case 4   *258*
   Case 5   *260*
   Case 6   *261*

  APPENDIX II SUMMARY OF I CHING ACUPUNCTURE—THE BALANCE
  METHOD 263
   Balance Method 1   *263*
   Balance Method 2   *263*
   Balance Method 3   *264*
   Balance Method 4   *264*
   Balance Method 5   *264*
   Balance Method 6   *264*
   Summary Table   *265*

CONCLUSION. 267

BIBLIOGRAPHY 269

List of Figures and Tables

Figures

3.1	Classical Diagram of Ancient Chinese Cosmology	39
3.2	The Early Heaven Ba Gua	42
3.3	The Eight Trigrams Grouped by their Yang-Yin Polarity	43
3.4	The Eight Trigrams: Their Names and Positions in the Ba Gua	44
3.5	The Eight Trigrams: The Number of Strokes in each Trigram	45
3.6	The Early Heaven Ba Gua and Nine	46
3.7	The Early Heaven Ba Gua and the Human Body	48
4.1	The Five Phases	50
4.2	The Five Phase Promotion Cycle	51
4.3	The Five Phase Controlling Cycle	52
4.4	The Five Phase Reduction Cycle	53
5.1	The He Tu Diagram	66
5.2	The He Tu Diagram with Numbers	66
5.3	The He Tu Pairings	68
5.4	The He Tu and the Human Body	69
6.1	The Nine Palaces	72
6.2	The Nine Palaces and the Human Body	74
7.1	The Later Heaven Ba Gua	75
7.2	The Later Heaven Ba Gua and the Five Phases	76
7.3	The He Tu	80
7.4	The He Tu Expanded to the Nine Palaces	80
7.5	The Later Heaven Ba Gua	80
7.6	The Later Heaven Ba Gua with Numbers and Five Phases	80
7.7	The Early Heaven Ba Gua and Trigrams Positions	81
7.8	The Nine Palaces Numbers for the Later Heaven Ba Gua Trigrams	82
7.9	The Five Phases are Integrated into the Nine Palaces and Each Palace Contains an Element	83
7.10	The Geographical Locations are Integrated into the Nine Palaces	84
7.11	The Nine Palaces Combines Numbers, Five Phases and Geographical Directions	85
7.12	The Integrated Nine Palaces	86
7.13	The Nine Palaces: Early Heaven Ba Gua	87
7.14	The Nine Palaces: Later Heaven Ba Gua	88
7.15	The Nine Palaces: Early and Later Heaven Ba Gua Combined	89
7.16	The Early Heaven and Later Heaven Ba Gua Combined	90
8.1	The Twelve Earthly Branches	93
8.2	The Twelve Branches	98
8.3	The Branches and Hidden Elements	101
8.4	The Twelve-Stage Growth Cycle	103
8.5	The Nine Palaces and He Tu	109
8.6	Nine Palaces Showing Acupuncture Channel Correspondences	110
8.7	The Twelve Branches, Elements and Directions	125
8.8	The Twelve Branches and the Times of Day	126

8.9	The Twelve Branches, Channels and Internal Organs	127
8.10	The Fire Branch Trinity	129
8.11	The Wood Branch Trinity	130
8.12	The Metal Branch Trinity	131
8.13	The Water Branch Trinity	132
9.1	The Nine Palaces	145
9.2	The Early Heaven Ba Gua	151
10.1	The Ba Gua with the 12 Acupuncture Channels	161
12.1	The Daily Meridian Clock in a Circular Format	173
12.2	The Daily Meridian Clock in a Grid	174
13.1	Two Trigrams and their Corresponding Lines	175
13.2	Hexagram Composed of Two Trigrams	176
13.3	Hexagram with the Six Stages	176
14.1	The Favorable Hexagrams	190
14.2	The Later Heaven Ba Gua	193

TABLES

I.1	Chinese Dynasties	17
2.1	Yin-Yang Correspondences	19
4.1	The Five Phases Table	54
4.2	The Eight-Trigram Correspondences	63
8.1	The Ten Heavenly Stems	92
8.2	The Twelve Earthly Branches	94
8.3	The Stem and Branch Cycle of 60	96
8.4	The Twelve Branches and their Name, Element, Season, Time of Day and Direction	99
8.5	The Branches and Hidden Elements	100
8.6	The Five Phases Elements and Seasons	102
8.7	The Twelve-Stage Growth Cycle	104
8.8	The 24 Seasons	106
8.9	The Arm and Leg Channels	133
9.1	The 12 Joints and Acupuncture Channels	144
9.2	The Six Channel Pairings	152
10.1	The Body and the Yin–Yang Acupuncture Channels	161
11.1	The Yang Channels: Hexagram Lines and Acupuncture Points	164
11.2	The Yin Channels: Hexagram Lines and Acupuncture Points	165
11.3	The Stream and Sea Points	166
13.1	The Yang Channels: Hexagram Lines and Acupuncture Points	177
13.2	The Yin Channels: Hexagram Lines and Acupuncture Points	177
13.3	Hexagrams and the Six Channels: Application 1	178
14.1	Hexagrams and Primary Channels	183
14.2	The Yang Channels: Hexagram Lines and Acupuncture Points	183
14.3	The Yin Channels: Hexagram Lines and Acupuncture Points	184
14.4	The 64 Hexagrams	188

Disclaimer

The information in this book is based on the author's knowledge and personal experience. This information is presented for educational purposes to assist the reader in expanding his or her knowledge of Chinese philosophy and Chinese medicine. The techniques and practices are to be used at the reader's own discretion and liability. The author is not responsible in any manner whatsoever for any physical injury that may occur by following instructions in this book.

ACKNOWLEDGEMENTS

I would like to thank Dr. Chao Chen. A legend in the acupuncture community, Dr. Chen combined aspects of *I Ching*, Chinese medical theories and his clinical experience and wrote a thesis in 1976: *Essence of Acupuncture Therapy as Based on Yi King and Computers*. In the text, Dr. Chen outlines his theory and clinical practice of corresponding balance. I was fortunate to meet Dr. Chen and learn directly from him and his son Yu Chen. I want to thank both of them for sharing their knowledge and experience with me. Dr. Chen has made a significant contribution to the practice of acupuncture.

I would like to thank Molly Maguire for her friendship, inspiration and editorial guidance. Your contributions helped make this book a reality; for this I will always be grateful.

Thank you, Jessica Kingsley, for sharing my vision of this book and supporting my dream of having it published. Your guidance was invaluable to this book's creation. My deepest appreciation to you for making this book available to anybody interested in learning these ancient theories, principles and applications.

AUTHOR NOTE

For the past 30 years I have studied, practiced and taught Chinese metaphysics and Chinese medicine. The arts I have studied include Taoist philosophy, *I Ching*, feng shui, Chinese astrology, qi men dun jia, Tai Chi Chuan, Qi Gong, nei gong, acupuncture and herbal medicine. The philosophies and models within those systems comprise many of the theories for the practice of Chinese medicine. In this text, these classic theories and models are presented to provide you the key to unlock the mysteries behind many applications in Chinese medicine, especially the practice of acupuncture.

INTRODUCTION

Chinese medicine is based on principles, theories and applications of Chinese metaphysics. The fundamental theories of Chinese medicine can be traced back to the Zhou dynasty, the second historic period of China. Understanding Chinese medicine and its theoretical bases requires a deep understanding of Chinese metaphysics, which is a major objective of *I Ching Acupuncture—The Balance Method*. The central goal of this text is to present acupuncture applications based on Chinese metaphysical theories. A clear understanding of these theories, which are unified in *I Ching* theory, increases intention and clinical effectiveness, which are the primary goals of medicine. Intention holds a special place in Chinese arts, whether martial arts, Qi Gong or medicine.

The Chinese have a unique understanding of the body and mind. In Chinese creative, martial and healing arts, there is a saying: "Where the mind goes, Qi will follow." Another way to say this is: mind leads Qi. The aspect of the body-mind that can focus one's attention is called *Yi*. Aspects of Yi include focus, concentration and intention. Wherever intention is focused, Qi is directed to that area. With practice or cultivation, the ability to direct Qi is developed to higher levels. Cultivating this skill is a major aspect of martial arts and Qi Gong practice. As a person builds their personal energy or Qi with meditation, Qi Gong, Tai Chi Chuan or other practices, it can be directed internally throughout their body, promoting health and vitality. When a person learns more about their body, especially the locations of the acupuncture channels, they can direct Qi in the channels and the areas in which they flow throughout the body. The knowledge of the body provides the terrain for Yi to focus, and Qi will flow where the Yi is directed. The quantity of Qi a person has, and the knowledge where to direct it, are keys to using Yi effectively.

Having a deep understanding of the principles and theories of Chinese philosophy and *I Ching* theory increases intention, because such understanding allows for a comprehensive foundation of why a method works, which increases the ability of the practitioner to select effective treatments. Knowing how a method works within a human body allows the practitioner to visualize the system or method being applied; Yi can be focused on the areas to be treated. Naturally, this creates an exchange of Qi between practitioner and patient. The level of the practitioner's Qi creates the amount of the Qi exchange, and this Qi exchange increases the healing effect. Practitioners can develop intention by practicing Qi Gong and meditation, which are branches of Chinese medicine.

The Balance Method integrates Chinese metaphysics and Chinese medical classics, thereby *balancing* the underlying philosophy of Chinese medicine with practical applications of acupuncture technique. Both are referenced to trace the path of the originators of acupuncture. The first part of this book introduces fundamentals of Chinese philosophy, including Qi, Yin–Yang, Five Phases, Eight Trigrams, Ba Gua, 64 Hexagrams, Luo Shu, He Tu and the Chinese calendar. The second part of the book presents clinical applications for acupuncture.

Chinese Metaphysics Models

There are four major models and two significant philosophies that comprise the main aspect of Chinese metaphysics; all of them contain applications for divination and healing arts. The major models are the Early Heaven Ba Gua, Later Heaven Ba Gua, He Tu and Luo Shu. The major philosophies are Yin–Yang and Five Phases. Chinese culture attributes the origin of these classic models to pre-historic figures, with the exception of the Later Heaven Ba Gua. There is no consensus regarding the origins of Yin–Yang and Five Phases theory; however, historians agree that these two ideas were integrated with other major models of Chinese metaphysics during the Warring States Period of the Zhou dynasty, marking the origin of the common Chinese medicine practiced today. This book explains how fundamental aspects of Chinese philosophy became integrated, creating guiding principles for modern Chinese medicine.

Chinese literature contains the "Five Classics," attributed to Confucius and his students, a record of their views from pre-historic time through the early historic period. The Five Classics comprise the *Classic of Poetry, Classic of History, Classic of Rites, Classic of Changes* and *Spring and Autumn Annals*. The four major models presented in this book are listed in the Five

Classics, but their forms, theories and applications are minimal compared to the depth of common knowledge found from the Han dynasty to modern times.

TABLE I.1 CHINESE DYNASTIES

Dynasty	Years
Pre-historic period	
Yangshao	5000 BC
Longshan	2500 BC
Xia	2100–1600 BC
Historic period	
Shang	1600–1045 BC
Zhou	1045–221 BC
Western Zhou	1045–771 BC
Eastern Zhou	770–256 BC
Spring and Autumn Period	722–481 BC
Warring States Period	403–221 BC
Qin	221–206 BC
Han	206 BC–AD 220
Western Han	206 BC–AD 24
Eastern Han	25 AD–AD 220
Three Kingdoms	220–280
Jin (Western and Eastern)	265–420
Southern and Northern	420–589
Sui	581–618
Tang	618–907
Five Dynasties and Ten Kingdoms	907–960
Song	960–1279
Liao	916–1125
Jin	1115–1234
Yuan	1271–1368
Ming	1368–1644
Qing (Manchu)	1644–1911
Republic of China	1912–1949
People's Republic of China	1949–present

PART I

ORIGINS, PRINCIPLES AND THEORY

Chapter 1

QI

The ancient Chinese had a profound understanding of the changing nature of their world. Living close to nature, the indigenous Chinese people observed stars and planets and the unique qualities of the four seasons and perceived how humanity responded to these natural phenomena and cycles. Nature's patterns include daily, monthly, seasonal and lifetime cycles, and with keen insight they perceived the singular, primary influence contained in every cycle and aspect of life: change.

Two classic Chinese books, the *I Ching* (*The Book of Changes*) and the *Nei Jing* (*The Inner Classic of Chinese Medicine*), both highlight change as their central theme. The *I Ching* presents life *as* change and provides guidance and advice on how to live in harmony with change.

Life Cycles

The first chapter in the *Nei Jing Su Wen* presents a major cycle of change: women and men's transitions through life cycles of seven and eight years. Each stage brings unique, yet natural, qualities each person will experience. The following is a summary of the seven- and eight-year cycles for males and females found in the *Nei Jing Su Wen*. Males have eight-year cycles, and women have seven-year cycles. These cycles are examples of the Chinese insight that change is a central part of life.

The female cycles of seven years are as follows:

- A woman's Kidney energy becomes prosperous at seven years of age (1×7).

- Her menstruation appears as the *Ren* (Sea of Yin) Channel flows and the *Chong* (Sea of Blood) Channel becomes prosperous at the age of 14 (2×7).

- Her Kidney Qi reaches a balanced state, and her teeth are completely developed at the age of 21 (3×7).

- Her vital energy and blood are substantial, her four limbs are strong and her body is at optimal condition at the age of 28 (4×7).

- Her peak condition declines gradually. The Yang Ming Channel is depleted, her face withers and her hair begins to fall out at the age of 35 (5×7).

- Her three Yang Channels, Tai Yang, Yang Ming and Shao Yang, begin to decline. Her face complexion wanes and her hair turns white at the age of 42 (6×7).

- The Ren and Chong Channels are both declining, her menstruation ends, her physique turns old and feeble, and she can no longer conceive at the age of 49 (7×7).

The male cycles of eight years are as follows:

- A man's Kidney energy is prosperous, his hair develops and his teeth emerge at the age of eight (1×8).

- His Kidney energy grows and is filled with vital energy, and he is able to let his sperm out at the age of 16 (2×8).

- His Kidney energy is developed, his extremities are strong, and all of his teeth are developed by the age of 24 (3×8).

- His body has developed to its best condition, and his extremities and muscles are very strong at the age of 32 (4×8).

- His Kidney energy begins to decline, his hair falls out and his teeth begin to wither at the age of 40 (5×8).

- His Kidney energy declines more, the Yang energy of the entire body declines, his complexion becomes withered and his hair turns white at the age of 48 (6×8).

- His Liver energy declines as a result of Kidney deficiency; the tendons become rigid and fail to be nimble at the age of 56 (7×8).

- His essence and vital energy is weak, as are his bones and tendons; his teeth fall out and his body becomes decrepit at the age of 64 (8×8).

These cycles are nature's cycle of human development. The *Nei Jing Su Wen* suggests that if we do not live in harmony during these life cycles, we can suffer from self-created stress and illness and prematurely age, as we will be acting against the natural rhythmic unfolding of our lives. This classic book offers guidance on how to live in harmony during the seven- and eight-year cycles, with the twin goals of longevity and the satisfaction of living out our destined lifetime.

The second chapter of the *Nei Jing Su Wen* presents the four seasons of the year, their seasonal qualities, and their influences on people. It describes conditions that may occur if we live lifestyles out of tune with seasonal energetics, and offers guidance about how to live in balance with each season. When we live in harmony with a season we benefit not only from that season's energy, but also from the next season's energetics. When we obtain a benefit from one season, it prepares us to benefit from the next season, building a synergistic influence throughout a year. The Chinese studied this influence deeply and perceived a force not only inside cycles of time, but within everything in life. They named this influence *Qi*. Chinese philosophy and medicine is a profound study of Qi.

Qi

Qi comprises all of life. The solar system, mountains, oceans, plants and humanity are comprised of Qi of different densities, moving through endless flows of transformation. Qi includes both matter and energy. It is the force that allows the transformation from energy to matter and matter to energy. For example, water, a type of Qi, is a perfect example of how Qi transforms. Water can exist in the form of ice, which can transform into water, while water can transform into steam. Qi is ice, Qi is water, Qi is steam and Qi is the heat that allows the transformation to occur: Qi is all of life. It takes form to become the densest substances as well as the subtlest substances. Every part of the universe is a blend of different types of Qi. To understand this blending is to understand the energies of life. Knowing the rhythms and expressions of Qi is to be able to both predict and transform life. Chinese philosophy and metaphysics is, essentially, a study of the variations and patterns of Qi. Chinese medicine can be considered applied Chinese philosophy—in effect, a complex study of the transformations and stages of Qi. All of the arts in Chinese culture, including Chinese medicine, feng shui, Chinese astrology and Qi Gong, are based on a deep study of Qi.

Stages of Qi

The Chinese description of Qi is steam rising from rice being cooked: the cooking process creates Qi, the result of three elements: rice, water and heat. Qi is the result of interactions, and the stages of interactions are defined by unique names to clearly identify the specific processes involved, allowing analysis, diagnosis and treatment for each stage or situation. In Chinese medicine, prenatal essence or energies is called Jing. From a Western perspective Jing would be similar to DNA. Jing contains our genetic code or the blueprint of our life, and it unfolds in many patterns. The longest patterns are the cycles of seven and eight years of unfolding for females and males.

In Chinese medical theory, the body is viewed in three major sections, which are called the three Jiao (San Jiao). These Jiao are the lower, middle and upper Jiao. The lower Jiao ranges from the perineum to the Kidneys, the middle Jiao is from the Kidneys to the diaphragm area, and the upper Jiao is from the heart area and above. The lower Jiao and the Kidneys contain what the Chinese call Jing. The original spark of life from a Chinese medical perspective is when Jing, which is Yin, is ignited by the body's Yang, or heat. This Yang cooks the Jing to create the first Qi in the body. The Chinese name for "original" is Yuan. Original or Yuan Qi is created when Jing is cooked by Yang. The image is seen as Yang-cooks-Yin (Jing) to create steam, which is Yuan Qi. This Yuan Qi ignites all the body's organs and functions, and continually replenishes them throughout our life.

The lower Jiao is the first stage in the transformation of Qi, from Jing to Yuan Qi. The middle Jiao includes the Stomach and Spleen. In Chinese medical theory, a person consumes food and water and these organs break them down and transform them into Qi. This Qi produced from the transformation of food and drink is called Gu Qi. The Spleen then

transports the Gu Qi to the Lungs, where it mixes with breath or o
to create what the Chinese call Zhong Qi. This Zhong Qi is transp
through the body in the upper Jiao: a portion moves into the acupun
channels, and another portion is transported to the external layers o
body.

The transformations in the lower, middle and upper Jiao, as described
above, show how each Jiao produces different Qi. When imbalances
exist within one of the Jiao or organ systems, they display unique signs
and symptoms, which become the basis for analysis and treatment. Qi
continually transforms throughout the body as it moves from the three
Jiao or areas of the body, and their corresponding organs, glands and
anatomical structures.

Qi is contained in every model of Chinese metaphysics: Yin–Yang,
Eight Trigrams, Ba Gua, 64 Hexagrams and Five Phases. Therefore,
understanding Qi, its transformations and stages is essential for
understanding all aspects of Chinese philosophy and Chinese medicine.

Chapter 2

YIN–YANG

Chinese medicine and healing is applied philosophy. Chinese philosophy is based on the direct experience of nature, and from this experience philosophical models were developed reflecting the realities of life. The models and philosophical ideas within them are applied to the human body and healing, creating applied philosophy. Originally, the philosophies were simple. Over time they were expanded to elegant and seemingly complex theories and principles that would be applied to most every aspect of Chinese culture. In China, a model of understanding nature evolved that would form the building blocks of Chinese philosophy, acupuncture, herbal medicine, Qi Gong, nutrition, martial arts, feng shui and astrology: the model is Yin–Yang.

The first reference to Yin–Yang was in the classic book *I Ching*. Yin–Yang theory grew for centuries into a highly sophisticated system and became its own school, the Yin–Yang School, which in turn became part of the Naturalist School. This school viewed nature as a positive force and promoted living in harmony with nature's laws, Yin–Yang being a way to understand them. This theory becomes a model to facilitate deeper understanding of nature and ourselves. Yin–Yang theory is eventually applied to the human body and becomes a primary principle in the *Nei Jing* (*The Inner Classic of Chinese Medicine*). A deep understanding of Yin–Yang allows a deeper understanding of Chinese medicine.

Early writings on Yin–Yang are based on the image of a hill, where the sunny side is Yang and the dark side is Yin. This initial view expands to light and darkness, day and night, and to all of life; every aspect of life is categorized into Yin–Yang. Yin–Yang is a relationship-based theory. When two things are compared to each other, one will be Yin and the other will be Yang. For example, to experience cold we must have the experience of heat; each of these experiences gives life to the other. Every aspect of life can be compared to another aspect within the Yin–Yang model. The most complex situations can be reduced to Yin–Yang theory, providing the basis for diagnosis and treatment. Yin–Yang is a major aspect of systems of correspondences, a primary theory of Chinese medicine. Systems of correspondences are the guiding principle in classical Chinese medicine; it is a systematic method to identify the relationships between two or more things, and is a major aspect of the Balance Method.

Yin–Yang includes viewing the universe as one integrated whole, as well as two opposing but interdependent aspects. The smallest and largest can be categorized into Yin–Yang. For example, heaven–earth, man–woman, hot–cold, left–right, light–dark, front–back, hard–soft, North–South, East–West, top–bottom, fast–slow, waxing–waning, timely–untimely, empty–full and auspicious–inauspicious are Yin–Yang correspondences. Yin–Yang theory categorizes any situation into two parts; each part is inseparable from its opposite. For example, there must be a left to have right, a strong to have weak, and a front to have a back; they are not two separate entities but two sides of the same situation. Yin–Yang is a model which views a situation as consisting of two parts while simultaneously existing as one inseparable whole. This dynamic is integral to understanding Yin–Yang.

A major application of Yin–Yang theory is based on Yang representing a growing or expanding phase and Yin a declining phase. The daily cycle of sunlight and darkness, and the yearly cycle of the four seasons, are examples of natural expanding and declining cycles. Sunrise represents the expansion stage and nighttime reflects the declining stage. Spring and summer reflect the growth cycle and the fall and winter the declining cycle. All of life flows through this basic model of rising and declining. Each expansion leads to a decline, leading to another expansion and decline, in an endless cycle. Table 2.1 lists major Yin–Yang correspondences.

Within a cycle Yin–Yang contains four major interactions: opposition, interdependence, mutual consumption and inner transformation. Each of these four Yin–Yang interactions is a way to influence a situation. These interactions are the foundation relationships of the methods and applications described in this book.

TABLE 2.1 YIN–YANG CORRESPONDENCES

Yang	Yin
Positive	Negative
Sunny	Shady
Light	Dark
Sun	Moon
Day	Night
Heaven	Earth
East	West
Left	Right
South	North
Round	Flat
Movement	Stillness
Exterior	Interior
Expansion	Contraction
Fire	Water
Wood	Metal
Spirit	Matter
Hot	Cold
Large	Small
Wide	Narrow
Rising	Declining
Male	Female
Summer	Winter
Intuitive	Logical
Above	Below
Active	Rest
Son	Daughter
Back	Front
Top	Bottom
Happy	Sad
Hun	Po
Yang	Yin

;ition

)n contains the relationship of opposing aspects of life. All
‎ life have an opposite relationship, in that there are always two
‎ e same condition, which are inseparable. Because opposites are
two sides of the same situation, when one side is influenced, the other is
also influenced. There is no exception to this dynamic. This theory is a
guide for treating the opposite anatomical area of imbalance.

Interdependence

Interdependence contains the dynamic that there is an inseparable
relationship between two parts of a whole: each part requires the other to
exist and each influences each other. This is a guiding theory to identify
and treat acupuncture channels or anatomical areas that are interdependent.

Mutual Consumption

Yin–Yang is in dynamic interaction and naturally adjusts to maintain
balance by one area consuming the other, maintaining homeostasis. This
is a guiding theory to find and treat the mutually consuming acupuncture
channel to treat an imbalance of excess or deficiency.

Inner Transformation

Yin–Yang is a cyclical pattern where one aspect changes into the other,
as night transforms into day and day transforms into night. There is
an inner force that drives this natural movement. This transformation
requires two conditions: the first is when innate conditions are ready or
ripe (for example, when an egg becomes a chick). The second is timing:
transformation occurs when the time is ready for change to occur. This is
a guiding principle for understanding the nature of a condition and the
duration of a treatment, and for perceiving the response of the patient.

These four dynamics of Yin–Yang are integrated and exist at all times;
they are major principles in the *Nei Jing* and *I Ching Acupuncture—The
Balance Method*.

Tai Chi Theory

Yin–Yang theory extends into every Chinese philosophical system, including Tai Chi theory. The Tai Chi diagram and its theory is an integral aspect in Chinese philosophy, and its principle is contained in all Chinese metaphysical arts. The Tai Chi symbol contains the principle of Yin–Yang, and it explains how Yin–Yang is inseparable; it is the force that drives unity and dynamic interaction of Yin–Yang.

The Tai Chi symbol is shown below, which symbolizes the interactions of Yin–Yang: opposition, interdependence, mutual consumption and inner transformation. This classic symbol contains three, not two, forces or energies:

- The first is Yang, the white area.

- The second is Yin, the black area.

- The third is the center curving line and it is called the Yuan line or force; it is the glue or force that contains Yin–Yang as one inseparable whole.

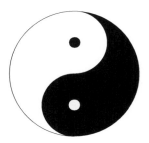

The white circle in the black area reveals how the seeds of Yang exist in Yin, and the black circle in the white area reveals how the seeds of Yin exist in Yang.

The Tai Chi symbol includes the center force: this is the curve in the center of the symbol, and it unifies Yin–Yang. It is the balancing energy and glue for the inseparable nature of Yin–Yang. From a medical perspective, it is the guiding principle to find balance when there is an imbalance. Tai Chi theory contains the principle that within each situation there is a balancing or harmonizing situation. Notice in the Tai Chi diagram how the curving line in the center extends to both Yin and Yang areas, and how it curves, implying a dynamic force, a changing force; life is not static. Yin–Yang flows in a dance up and down, left to right, front to back and side to side. Yin–Yang contains a range, and as long as we stay within the range of the circle, we have balance. Tai Chi is the center force that maintains a balancing force to maintain harmony.

If the balance of Yin–Yang is altered, something new is created and the integrity of the original pattern is changed. For example, if a person sits in the sun she will obtain healing properties of the sun, but if she stays too long in the sun it can burn her body, creating pain and possible sunstroke; this condition breaks Yin–Yang balance.

Yin–Yang implies a range of dynamic play, it is not a fixed range. Each person has a unique range of balance, and Chinese medicine provides tools to identify imbalances, while *I Ching* acupuncture offers strategies for clinical point selection to restore balance.

Chapter 3

EIGHT TRIGRAMS AND THE EARLY HEAVEN BA GUA

Three Forces

The Tai Chi symbol embodies three forces. There is another important symbol and code in Chinese culture that also contains three forces: a trigram. In Chinese, a trigram is called a *gua*.

A trigram:

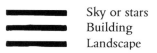

The three lines can be viewed in a similar way to the three forces in the Tai Chi symbol, and can be applied to all aspects of life. For feng shui purposes, the top line represents the sky, the middle line a building and the bottom line the landscape.

Sky or stars
Building
Landscape

Yin and Yang Lines

Shade or *darkness* is Yin, and there are two dashes or two strokes for a Yin line. This two-lined image is Yin. Two is an even number, and all even numbers are Yin.

▬ ▬

Light or *brightness* is Yang, and Yang is an unbroken line. One is an odd number, and all odd numbers are Yang.

▬▬▬

Yin and Yang lines are images that reflect life. A trigram can be viewed as heaven, human and earth or, in Chinese medicine, as Shen (spirit), Qi and Jing:

Heaven
Human
Earth

Shen
Qi
Jing

This image of life, composed of three lines representing the influences of heaven, human and earth, is based on San Qing, a key concept for understanding Chinese philosophy. San Qing can be translated as "the three forces," and is a guiding principle for the Eight Trigrams and *I Ching* theory. A trigram reflects the three forces and the basic theory of San Qing.

Eight Trigrams

A circle represents the oneness of life; from this oneness we can view life in two major parts: Yin and Yang. Yin–Yang can expand in many ways. One is the trinity of life: heaven, human and earth, represented in a trigram, as shown above. Yin and Yang lines can be combined in a trigram in eight different ways: the Eight Trigrams.

A trigram reflects the concept of integration, whereby each line influences the other two lines. It is an expansion of Yin–Yang theory into three forces or three influences, and because these three forces are interdependent, evaluation of all three lines is required to obtain a complete understanding of a situation.

The early *I Ching* contained Yin–Yang theory and symbolism. The images of the trigrams, for example Lake, Wind, Mountain and Water, are symbols or metaphors for areas of life to which they correspond. For example, in Chinese medicine Water relates to the Kidneys and Bladder; therefore the Water trigram would imply that those organs are involved in a particular condition. Each trigram is a code that holds a variety of related information about every aspect of life, and is a microsystem for understanding areas of disharmony and imbalance. All of life can be categorized into Yin–Yang, as well as trigrams.

The Eight Trigrams are codes that reveal information about every aspect of life. The Eight Trigrams have unique formations—the Early Heaven and Later Heaven formations, which are described later in this chapter and in Chapter 7. Each of these formations is called a Ba Gua. Each Ba Gua is based on natural logic and one of the most influential mathematical models in the modern world, the binary system.

One way the Chinese view the energetics of life is based on Yin–Yang theory. The *I Ching* begins with Yin–Yang theory and expands into Eight Trigrams; this process of unfolding is a foundation theory for the Balance Method. The following introduces the unfolding of *I Ching* theory and the creation of the Eight Trigrams and the Early Heaven Ba Gua.

I Ching theory uses a line system to explain how life unfolds through origin, growth and completion, and it follows a three-step energetic pattern, as follows:

- One gives life to two: Yin–Yang.

- Two give life to three: Tai Chi or a trigram.

- Three, or Tai Chi, gives life to all things.

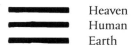 Heaven
Human
Earth

I Ching Numerology

In *I Ching* theory, there are numerous numerological systems. One system is based on Yin–Yang, and in this system the number one is excluded. (The number one represents the inclusion of all things as one inseparable whole.) The numbers two and three set the theory for Yin–Yang.

Odd numbers are Yang and even numbers are Yin. The polarity of a number is based on this pattern of odd and even numbers. According to *I Ching* theory:

- Heaven is symbolized by the number three, and Yang numbers.

- Earth is symbolized by the number two, and Yin numbers.

In other words, Yang numbers are odd and represent heaven, and even numbers are Yin and represent earth.

When integrating a trigram and this numerical theory, a unique pattern and polarity of numbers appears. The method is to place the number two with each line in a trigram, which creates the number six; as an even (Yin) number, six represents earth.

$$
\begin{array}{c}
\underline{} \quad 2 \\
\underline{} \quad 2 \\
\underline{} \quad 2
\end{array}
$$

The total for the three lines in this trigram is six, a Yin number and a *reducing* or *declining* pattern.

The number three is placed at each line in a trigram, which sums to nine; as an odd (Yang) number, nine represents heaven.

$$
\begin{array}{c}
\underline{} \quad 3 \\
\underline{} \quad 3 \\
\underline{} \quad 3
\end{array}
$$

The total for the three lines in this trigram is nine, a Yang number and an *increasing* or *reinforcing* pattern. The three levels represent the aspects of a person: physical, mental and spiritual. Applying numbers at each level creates a number that influences each aspect of a person. Six influences Yin and all levels of a person, and nine influences Yang and all levels of a person.

Chinese philosophy contains a primary principle: Humans are part of an inseparable trinity of heaven, human and earth. Trigrams reflect this trinity. Placing numbers next to each line creates the influences of these three dimensions on a person. This process of assigning numbers to lines in a trigram is an example, and sets a model, for integrating multiple methods. The result of this type of integration is the basis for many applications in Chinese healing and divination arts. This book presents a variety of these methods.

In *I Ching* theory, numbers are a substitute for saying "Yin" or "Yang." In the practice of acupuncture, a common way to *reinforce* is to twist the needle nine times, and to *reduce*, twist the needle six times. This method applies the six and nine theory just presented: odd numbers are Yang, and they reinforce or increase; even numbers are Yin, and decrease. This is an example of how *I Ching* numerology and Yin–Yang polarity are applied to trigrams and acupuncture.

In traditional *I Ching* books pairs of trigrams are combined to form hexagrams, which are made up of the six lines of the two trigrams. There are 64 different hexagrams. Each line of a hexagram contains a particular numerical description. For example, the lines may say:

- Six on line 6.

- Six on line 5.

- Nine on line 4.

- Nine on line 3.

- Nine on line 2.

- Nine on line 1.

"Nine" means a Yang line and "six" means a Yin line, so these line descriptions tell us if there is a Yin or Yang line at each of the lines in the hexagram. The polarity of the six lines given above can be presented in the form of a hexagram like this:

This method of numerology can be expanded to *all* numbers. For example, 2, 4, 6, 8, 88, 98, 108 and 200 are all even numbers, and so are Yin numbers. Numbers 1, 5, 9, 15, 27, 109 and 289 are all odd numbers, and so are Yang numbers.

Formation of the Eight Trigrams and the Early Heaven Ba Gua

I Ching is a system that reflects universal correspondences. This classic book reveals patterns and relationships of anatomy and acupuncture channels that are the basis for the clinical applications of *I Ching* acupuncture. In Chinese philosophy the universe has a pre-heaven and post-heaven or un-manifest and manifest aspects. The un-manifest realm is called Wu Ji. In this Wu Ji state all potentiality for creation exists; any possibility within creation can occur in the Wu Ji state. Wu Ji is challenging to explain. The term is often translated as "mystery," "void," "primordial," "invisible," "formless," "limitless" and "unconditioned." It refers to a state or place beyond the intellectual comprehension linked to our normal perception of life. Wu Ji also includes the place to which we return after our life is physically completed; it is a mystery. Wu Ji is a non-polar, non-separate state; it is the origin of creation.

Out of this un-manifest field, seeds of polarity or Yin–Yang manifest, and movement manifests from stillness. Wu Ji manifests post-heaven life, and this unfolding follows a pattern. The *I Ching* reflects this pattern and provides a model to understand patterns and relationships for many aspects of our life. Figure 3.1 is a classical model of how the ancient Chinese viewed creation.

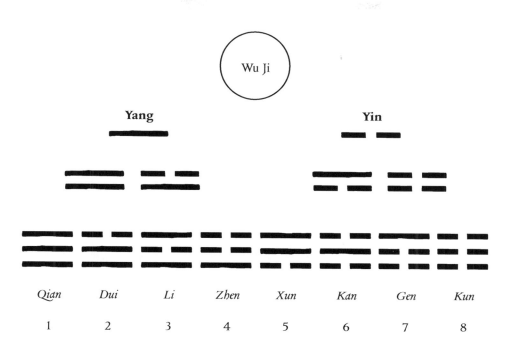

Figure 3.1 Classical Diagram of Ancient Chinese Cosmology

From a Chinese metaphysical viewpoint, this classical diagram explains creation and contains a profound pattern and logic that predates one of the most important discoveries in mathematics, the binary system. Yin–Yang is the binary system, and it is this theory that forms the Early Heaven Ba Gua; it is the basis of the *I Ching*. Wu Ji theory reflects before creation, before polarity or Yin–Yang. From the un-manifest state, movement occurs. Yin–Yang is activated as Wu Ji unfolds; this is the One birthing Two. As will be explained below, as Yin–Yang mingle and interact, four forces are created, and as these four forces mingle, eight forces manifest. This is a natural unfolding, based on Yin–Yang and binary theory. The logic and unfolding will now be explained using Chinese metaphysical theories.

Wu Ji

From the non-polar or un-manifest Wu Ji, manifestation and polarity emerge. This process is the One giving birth to the Two, or Yin–Yang. This is one force interacting with itself in an opposing, interdependent, mutual consuming and inner-transforming way. In *I Ching* language, these two forces are expressed in a system of lines.

Yang is represented as a simple line and odd numbers, and Yin as a broken line and even number.

Yang   **Yin**

Yang and Yin both expand, as each interacts with itself.

Yang   **Yin**

Adding a Yang and Yin line to each produces the four forces.

Four produces eight; each of the four forces is doubled.

A Yang and Yin line added to each creates the eight forces (Eight Trigrams).

1   2   3   4   5   6   7   8

According to this pattern the eight forces or Eight Trigrams are created, and this formation, called the "Early Heaven Ba Gua," is the basis of the Balance Method.

There is also another theory that can explain this formation of the Early Heaven Ba Gua, and which follows the binary theory, as described below.

Wu Ji represents One; alternating Yang and Yin reflects this pattern.

Yin–Yang represents Two; alternating pairs of Yang and pairs of Yin two times reflects this pattern.

The four forces represent Four; alternating four Yang lines and four Yin lines reflects this pattern.

Combining the three lines from the three series above creates the Eight Trigrams; this specific order or formation of the Eight Trigrams creates the Early Heaven Ba Gua.

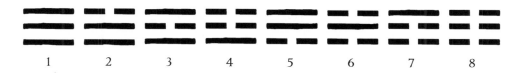

The formation of the Eight Trigrams can be explained with either cosmological or mathematical theory; both methods explain the same situation.

The Eight Trigrams can be arranged in an octagon formation, which is called a Ba Gua. Figure 3.2 shows the Early Heaven Ba Gua.

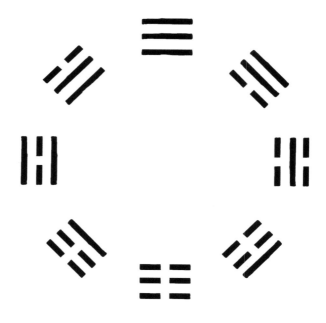

Figure 3.2 The Early Heaven Ba Gua

Structure of the Eight Trigrams

The natural school of philosophy, including Yin–Yang and Five Phases theory, which was developed in the Zhou dynasty, reached a high level of sophistication a few centuries later in the Han dynasty. Most scholars and historians believe the *Nei Jing* was written in the Han dynasty. The *Nei Jing* is a collection of theories and clinical experiences from centuries before the book was written. It was during the Han dynasty that many systems of correspondences and commentaries were added to the Eight Trigrams and the 64 Hexagrams, specifically the "Ten Wings" of the *I Ching*.

The early understanding and applications of the Ba Gua were based on symbolism and Yin–Yang theory. The foundation method of the Balance Method is based on Yin–Yang theory and body imaging.

There are two main approaches to understanding the *I Ching*. The first method is by means of symbolism, which includes systems of correspondences and imaging. These correspondences are models that categorize and connect all of life into Yin–Yang, Five Phases, trigrams, Ba Gua and hexagrams. The second method uses numbers, and includes the mathematical aspect of the *I Ching*. The Balance Method includes both methods in the practice of acupuncture.

Figure 3.3 shows the Eight Trigrams grouped by their Yang and Yin polarity. Trigrams that are made up of an odd number of strokes are Yang, as odd numbers are Yang, and trigrams that are made up of an even number of strokes are Yin, as even numbers are Yin.

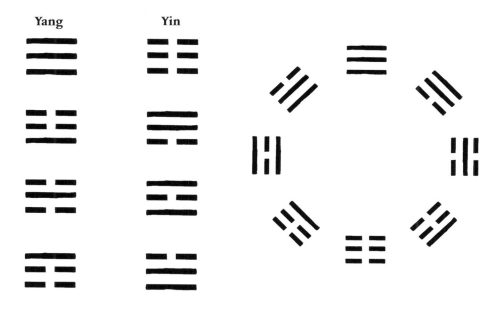

Figure 3.3 The Eight Trigrams Grouped by their Yin–Yang Polarity

There are many ways to evaluate trigrams, hexagrams and the Ba Gua. The following is an introduction to evaluating these models.

Trigrams are evaluated from the bottom line to the top line.

- Odd numbers are Yang.

- Even numbers are Yin.

- Odd or Yang numbers consist of one stroke: ▬▬▬

- Even or Yin numbers consist of two strokes: ▬▬ ▬▬

- The number following the name of each trigram in Figures 3.4 and 3.5 indicates the trigram's position maintained in the Early Heaven Ba Gua formation; it is not the number of the trigram. (Other diagrams do have numbers for each trigram, and they will be presented later in this book.)

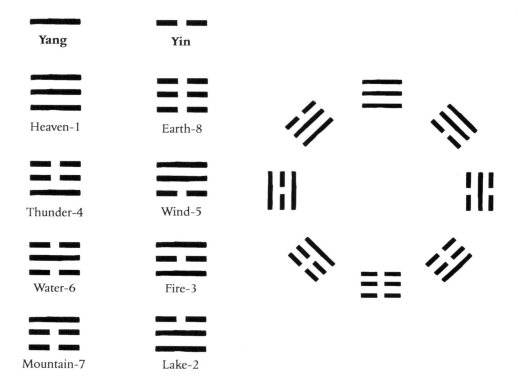

Figure 3.4 The Eight Trigrams: Their Names and Positions in the Ba Gua

There is an inner structure of trigrams that reveals the balanced nature of life. The following section explains important patterns that comprise this balance within the Eight Trigrams, the Ba Gua and the practice of acupuncture.

- Yang trigrams contain either all Yang lines, or one Yang line. Yang trigrams are Heaven, Thunder, Water and Mountain.

- Yin trigrams contain either all Yin lines, or one Yin line. Yin trigrams are Earth, Wind, Fire and Lake (Figure 3.5).

- The total number of Yang trigrams' lines or strokes is 18.

- The total number of Yin trigrams' lines or strokes is 18.

- The total of the Yang trigrams' numerical positions is $1 + 4 + 6 + 7 = 18$.

- The total of the Yin trigrams' numerical positions is $2 + 3 + 5 + 8 = 18$.

- The sum of the strokes for each set of trigrams is 18, so the total sum of the strokes for Yin and Yang trigrams combined is 36. Both these patterns reflect Yin–Yang balance.

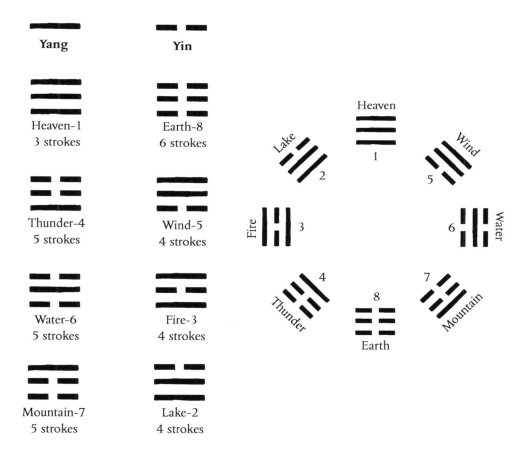

Figure 3.5 The Eight Trigrams: The Number of Strokes in Each Trigram

Structure of the Early Heaven Ba Gua

The Early Heaven Ba Gua is depicted in Figure 3.6; it has many applications in Chinese metaphysics. The structure of patterns within this Ba Gua embodies many forms of balance, and contains guiding principles of the Balance Method.

1. *The first analysis of the Ba Gua* is comparison of pairs of opposite trigrams, which includes the sum of their lines or strokes.

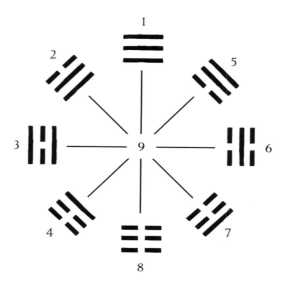

Figure 3.6 The Early Heaven Ba Gua and Nine

- o The sum of the lines or strokes of Heaven-1 and Earth-8 is nine: Heaven has three strokes and Earth has six.

- o The sum of the lines or strokes of Mountain-7 and Lake-2 is nine: Mountain has five strokes and Lake has four.

- o The sum of the lines or strokes of Thunder-4 and Wind-5 is nine: Thunder has five strokes and Wind has four.

- o The sum of the lines or strokes of Water-6 and Fire-3 is nine: Water has five strokes and Fire has four.

2. *The second analysis of the Ba Gua* shows that opposite trigrams are inverted images. For example, Heaven-1 has three Yang lines and its opposite trigram, Earth-8, has three Yin lines: they are opposite Yin–Yang polarities.

All opposite trigrams are mirror images: when there is a Yang stroke in a trigram there is a Yin stroke in the same line of its corresponding trigram. The trigrams Heaven and Earth (below) illustrate this correspondence.

The Ba Gua, then, contains the Yin–Yang dynamic that opposites are inverted images of polarity. Applying this inverted imaging of opposites theory to the human body reveals that corresponding areas in the body are related and can influence or treat each other.

Application of the Early Heaven Ba Gua in Acupuncture

The Ba Gua is a model of correspondences that reveal relationships between locations or positions in a situation. When superimposing the Ba Gua on the human body and applying the fundamental principles of Yin–Yang theory, it becomes clear that opposite anatomical areas balance each other. Treating opposite or corresponding areas of a condition is a fundamental principle in clinical practice. Chapter 25 of the *Nei Jing Su Wen* presents the following guidance: "Man corresponds with nature: In heaven, there are Yin and Yang; in man there are 12 large joints of the limbs," and "When one understands the principles of the 12 joints, a sage will never surpass him." In Chapter 27 it states: "Diverse pricking to the right side or to the left, contralateral insertion of pricking the upper part to cure the lower disease, and pricking the left side to cure the right."

These *Nei Jing Su Wen* references demonstrate that the 12 joints and the limbs are similar to the Ba Gua, and opposite joints are connected and balance each other. When the Ba Gua is superimposed on the human body, both Ba Gua and Twelve Joint theory reveal the basis of Balance Method 1, balancing the Six Channel pairs (see Chapter 9).

Figure 3.7 represents the correlation between the human body and the Early Heaven Ba Gua. It contains guiding principles for selecting acupuncture points, based on the relationships between anatomy and acupuncture channels. *Nei Jing Su Wen* theories and applications are contained in the Early Heaven Ba Gua. The applications emphasize the relationship between the hand and foot and foot and hand (i.e. we select points on the foot to treat the hand, and vice versa), as well as the 12 joints: ankle–wrist, knee–elbow and hip–shoulder. Acupuncture treatments using those relationships are presented in the acupuncture applications in Part II of this book.

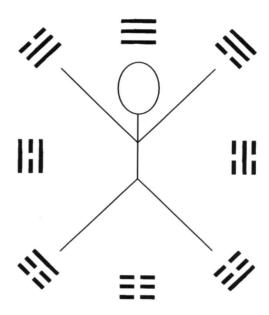

Figure 3.7 The Early Heaven Ba Gua and the Human Body

Chapter 4

FIVE PHASES

The Five Phases, or Wu Xing, is an integral aspect of Chinese metaphysics and permeates many aspects of Chinese culture. Though the origin of the Five Phases is not known, it is believed to have originated in a different part of China than the Yin–Yang tradition. From a historical perspective, the philosopher Zou Yan integrated and presented the Yin–Yang and Five Phases schools during the Warring States Period of the Zhou dynasty, and then began a process of refinement and further development of the theories. Yin–Yang and Five Phases became so influential that they were thought to be heaven's hand in human life, and were used to predict the trends of Chinese dynasties.

Dong Zhongshu, a famous philosopher in the Western Han dynasty, applied the Five Phases to human society and affairs. He presented the following aspects of Five Phases interactions that evolved into the major ways the Five Phases are used in many Chinese arts, including acupuncture:

- the parent and child or 'promotion' cycle

- the grandparent and grandchild or 'controlling' cycle

- correspondences of many aspects of life, including geographical, seasonal, body styles, planets, foods and colors.

Figure 4.1 on the following page depicts the Five Phases. The Five Phases model is a system of correspondences, a way to organize and evaluate any condition from a Five Phases perspective.

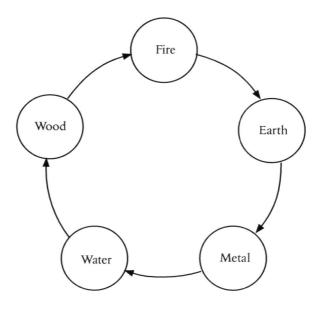

Figure 4.1 The Five Phases

The circular pattern of the Five Phases illustrates the position of each phase within the circle:

1. Wood is positioned where the circle begins to move upward, and represents growth, or spring.

2. Fire is located where the portion of the circle reaches its peak, symbolizing summer.

3. Earth is positioned where harvesting takes place, at the upper right, between Fire and Metal. It represents harvesting and Indian summer.

4. Metal is located at the lower right, between Earth and Water. It represents turning inward and the fall.

5. Water is at the lower left, between Metal and Wood. Water is where the circle turns completely inward to regenerate. It represents Winter and the preparation for spring, which is the beginning of a new cycle.

This cycle continues infinitely and reflects self-generation and the eternal nature of life.

Five Phases Cycles

The Five Phases interact in a variety of ways or cycles. Three major cycles are the *promotion, controlling* and *reduction* cycles. The following diagrams and tables list information for the Five Phases.

The Promotion Cycle

The promotion cycle is the parent-to-child relationship. When balanced the cycle nourishes, supplements or strengthens its child element.

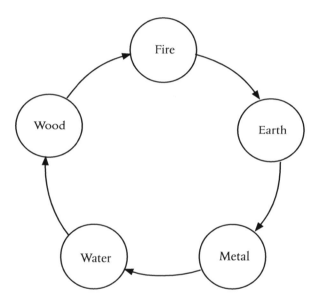

Figure 4.2 The Five Phase Promotion Cycle

The diagram illustrates the promotion cycle. Some of the basic interactions of this cycle are as follows:

- Water placed on Wood promotes growth; Water is the mother of Wood.

- Wood placed in Fire promotes growth; Wood is the mother of Fire.

- Fire transforms substances into ashes or Earth; Fire is the mother of Earth.

- Metal is found within Earth; the Earth element is the mother of Metal.

- Metal can be liquified into Water; Metal is the mother of Water.

The Controlling Cycle

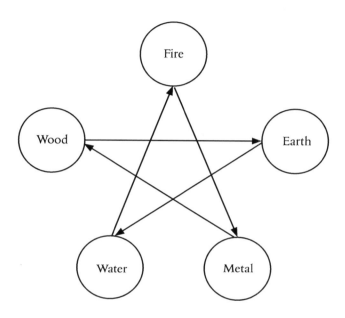

Figure 4.3 The Five Phase Controlling Cycle

Figure 4.3 represents the controlling cycle of the Five Phases. The controlling cycle is the grandparent-to-grandchild relationship. Some of the basic interactions of this cycle are as follows:

- Fire melts Metal or controls Metal; this is the grandparent and controlling relationship.

- Metal cuts Wood or controls Wood; this is the grandparent or controlling relationship.

- Wood absorbs nutrients from the Earth and controls Earth; this is the grandparent or controlling relationship.

- Earth absorbs Water or controls Water; this is the grandparent or controlling relationship.

- Water puts out Fire or controls Fire; this is the grandparent or controlling relationship.

The Reduction Cycle

The reduction cycle, like the promotion cycle, is the relationship between the parent and child, but in this cycle, the parent wants to give to the child and the child wants to take from the parent. The child takes from the parent; it reduces, diminishes, drains or sedates the parent. This cycle is often used when there is an excess of the parent phase.

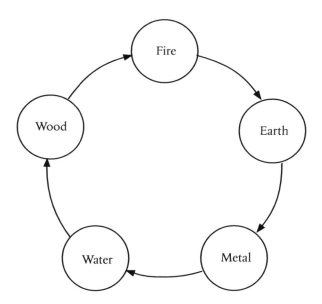

Figure 4.4 The Five Phase Reduction Cycle

Table 4.1 lists major correspondences for each phase, and is the basis of many applications of Five Phases theory.

Table 4.1 The Five Phases Table

	Wood	Fire	Earth	Metal	Water
Stage	Birth	Growth	Transformation	Harvest	Storage
Planet	Jupiter	Mars	Saturn	Venus	Mercury
Color	Green	Red	Yellow	White	Black
Direction	East	South	Center	West	North
Season	Spring	Summer	Indian summer	Fall	Winter
Climate	Wind	Heat	Damp	Dry	Cold
Taste	Sour	Bitter	Sweet	Pungent	Salty
Yin–Yang	Lesser Yang	Utmost Yang		Lesser Yin	Utmost Yin
Stems	1-Yang Wood 2-Yin Wood	3-Yang Fire 4-Yin Fire	5-Yang Earth 6-Yang Earth	7-Yang Metal 8-Yin Metal	9-Yang Water 10-Yin Water
Branches	Tiger, Rabbit	Snake, Horse	Ox, Dragon, Sheep, Dog	Monkey, Cock	Pig
He Tu numbers	3, 8	2, 7	5, 10	4, 9	1, 6
Luo Shu numbers	3, 4	9	2, 5, 8	6, 7	1
Later Heaven trigram	Thunder, Wind	Fire	Earth, Mountain	Lake, Heaven	Water
Yin organs	Liver	Heart	Spleen	Lungs	Kidneys
Yang organs	Gallbladder	Small Intestine	Stomach	Large Intestine	Bladder
Sense organs	Eyes	Tongue	Mouth	Nose	Ears
Tissues	Sinews	Vessels	Muscles	Skin	Bones
Emotions	Kindness, anger	Joy, hastiness	Openness, pensiveness	Courage, sadness	Gentleness, fear
Sounds	Shouting	Laughing	Singing	Crying	Groaning

Animals	Fish	Birds	Humans	Mammals	Shell-covered
Domestic animals	Sheep	Fowl	Ox	Dog	Pig
Grains	Wheat	Beans	Rice	Hemp	Millet
Spirit	*Hun*	*Shen*	*Yi*	*Po*	*Zhi*
Sounds	Shhh	Haw	Ho	Ssss	Chuii (wave sound)

Five Phases Correspondences

The Five Phases is a significant system of correspondences and is a method to categorize all aspects of life. Important correspondences of each phase are listed below. These attributes play an important role in Chinese astrology, feng shui and Chinese medicine.

Wood—Mu

- Growth, movement upward, expansion, budding, opening up.

- Initial rise of energy, new energy cycle.

- Vitality, active, free-flowing, new.

- Germinating, bending, reaching above.

- Liver and Gallbladder, tendons, smooth flow of emotions.

- Sexuality.

Fire—Huo

- Illumination, warmth, light, burning, joy.

- Heat, fire, flame, climax, zenith, expansion, rising.

- Excitement.

- Peak of Yang cycle.

- Heart, blood, circulation.

- Shen (spirit).

Earth—Di

- Earth, ground, clay, soil.

- Foundation, nourishing, supporting, maintaining.

- Transformation, cauldron, yielding, center, middle, harvesting.

- Place of interaction.

- Spleen, Stomach, Transporting.

Metal—Jin

- Metals, gold, silver, bronze.

- Crystallization, coagulation, melting, concentration, insight, concepts.

- Inward, introvert, withdrawing.

- Melancholy, sadness, depression.

- Begins Yin cycle.

- Restrains, downward movement.

- Lungs, mouth, skin, exterior, connects to exterior.

Water—Shui

- Fluid, flowing, cascading, downward movement.

- Adapting, adjusting.

- Dissolving, changing.

- Emotions, feeling, metaphysics.

- Mystery, hidden, womb, renewal, rejuvenation, healing.

- Kidneys, Jing (essence), bones, prenatal, primordial, ancestral.

Five Phases Shapes

All shapes or forms are categorized into the Five Phases and the following introduces these and other related correspondences. The Five Phases shapes have a significant influence in Qi Gong and feng shui.

Wood

- Wood is a beam or a rod-shaped item.

- Wood is the color green.

- Wood includes plants and flowers.

- Direction is East and Southeast.

- Remedies for enhancing are Water and Wood.

Fire

- Fire is a pyramid shape.

- Fire includes the colors red, pink and purple.

- Fire includes red candles, red lampshades, red lights and pyramid shapes.

- Direction is South.

- Remedies for enhancement are Wood and Fire.

Earth

- Earth is a rectangle, square or flat shape.

- Earth includes the colors yellow, beige and tan.

- Earth includes rocks, crystals, ceramics and porcelain.

- Directions include the Center, Northeast and Southwest.

- Remedies for enhancement are Fire and Earth.

Metal

- Metal is round, spherical or circular shapes.

- Metal includes white, gold and silver colors.

- Metal includes metal chimes, metal coins and grandfather clocks.

- Directions include Northwest and West.

- Remedies for enhancement are Earth and Metal.

Water

- Water is cascading, wavy or curved shapes.

- Water flows downward.

- Water includes blue, blue-green and black colors.

- Water includes aquariums, fountains, cascading structures, lakes and streams.

- Direction is North.

- Remedies for enhancement are Metal and Water.

Integrating Eight Trigrams and Five Phases

The Han dynasty was one of the renaissance periods in Chinese culture, occurring after the unification of China during the Qin dynasty. The emperor promoted an environment of free thought and interaction, which allowed the development of the best of Chinese theories and applications. The Han dynasty was a significant time for the refinement of the *I Ching*. Systems of correspondences were integrated into the *I Ching*, including the "Ten Wings," which is a major commentary. The *Shou Gua* or "Eighth Wing" is a particularly significant work on the Eight Trigrams. It is the basis of much knowledge used in modern texts and has important relationships to Chinese medicine, acupuncture and feng shui.

The following is a selection of valuable information from the "Ten Wings" of the *Book of Changes* that forms the building blocks of *I Ching* acupuncture:

- Heaven is symbolized by three (and all odd numbers) and Earth by two (and all even numbers).

- The Sages perceived the changes of Yin and Yang and created the Eight Trigrams.

- The trigrams are a tool reflecting the changes of Yin–Yang in life, as well as images expressing the successive transformations of Yin–Yang.

- The following trigrams and their corresponding anatomical structures are the foundation components for medical predictions and applications:

  ○ **Qian/Heaven** functions like the *head*.

  ○ **Kun/Earth** functions like the *Stomach*.

  ○ **Zhen/Thunder** functions like the *foot*.

  ○ **Xun/Wind** functions like the *thigh*.

  ○ **Kan/Water** functions like the *ear*.

  ○ **Li/Fire** functions like the *eye*.

  ○ **Gen/Mountain** functions like the *hand*.

  ○ **Dui/Lake** functions like the *mouth*.

- ○ **Qian** is Heaven, the father and Metal.

- ○ **Kun** is Earth, the mother and Earth.

- ○ **Zhen** is Thunder, the first/eldest son and Wood.

- ○ **Xun** is Wind, the first/eldest daughter and Wood.

- ○ **Kan** is Water, the second son and Water.

- ○ **Li** is Fire, the second daughter and Fire.

- ○ **Gen** is Mountain, the youngest son and Earth.

- ○ **Dui** is Lake, the youngest daughter and Metal.

The Eight Trigrams and Corresponding Areas of Life

The following "Ten Wings" information provides the basis for predicting potential health problems.

TRIGRAM: KAN

Direction: North
Person: Middle son
Quality of life: Wealth
Body or disease: Kidneys, ears, blood
Five Phases: Water

TRIGRAM: KUN

Direction: Southwest
Person: Mother, older females
Quality of life: Love, relationships and marriage
Body or disease: Spleen, Stomach
Five Phases: Earth

TRIGRAM: **ZHEN**

Direction: East
Person: Eldest males, older males
Quality of life: Family, superiors and mentors
Body or disease: Feet, legs
Five Phases: Wood

TRIGRAM: **XUN**

Direction: Southeast
Person: Elder females
Quality of life: Prosperity, money, property and material possessions
Body or disease: Thighs, wind and colds
Five Phases: Wood

TRIGRAM: **DUI**

Direction: West
Person: Youngest daughter, young females, students
Quality of life: Creativity
Body or disease: Lungs, mouth
Five Phases: Metal

TRIGRAM: **QIAN**

Direction: Northwest
Person: Father, elder males, elders
Quality of life: Travel, movement and helpers
Body or disease: Head
Five Phases: Metal

Trigram: Gen

Direction: Northeast
Person: Youngest daughter, young females
Quality of life: Knowledge, wisdom
Body or disease: Hands, fingers and spine
Five Phases: Earth

Trigram: Li

Direction: South
Person: Middle females
Quality of life: Fame, reputations and professional position
Body or disease: Heart, eyes
Five Phases: Fire

Summary of Eight-Trigram Correspondences

Table 4.2 contains basic information about each trigram that can be used for a variety of Chinese metaphysical systems.

Integrating the Five Phases and the Eight Trigrams makes a connection between a major theory and a Chinese metaphysical model; the unified model provides insights and applications in a variety of divination and healing arts.

TABLE 4.2 THE EIGHT-TRIGRAM CORRESPONDENCES

Trigram	Name	Number	Element	Color	Location	Family	Disease	Life aspirations
☵	*Kan*	1	Water	Blue, black	North	Second son	Kidneys, ears, blood	Career
☷	*Kun*	2	Earth	Yellow, beige	Southwest	Mother, Elderly woman	Stomach, Spleen, abdomen, digestion	Relationships
☳	*Zhen*	3	Wood, Thunder	Green	East	Eldest son	Feet, lungs, throat	Family
☴	*Xun*	4	Wood, Wind	Green	Southeast	Eldest daughter	Buttocks, thighs, colds	Wealth
☱	*Dui*	7	Metal, Lake	White, gold	West	Youngest daughter	Pulmonary disease, headaches	Creativity
☰	*Qian*	6	Metal, Heaven	White, gold	Northwest	Father, Elderly male	Head, lungs, mouth	Travel
☶	*Gen*	8	Earth, Mountain	Yellow, beige	Northeast	Youngest male	Hands, fingers, back	Knowledge
☲	*Li*	9	Fire	Red, purple	South	Second daughter	Heart, eyes	Fame, reputation

Chapter 5

THE HE TU DIAGRAM

The He Tu is a profound diagram with many applications in Chinese arts, and it contains guiding principles in *I Ching* and *Nei Jing* theory. This chapter presents important principles contained in this ancient diagram.

The He Tu Diagram

According to Chinese legend, Fu Xi found the He Tu diagram in pre-historic time; its origin is unknown. We do know it is a very old diagram, which probably originated during early Chinese culture. The essence of its meaning was not commonly known until the legendary *I Ching* master Shao Yong analyzed it during the Song dynasty. Shao Yong did what now seems like an obvious thing: he converted the He Tu dots into a number system. Shao Yong counted the dots and assigned odd numbers to Yang and even numbers to Yin. Additionally, he noticed that dark dots are Yin and lights dots are Yang. He combined these two patterns to reveal that the He Tu contained a code: odd numbers and light dots are Yang and even numbers and dark dots are Yin. Figure 5.1 presents the standard He Tu diagram.

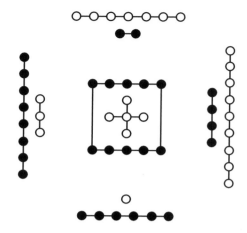

Figure 5.1 The He Tu Diagram

Figure 5.2 shows the ancient number system of the He Tu. Count the dots to find their number: dark dots are Yin and light dots are Yang.

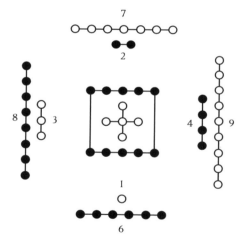

Figure 5.2 The He Tu Diagram with Numbers

One essential principle in the He Tu is that each of the four directions has a pair; nothing is in isolation. Notice that each area, top and bottom and left and right, contains two sets of numbers. Each area contains the fundamental principle of Yin–Yang: there is an odd or Yang number and an even or Yin number. Additionally, there are light dots and dark dots in each direction, which represent Yang and Yin. These relationships are the basis of a guiding principle: all things in life contain their Yin or Yang pairing.

Five phases were identified within the He Tu: the bottom is Water, the left is Wood, the top is Fire, the right is Metal and the center is Earth (see Figure 5.3). These five dimensions within the He Tu contain a code that is applied to methods from feng shui to Chinese medicine.

It is believed that the He Tu diagram predates Yin–Yang theory, but contains the principles of Yin–Yang. In the He Tu diagram there are eight directions or areas grouped into four sets of two pairs. This grouping is the guiding principle for pairing areas of the body and the acupuncture channels. For example, the limbs contain correspondences or pairs—the ankle and wrist; the knee and elbow; and the hip and shoulder. Because these anatomical structures are pairs, they treat each other; for example, for conditions at the wrist, treat the ankle. The He Tu contains the seeds of the eventual grouping of the 12 acupuncture channels into six pairs of channels: the Yin–Yang pairs.

Structure of the He Tu

In each of the cardinal directions there are two numbers: one is an odd number which is Yang, and one is an even number which is Yin, reflecting Yin–Yang in each direction.

At the center there are five dots. Five represents the center, the core, Yuan or primordial. Five is also the Earth element, and this diagram reveals that all elements, numbers and directions originate in the center, or earth. Each He Tu combination is related to the number five: for example, $6 - 1 = 5$; $9 - 4 = 5$; $8 - 3 = 5$ and $7 - 2 = 5$. All these combinations originate from the center of the He Tu.

This is one theory that supports the Earth School of Chinese medicine. The functions of the Spleen and Stomach play a key role in the theory underpinning the Earth School. The digestion of food and drink and the transformation of it into Qi, blood and nutrients is a major function of the Spleen and Stomach, the Earth organs. When the Earth organs do not function properly the entire body is affected because the whole body requires Qi, blood and nutrients. According to the Earth School theory, the Spleen and Stomach influence the entire body and all conditions of the organs and vital substances, so they should be treated in all conditions. In the He Tu, the center is Earth and reflects the Spleen and Stomach. Each of the four pairs has a difference of the number five, which is the center. The He Tu model underpins the principle that the Earth organs are affected in all conditions, and that the Earth organs in turn have influence over the entire body.

Each of the directional numbers shares an element:

- 1–6 combine to create Water.

- 2–7 combine to create Fire.

- 3–8 combine to create Wood.

- 4–9 combine to create Metal.

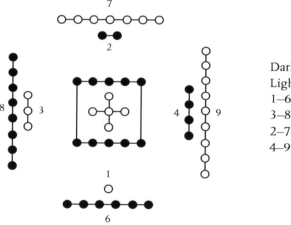

Dark dots are Yin
Light dots are Yang
1–6 is North and Water
3–8 is East and Wood
2–7 is South and Fire
4–9 is West and Metal

Figure 5.3 The He Tu Pairings

The Yin–Yang pairs are the basis for the Guest and Host acupuncture treatments. "Guest and Host" means combining Yin–Yang paired channels in a treatment—combining the Large Intestine and the Lungs in a treatment, or combining the Spleen and Stomach in a treatment are examples of a Guest and Host treatment. Chapter 9 of the *Nei Jing Ling Shu* (*Spiritual Pivot*) deals with using Yin–Yang pairs in every treatment for acupuncture channel conditions. By combining two channels that are connected, a stronger influence occurs; this is an example of the benefit of applying the principle of Yin–Yang.

When a He Tu diagram is superimposed on a human body it provides guiding principles for treating anatomical areas and acupuncture channels: it reveals relationships between opposite areas. For example, numbers 1 and 2, or 6 and 7, indicate that the lower limbs can treat the top of the head. Additionally, numbers 3 and 4, or 8 and 9, relate to the arms on each side of the body: they are related and can treat each other. Figure 5.4 shows these relationships. The He Tu contains a Yin and Yang influence in each area, reflecting the inseparable relationships between Yin–Yang paired channels and organs. Each of the areas also contains a relationship to the number five, which relates to the center, the abdomen or the origin of five. The center relates to internal organs, and Figure 5.4 indicates that the points on the limbs—for example, the five Transporting (Antique) points (see pages 164–165)—can influence the internal organs.

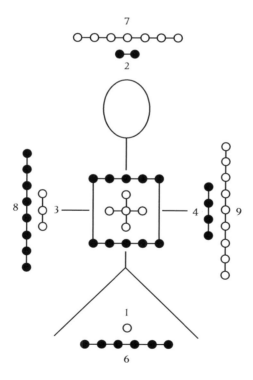

Figure 5.4 The He Tu and the Human Body

Chapter 6

NINE PALACES

The Nine Palaces Diagram

The Nine Palaces (Luo Shu) is one of China's oldest diagrams. The classic diagram has applications in feng shui, nine-star astrology, qi men dun jia and acupuncture. Chinese legend tells us that Yu the Great, one of China's pre-historic leaders, was rewarded by the Heavens with the Luo Shu Nine Palaces diagram for his many positive contributions to humanity. Figure 6.1 shows the Nine Palaces.

In cultures around the world there are many magic squares which are composed of a number of boxes or squares ("palaces"). The Chinese have a particularly unique understanding concerning the influence of the number three. Numerous Chinese energy models include the number three, including Tai Chi, a trigram and the Three Treasures. The Nine Palaces are composed of three "palaces" multiplied by three.

In the practice of Chinese medicine, this understanding is applied to a common pulse method. The common wrist pulse method practiced has three *positions*—*cun*, *guan* and *chi*—with three *depths*—the superficial, middle and deep *levels*. The three positions, each with its three levels, create nine positions to palpate. This is an example of the Nine Palaces placed on the human body, at the wrist. If you view the Nine Palaces as a three-dimensional field, 4-9-2 indicates the superficial layer close to the skin; 8-1-6 indicates the deep layers, when pressing firmly at the wrist, and 3-5-7 represents the region in between the superficial and the deep layers.

The numbers in the Nine Palaces have no significance for the pulse, but only the three layers and three positions, which constitute the nine pulse positions. This pulse method is an example of applied philosophy—a theory that is applied to the human body and medicine. It also reflects the concept of how the body functions according to this model of correspondences.

4	9	2
3	5	7
8	1	6

Figure 6.1 The Nine Palaces

Structure of the Nine Palaces

The Nine Palaces is a model of systems of correspondences. This model has affinities with major theories of Chinese metaphysics, including Yin–Yang, Tai Chi and Five Phases, the fundamental principles of which are applied to the Nine Palaces to interpret and enhance many aspects of our lives. The systems that use the Nine Palaces include feng shui, Chinese astrology and acupuncture. Analyzing theories of the Nine Palaces, which were eventually applied to the human body and contributed to the development of Chinese medicine during the Han dynasty, reveals guiding principles for the *Nei Jing*.

Analysis of the Nine Palaces begins with numbers and their unique patterns:

- There are three rows and three columns.

- The smallest number is at the bottom, in the Yin position, and the largest number is at the top, in the Yang position.

- Horizontal, vertical and diagonal patterns are related. The total of all three numbers in any of the patterns, vertical, horizontal or diagonal, is 15.

- Directional opposites total to the same number, ten; therefore opposites are related to each other and complete each other.

The relationships within the Nine Palaces are similar to the Early Heaven Ba Gua, where opposite trigrams are related like lock and key, and represent two sides to the same condition. Superimposing the Nine Palaces on the human body indicates that opposite anatomical areas relate to each other and can treat each other. As a theory, Nine Palaces indicates that opposites are inseparably connected. This is the theoretical basis for a main acupuncture treatment strategy that is found in Chapter 9 of the *Nei Jing Ling Shu*: this strategy is always to include Yin–Yang paired channels in treatments. These channel pairs are treated in order to create balance between the two; they are in effect one inseparable channel.

The sequential number pattern in the Nine Palaces is profound. Following the pattern from the center, or the number 5, and moving to 6, 7, 8, 9, 1, 2, 3 and finally 4, a major formula is traced. There is a Qi Gong form called the "Dance of Yu." This is a shamanic form in which the practitioner performs a dance following the ascending numerical pattern found in the Nine Palaces to attune himself with cosmic forces. To visualize the dance, imagine you are standing in sand with the diagram from Figure 6.2 drawn in the sand. Stand in the center at the number 5. Walk in the Nine Palaces by moving in ascending order of the numbers. Move to number 6, then 7, then 8, 9, 1, 2 3 and 4. Follow the order of the numbers.

The Nine Palaces and its numerical pattern is one model that explains the exact order of the Ying Qi cycle presented in Chapter 16 of the *Nei Jing Ling Shu*. The Ying Qi cycle is also called "the daily cycle" or "the daily meridian clock." The theories behind this cycle are explained on page 108.

Chinese medicine applies numerous Chinese metaphysical models to the human body. For the practice of acupuncture, the Nine Palaces is a guiding theory for contralateral point selection, which is based on the principle that opposite areas and limbs influence each other and can treat each other. Figure 6.2 illustrates the Nine Palaces as a body-imaging model that reveals the images and relationships within the body. Following the fundamental theory that opposites are interrelated and can treat each other, Nine Palaces shows how it is that the upper area treats the lower area, while the lower area treats the upper area, and likewise the left and right sides reciprocally treat each other.

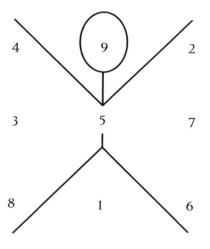

Figure 6.2 The Nine Palaces and the Human Body

Chapter 7

THE LATER HEAVEN BA GUA

Wen Wang was a leader of the Zhou state, during the Shang dynasty (1600–1045 BC). He became so powerful, and posed such a threat, that the emperor of the Shang dynasty imprisoned him. While in prison, it is believed, Wen Wang revealed a new variation of the Ba Gua: the Later Heaven Ba Gua. Figure 7.1 is the Later Heaven (Hou Tian) Ba Gua, which is also called the Wen Wang Ba Gua. In addition to his new arrangement, he combined the Eight Trigrams into pairs of two trigrams, creating the 64 Hexagrams and the *I Ching*. The *I Ching* at that time contained a basic image of each hexagram. Wen Wang's son, Wu, attached individual meanings to each of the six lines in the hexagrams. Wen and Wu mark the beginning of a long history of enhancements to the *I Ching*.

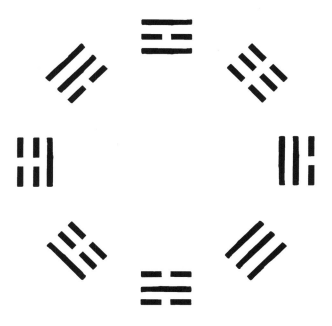

Figure 7.1 The Later Heaven Ba Gua

The Later Heaven Ba Gua represents a change from the trigram pattern of the Early Heaven Ba Gua (compare Figure 3.2 on page 42). The Later Heaven Ba Gua is driven by interactions between opposing trigrams and Five Phases. Figure 7.2 shows the Later Heaven Ba Gua with its Five Phases.

Whereas the Early Heaven Ba Gua begins with the Earth and Heaven trigrams in the bottom and top positions of the Ba Gua, the Later Heaven Ba Gua begins with Water and Fire in the bottom and top positions. Water and Fire thus become major metaphors for post-natal life in the Later Heaven Ba Gua. The interaction between these two phases identifies that balance is created through seeking harmony between opposite trigrams and their influences. The opposite Five Phases interaction can cause disharmonies, yet, with an understanding of the trigrams and their correspondences, a plan of action can be developed to promote balance.

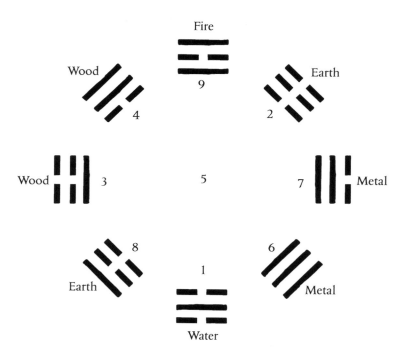

Figure 7.2 The Later Heaven Ba Gua and the Five Phases

The He Tu Diagram and the Nine Palaces as the Origins of the Later Heaven Ba Gua

Scholars and Chinese metaphysical practitioners believe that the Nine Palaces is derived from the He Tu (i.e. the He Tu is the terrain for extracting numbers to create the number sequence of the Nine Palaces) and that the Nine Palaces in turn are the origin of the Later Heaven Ba Gua numbers.

The following is a step-by-step explanation of this process.

1. The first step is to assign numbers to the original He Tu dot system.

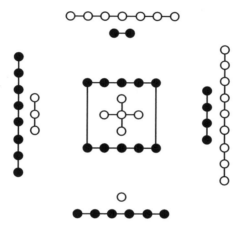

Counting and summing the dots in each area of the He Tu reveals the numbers shown below.

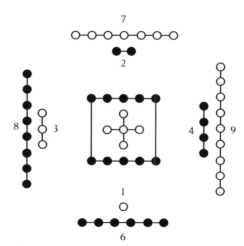

2. The second step is to follow the numerical pattern of *Yin* (even) *and Yang* (odd) *numbers* to find the *Nine Palaces numbers.* Beginning with 1 at the bottom, move upward to the left to 3. Then cut across the 5 to the right, to 7 (which replaces 9), then move upward to the top and place 9 there (instead of 7). Follow the pattern: A, B, C, D, E (pattern 1).

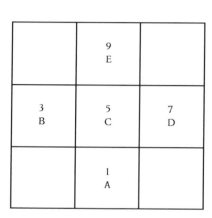

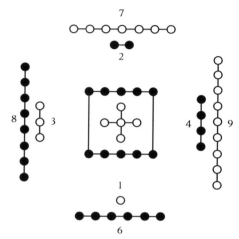

Pattern 1

3. The third step is to begin the Yin cycle. Start with 2 in the upper right corner. Move to 4 in the upper left corner, and then 6 in the lower right corner, then to 8 in the lower left corner, and then 10 in the center. This pattern (A, B, C, D, E) creates the Nine Palaces dot configuration for the Later Heaven Ba Gua (pattern 2).

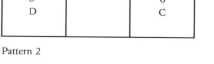

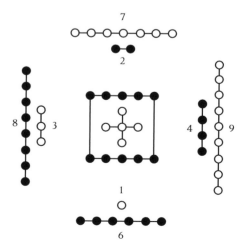

Pattern 2

4. Combining the two patterns into one grid creates the Nine Palaces.

	9 E	
3 B	5 C	7 D
	1 A	

Pattern 1

4 B		2 A
	10 E	
8 D		6 C

Pattern 2

4	9	2
3	5	7
8	1	6

The Nine Palaces

A reason for explaining this process is that other aspects of Chinese medical theory will be paired with Chinese metaphysical models that explain their meanings and applications. Combining and integrating multiple models explains some theories of unknown origin.

Figures 7.3 to 7.6 illustrate the unfolding of the He Tu and formation of the Later Heaven Ba Gua.

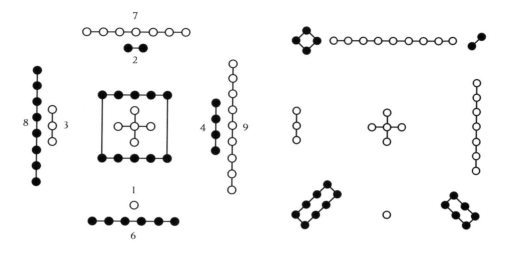

Figure 7.3 The He Tu

Figure 7.4 The He Tu Expanded to the Nine Palaces

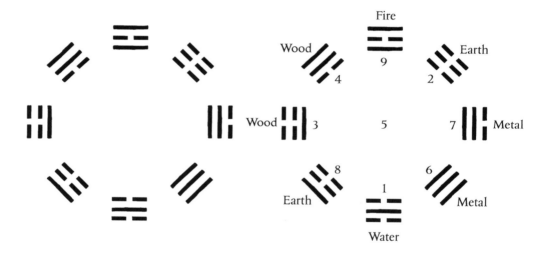

Figure 7.5 The Later Heaven Ba Gua

Figure 7.6 The Later Heaven Ba Gua with Numbers and Five Phases

Figure 7.6 shows the integration of the Nine Palaces numbers, Five Phases and the Later Heaven Ba Gua, and represents post-natal life. It has many applications in Chinese philosophy, healing and divination methods.

The full range of applications for the Later Heaven Ba Gua requires the integration of the Five Phases, Nine Palaces and the Eight Trigrams.

It was during the Han dynasty (206 BC–AD 220) that all these theories and diagrams became profoundly integrated. One of the first integrating actions is to transfer the Later Heaven Ba Gua trigrams into the Nine Palaces, with each trigram taking on the number and the palace.

Comparing the Later Heaven Ba Gua with the Early Heaven Ba Gua

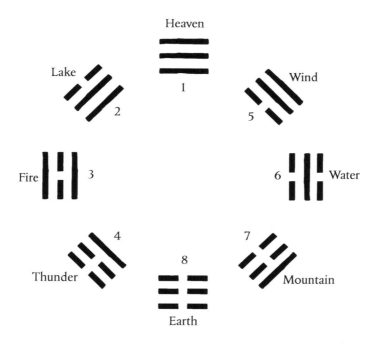

Figure 7.7 The Early Heaven Ba Gua and Trigrams Positions

One common area of confusion is the difference between the numbers associated with the Early Heaven Ba Gua, the Nine Palaces and the Later Heaven Ba Gua. The numbers for the Early Heaven Ba Gua are the positions of the trigrams within the Ba Gua, and indicate the flow of the trigrams: from the top, Heaven is the first position, Lake is the second, Fire is the third, Thunder the fourth, Wind the fifth, Water the sixth, Mountain the seventh and Earth the eighth position (see Figure 7.7).

The numbers in the Nine Palaces are the numbers for the trigrams in the Later Heaven Ba Gua. If a method includes moving the positions of the trigrams from the original order or pattern shown in Figure 7.8, the numbers stay with the trigrams. In other words, in the Later Heaven Ba Gua the number associated with a trigram is constant; it can be taken as the name of the trigram. Trigrams can move to different geographical palaces, but their number stays the same.

The series of Nine Palaces grids in Figures 7.8 to 7.12 shows how Five Phases and other essential information is added to the Nine Palaces. The purpose for these different Nine Palaces is to illustrate how numerous correspondences are integrated into the Nine Palaces; this method exists for numerous models of Chinese metaphysics.

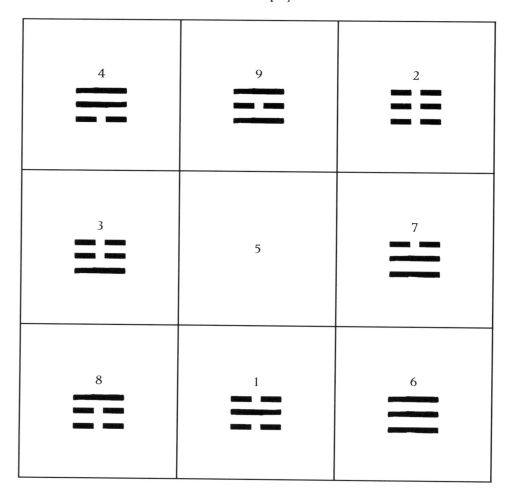

Figure 7.8 The Nine Palaces Numbers for the Later Heaven Ba Gua Trigrams

Wood 4	Fire 9	Earth 2
Wood 3	Center 5	Metal 7
Earth 8	Water 1	Metal 6

Figure 7.9 The Five Phases are Integrated into the Nine
Palaces, and Each Palace Contains an Element

Southeast 4	South 9	Southwest 2
East 3	Center 5	West 7
Northeast 8	North 1	Northwest 6

Figure 7.10 The Geographical Locations are Integrated into the Nine Palaces

Southeast Wood 4	South Fire 9	Southwest Earth 2
East Wood 3	Center 5	West Metal 7
Northeast Earth 8	North Water 1	Northwest Metal 6

Figure 7.11 The Nine Palaces Combines Numbers,
Five Phases and Geographical Directions

Southeast Wood Wind *Xun* 4	South Fire *Li* 9	Southwest Earth *Kun* 2
East Wood Thunder *Zhen* 3	5	West Metal Lake *Dui* 7
Northeast Earth Mountain *Gen* 8	North Water *Kan* 1	Northwest Metal Heaven *Qian* 6

Figure 7.12 The Integrated Nine Palaces

This Nine Palaces system contains foundational knowledge used in many of the Chinese metaphysical arts, and all corresponding relationships can be integrated into this model. A common issue when integrating different models is that it requires adjusting them to harmonize with each other. For example, there are nine palaces and only eight trigrams; here the adjustment is that the center does not have a trigram.

The Chinese integrated and compared many of their models. A particularly interesting one is the combining of the Early Heaven and Later Heaven Ba Gua. Figure 7.15 is the Early Heaven and Later Heaven Ba Gua combined. This combination is significant in feng shui and in a shamanic method of *I Ching* divination. The following diagrams present each of the models first individually, then integrated. Sometimes the numbers for the trigrams are included, sometimes they are not; when the trigrams are memorized, their numbers are not necessary.

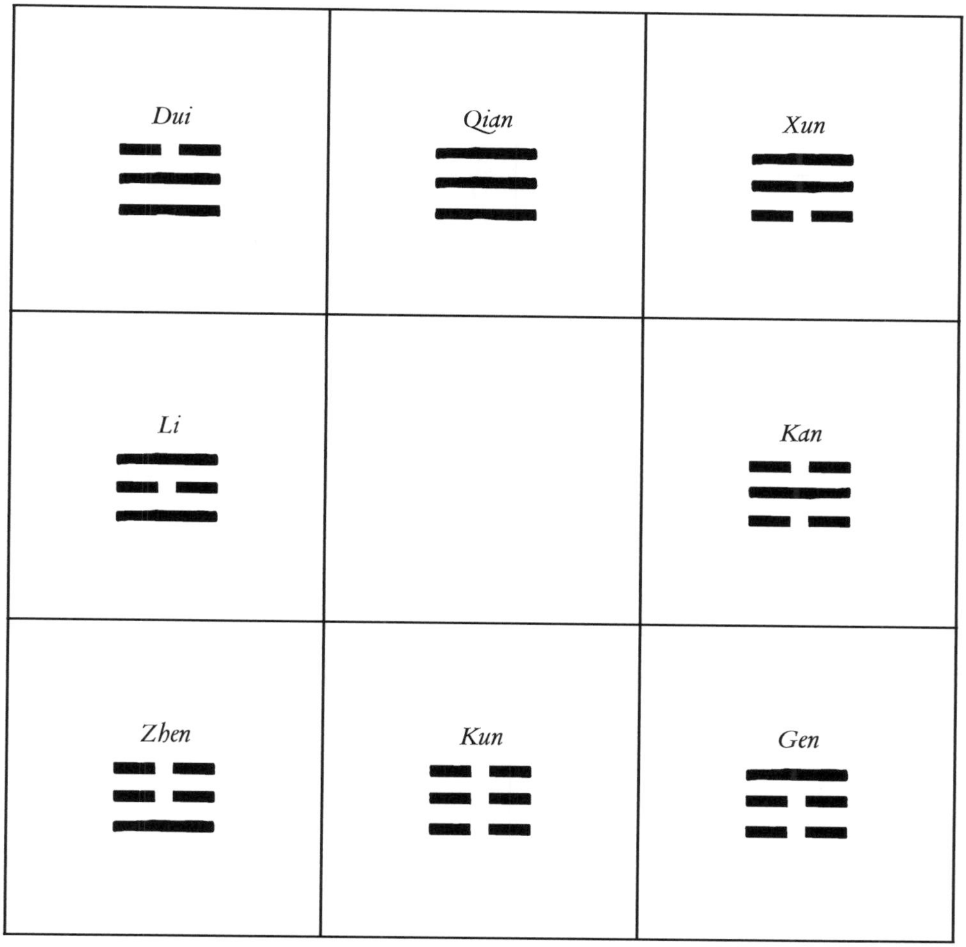

Dui	Qian	Xun
Li		Kan
Zhen	Kun	Gen

Figure 7.13 The Nine Palaces: Early Heaven Ba Gua

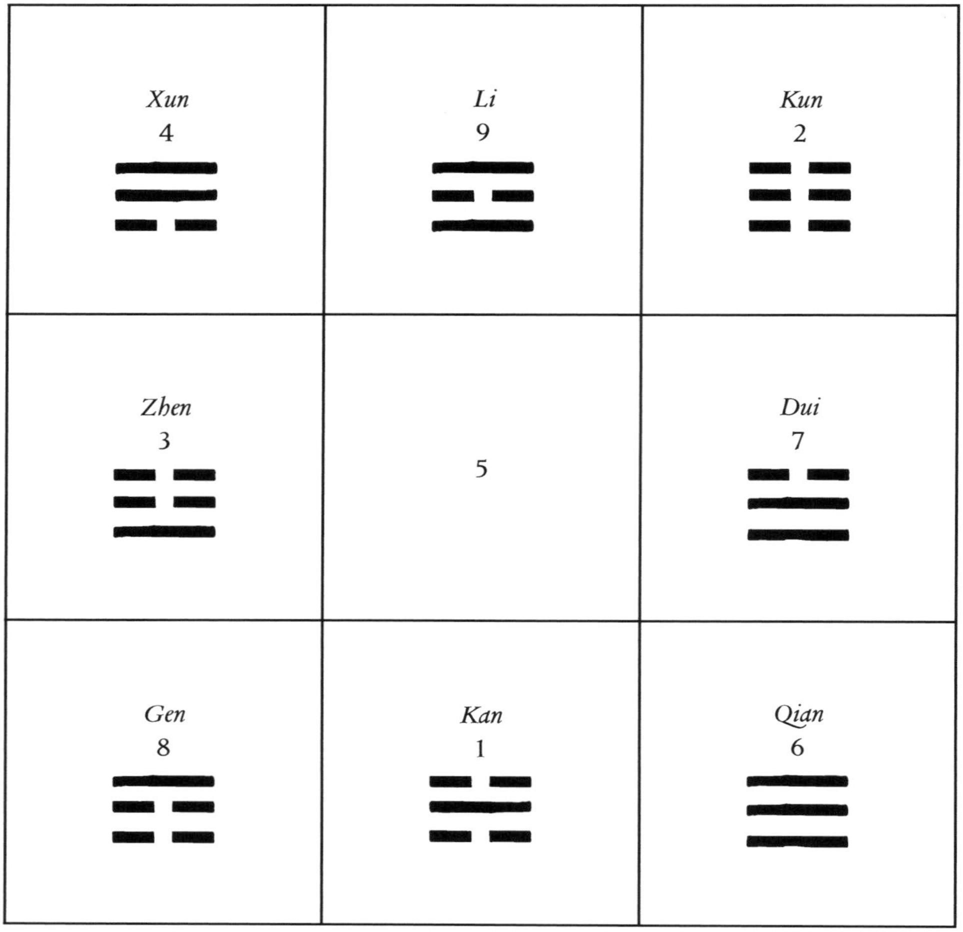

Xun 4	Li 9	Kun 2
Zhen 3	5	Dui 7
Gen 8	Kan 1	Qian 6

Figure 7.14 The Nine Palaces: Later Heaven Ba Gua

Southeast 7 *Dui* 4 *Xun*	South 6 *Qian* 9 *Li*	Southwest 4 *Xun* 2 *Kun*
East 9 *Li* 3 *Zhen*		West 1 *Kan* 7 *Dui*
Northeast 3 *Zhen* 8 *Gen*	North 2 *Kun* 1 *Kan*	Northwest 8 *Gen* 6 *Qian*

Figure 7.15 The Nine Palaces: Early and Later Heaven Ba Gua Combined

When studying and evaluating theories, systems and applications of Chinese arts, especially Chinese medicine, it is important to note that clinical applications are often based on multiple models. Knowing these models is often the key to unlocking the logic behind the method. The Early Heaven Ba Gua, He Tu, Yin–Yang, Five Phases, Later Heaven Ba Gua and Nine Palaces are six major diagrams, models and theories that contain principles and guiding logic for many applications in Chinese medicine, in the *I Ching* and the *Nei Jing*.

In addition to these profound models, the Chinese calendar is a significant contributor to Chinese metaphysics, especially the *Nei Jing*. The Chinese calendar is introduced in the next chapter.

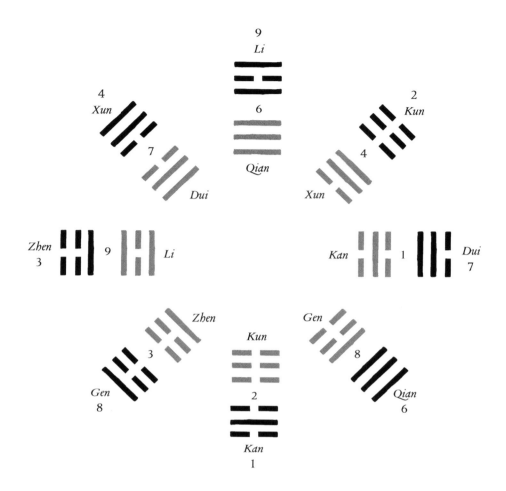

Note: The Early Heaven Gua is the inner Ba Gua.
The Later Heaven Gua is the outer Ba Gua.

Figure 7.16 The Early Heaven and Later Heaven Ba Gua Combined

Chapter 8

THE CHINESE CALENDAR

The Chinese view the universe as one integrated whole, and this whole can be viewed by using unique models, including Yin–Yang and Five Phases, which both play significant roles in *I Ching* and *Nei Jing* theory and their applications. The Chinese devised a method of calculating the influence of cycles of time based on Yin–Yang and Five Phases: these two combined create the Ten Heavenly Stems and Twelve Earthly Branches.

Yin–Yang is the fundamental principle in Chinese philosophy and is encapsulated in every theory. Regardless of the complexity of models and methods, each can be reduced to Yin–Yang. All aspects of time can be categorized as Yin–Yang, whether hourly, daily, monthly or yearly time cycles. Heavenly or celestial influences are Yang; they are often referred to as the Ten Heavenly Stems.

The Ten Heavenly Stems

Cycles of time correspond to the Five Phases (Water, Wood, Fire, Earth and Metal), and each element contains a Yin and Yang aspect, so that the resulting Ten Heavenly Stems (Tian Yuan) are: Yang Wood, Yin Wood; Yang Fire, Yin Fire; Yang Earth, Yin Earth; Yang Metal, Yin Metal; and Yang Water, Yin Water. Table 8.1 lists the Ten Heavenly Stems.

The flow or pattern of the Ten Stems is the Five Phases generating cycle, and they begin with the Wood phase. Number 1 is Yang Wood, and the pattern of the phases follows the generating cycle. Yang Wood is the beginning because Wood represents growth and springtime. Each element contains a Yin or Yang quality and this pattern of Yin–Yang and Five Phases flows into perpetuity, as all years, months, days and hours contain stems.

Table 8.1 The Ten Heavenly Stems

	Stem	Name
1	Yang Wood	*Jia*
2	Yin Wood	*Yi*
3	Yang Fire	*Bing*
4	Yin Fire	*Ding*
5	Yang Earth	*Wu*
6	Yin Earth	*Ji*
7	Yang Metal	*Geng*
8	Yin Metal	*Xin*
9	Yang Water	*Ren*
10	Yin Water	*Gui*

The Twelve Earthly Branches

The Twelve Earthly Branches comprise the Five Phases with their Yin–Yang qualities (ten branches), plus an extra Earth branch that also contains a Yin and Yang aspect.

Reading Figure 8.1 clockwise from Spring (in the East), the Twelve Branches are: Yang Wood, Yin Wood, *Yang Earth*; Yang Fire, Yin Fire, *Yin Earth*; Yang Metal, Yin Metal, *Yang Earth*; Yang Water, Yin Water, *Yin Earth*. Branches can also be referred to by their Chinese zodiac animal names. These branches, which reflect Earth energies, also correspond to the 12 months of the year and the daily pattern of 12 double-hour cycles.

Earth is a transformer, transforming one element into another, which explains the two extra Earth elements (one Yin and one Yang).

Figure 8.1 shows that when the Twelve Branches are placed in a 3×3 grid diagram, with three branches in each of the four cardinal directions (which relate to the four seasons), there is an Earth branch at each corner, where there is a change from one season to another or from one element to another.

	South Red Snake Horse Sheep + Fire − Fire − *Earth* 6 7 8 Summer	
East Green Dragon + *Earth* 5 Rabbit − Wood 4 Tiger + Wood 3 Spring		West Gold Monkey + Metal 9 Cock − Metal 10 Dog + *Earth* 11 Fall
	North Blue-Black Ox Rat Pig − *Earth* − Water + Water 2 1 12 Winter	

Note: + = *Yang*
          − = *Yin*

Figure 8.1 The Twelve Earthly Branches

The Earth branches are based on Yin–Yang and Five Phases theory. They follow earth's influences and are closely connected to the 12 months of a year, which are considered earth's pattern. It is common to refer to branches by their Chinese zodiac animal names, but significant applications are derived from their Yin–Yang and Five Phases qualities.

The Twelve Branches and their elements are presented in Table 8.2. Of the elements listed in the last column, the first one is the *main* element of the branch, and the others are *hidden* elements. The hidden elements explain certain relationships between branch pairings, and are important when explaining the acupuncture channel pairings of the arms and legs. Branch pairings and hidden elements are explained in detail in this and the next chapter.

TABLE 8.2 THE TWELVE EARTHLY BRANCHES

	Animal	Branch	Element	Main and hidden elements		
1	Rat	*Zi*	Yin Water	Yin Water *Gui*		
2	Ox	*Zhou*	Yin Earth	Yin Earth *Ji*	Yin Water *Gui*	Yin Metal *Xin*
3	Tiger	*Yin*	Yang Wood	Yang Wood *Jia*	Yang Fire *Bing*	Yang Earth *Wu*
4	Rabbit	*Mao*	Yin Wood	Yin Wood *Yi*		
5	Dragon	*Zhen*	Yang Earth	Yang Earth *Wu*	Yin Wood *Yi*	Yin Water *Gui*
6	Snake	*Si*	Yang Fire	Yang Fire *Bing*	Yang Earth *Wu*	Yang Metal *Geng*
7	Horse	*Wu*	Yin Fire	Yin Fire *Ding*	Yin Earth *Ji*	
8	Sheep	*Wei*	Yin Earth	Yin Earth *Ji*	Yin Fire *Ding*	Yin Wood *Yi*
9	Monkey	*Shen*	Yang Metal	Yang Metal *Geng*	Yang Earth *Wu*	Yang Water *Ren*
10	Cock	*You*	Yin Metal	Yin Metal *Xin*		
11	Dog	*Xu*	Yang Earth	Yang Earth *Wu*	Yin Metal *Xin*	Yin Fire *Ding*
12	Pig	*Hai*	Yang Water	Yang Water *Ren*	Yang Wood *Jia*	

The Stem and Branch Cycle of 60

Stems and branches represent a flow of energy. Each hour, day, month and year contains a stem and branch energy combination, and each specific stem and branch combination is called a "binomial." The binomials are organized in a cycle of 60, which includes every combination of stems and branches. Six cycles of ten stems and five cycles of 12 branches equals one cycle of 60. The 60-binomial cycle table, which is also called the JiaZi table, is shown in Table 8.3. (*Jia* is Yang Wood and *Zi* is the Rat.) This 60-year cycle contains every stem and branch pairing.

The first binomial contains Yang Wood, the second is Yin Wood, and so the Five Phases pattern continues until binomial 10. Yang Wood then reappears periodically at 11, 21, 31, 41 and 51, as the Ten Stems repeat for six cycles, completing the cycle of 60.

The branch Rat begins at binomial number one, and once completed the 12 animals or branches recur for another four cycles, beginning with the Rat at 13, 25, 37 and 49.

These cycles of stems and branches combine to create 60 individual stem–branch combinations.

The Heavenly Stems are in the top rows, and represent heavenly or Yang influences. They are always named according to Five Phases—for example, Yang Wood, Yin Wood, Yang Fire, Yin Fire. The lower rows contain the Earthly Branches, or Chinese zodiac animals. The branches can be named either as a Five Element or as an animal. I recommend using the animal name because it helps to differentiate branches from stems, and to distinguish among branches. The 60-binomial combinations recur during every hour, day, month and year cycle.

The "Four Pillars" are the Heavenly Stem and Earthly Branch for the hour, day, month and year being evaluated. In Chinese astrology, it is the Four Pillars that reflect a birth condition. Each pillar has a Heavenly Stem and an Earthly Branch, and each person has four branches or zodiac animals: one each for the hour, day, month and year of birth.

Table 8.3 The Stem and Branch Cycle of 60

Number	1	2	3	4	5	6
Stem	Yang Wood	Yin Wood	Yang Fire	Yin Fire	Yang Earth	Yin Earth
Branch	Rat	Ox	Tiger	Rabbit	Dragon	Snake
Number	**7**	**8**	**9**	**10**	**11**	**12**
Stem	Yang Metal	Yin Metal	Yang Water	Yin Water	Yang Wood	Yin Wood
Branch	Horse	Sheep	Monkey	Cock	Dog	Pig
Number	**13**	**14**	**15**	**16**	**17**	**18**
Stem	Yang Fire	Yin Fire	Yang Earth	Yin Earth	Yang Metal	Yin Metal
Branch	Rat	Ox	Tiger	Rabbit	Dragon	Snake
Number	**19**	**20**	**21**	**22**	**23**	**24**
Stem	Yang Water	Yin Water	Yang Wood	Yin Wood	Yang Fire	Yin Fire
Branch	Horse	Sheep	Monkey	Cock	Dog	Pig
Number	**25**	**26**	**27**	**28**	**29**	**30**
Stem	Yang Earth	Yin Earth	Yang Metal	Yin Metal	Yang Water	Yin Water
Branch	Rat	Ox	Tiger	Rabbit	Dragon	Snake
Number	**31**	**32**	**33**	**34**	**35**	**36**
Stem	Yang Wood	Yin Wood	Yang Fire	Yin Fire	Yang Earth	Yin Earth
Branch	Horse	Sheep	Monkey	Cock	Dog	Pig
Number	**37**	**38**	**39**	**40**	**41**	**42**
Stem	Yang Metal	Yin Metal	Yang Water	Yin Water	Yang Wood	Yin Wood
Branch	Rat	Ox	Tiger	Rabbit	Dragon	Snake
Number	**43**	**44**	**45**	**46**	**47**	**48**
Stem	Yang Fire	Yin Fire	Yang Earth	Yin Earth	Yang Metal	Yin Metal
Branch	Horse	Sheep	Monkey	Cock	Dog	Pig

Number	49	50	51	52	53	54
Stem	Yang Water	Yin Water	Yang Wood	Yin Wood	Yang Fire	Yin Fire
Branch	Rat	Ox	Tiger	Rabbit	Dragon	Snake
Number	55	56	57	58	59	60
Stem	Yang Earth	Yin Earth	Yang Metal	Yin Metal	Yang Water	Yin Water
Branch	Horse	Sheep	Monkey	Cock	Dog	Pig

The Twelve Earthly Branches and the Chinese Zodiac Animals

Sets of Correspondences

The Twelve Earthly Branches have many correspondences, including a main element, Chinese zodiac animal and geographical location. Figures 8.2 and 8.3 and Tables 8.4 and 8.5 show these correspondences. The animals or branches in the same geographical plane have an affinity for each other, as they share the same directional element, and therefore support or reinforce each other. In addition, a trinity/harmonic or elemental frame relationship links every fourth animal in a special relationship. (For example, Cock, Ox and Snake are four places apart from each other, and therefore are compatible from a basic astrological viewpoint, as explained later in this chapter.) These types of energetic relationships play an integral role in revealing fundamental theories within acupuncture.

The North, South, East and West are the *cardinal* or middle positions of the branches, as shown in the branch charts on the next few pages. They play a vital role in grouping the branches for Chinese astrology and the acupuncture channels. These pairings comprise the leg and arm channel combinations.

Figure 8.2 shows the Twelve Branches and their geographical positions, main element, direction and numerical position in the chart.

	South Red Snake Horse Sheep + Fire − Fire − *Earth* 6 7 8 Summer	
East Green Dragon + Earth 5 Rabbit − Wood 4 Tiger + Wood 3 Spring		West Gold Monkey + Metal 9 Cock − Metal 10 Dog + Earth 11 Fall
	North Blue-Black Ox Rat Pig − *Earth* − Water +Water 2 1 12 Winter	

Figure 8.2 The Twelve Branches

Table 8.4 summarizes additional correspondences of the branches, which include their name, main element, season, time of day and direction.

TABLE 8.4 THE TWELVE BRANCHES AND THEIR NAME, ELEMENT, SEASON, TIME OF DAY AND DIRECTION

Branch name	Main element	Season	Time of day	Direction
Pig *Hai*	Yang Water	Winter	9pm–11pm	North
Rat *Zi*	Yin Water	Winter	11pm–1am	North
Ox *Zhou*	Yin Earth	Winter	1am–3am	North
Tiger *Yin*	Yang Wood	Spring	3am–5am	East
Rabbit *Mao*	Yin Wood	Spring	5am–7am	East
Dragon *Zhen*	Yang Earth	Spring	7am–9am	East
Snake *Si*	Yang Fire	Summer	9am–11am	South
Horse *Wu*	Yin Fire	Summer	11am–1pm	South
Sheep *Wei*	Yin Earth	Summer	1pm–3pm	South
Monkey *Shen*	Yang Metal	Fall	3pm–5pm	West
Cock *You*	Yin Metal	Fall	5pm–7pm	West
Dog *Xu*	Yang Earth	Fall	7pm–9pm	West

Hidden Elements

Nine of the Twelve Branches or animals contain hidden elements, or Ren Yuan, which are Five Phases contained within a branch. The hidden element's Five Phases Qi is less powerful than that of the main element. The branches and their hidden elements are shown in Table 8.5 and Figure 8.3.

TABLE 8.5 THE BRANCHES AND HIDDEN ELEMENTS

Animal	Name	Main element	Hidden element
Pig	*Hai*	Yang Water	Yang Wood
Rat	*Zi*	Yin Water	
Ox	*Zhou*	Yin Earth	Yin Water, Yin Metal
Tiger	*Yin*	Yang Wood	Yang Fire, Yang Earth
Rabbit	*Mao*	Yin Wood	
Dragon	*Zhen*	Yang Earth	Yin Wood, Yin Water
Snake	*Si*	Yang Fire	Yang Earth, Yang Metal
Horse	*Wu*	Yin Fire	Yin Earth
Sheep	*Wei*	Yin Earth	Yin Fire, Yin Wood
Monkey	*Shen*	Yang Metal	Yang Earth, Yang Water
Cock	*You*	Yin Metal	
Dog	*Xu*	Yang Earth	Yin Metal, Yin Fire

	Snake Yang Fire Yang Earth Yang Metal	**Horse** Yin Fire Yin Earth	Sheep Yin Earth Ying Fire Yin Wood	
Dragon Yang Earth Yin Wood Yin Water				Monkey Yang Metal Yang Water Yang Earth
Rabbit Yin Wood				**Cock** Yin Metal
Tiger Yang Wood Yang Fire Yang Earth				Dog Yang Earth Yin Metal Yin Fire
	Ox Yin Earth Yin Water Yin Metal	**Rat** Yin Water	Pig Yang Water Yang Wood	

Figure 8.3 The Branches and Hidden Elements

The main element is the first listed under each animal, with the hidden elements in second and third place. The animals in bold print are the cardinal branches and are in central positions; they are also considered leaders in their geographical directions. Locate any branch or animal and count four spaces forward and backward (excluding blank squares). The three animals four spaces apart comprise a *frame* or *trinity*, and share an element in common. For example, Horse, Dog and Tiger are four spaces (or palaces) apart. Horse, as a cardinal position in the center of the South section, designates the elemental or phase frame as Fire. Note that Fire is contained in the hidden elements of both the Dog and Tiger. These frame or trinity groupings contain the same element, and so these animals resonate with each another. In Chinese astrology, this is a very basic method of identifying romantic attraction. In acupuncture, these frames correspond to the leg and arm pairings. The theoretical basis for these channels will be explained in this chapter.

The frame or trinity groups are as follows.

- Rat, Dragon and Monkey are the Water Frame.

- Rabbit, Sheep and Pig are the Wood Frame.

- Horse, Dog and Tiger are the Fire Frame.

- Cock, Ox and Snake are the Metal Frame.

The Twelve-Stage Growth Cycle

Chinese metaphysics views life as one integrated whole. Yin–Yang views the whole in two interdependent aspects, and the Twelve-Stage Growth Cycle views the same whole in 12 aspects or energetic phases. In these models each aspect has a relationship to the whole. Yin–Yang, Five Phases and the Twelve-Stage Growth Cycle can reveal different conditions within the same situation, thus offering a variety of analytical tools and treatment methods.

The Twelve-Stage Growth Cycle is an extension of Yin–Yang and the Five Phases cycle of expansion, peak, harvest, decline and regeneration, or waxing and waning. Each of the Five Phases represents a season, as well as months in a year. The Twelve-Stage Growth Cycle embraces the Twelve Branches or Chinese zodiac animals, which are tools that communicate the energetics of numerous patterns. Table 8.6 lists each of the Five Phases and their corresponding seasons.

TABLE 8.6 THE FIVE PHASES ELEMENTS AND SEASONS

Element	Season
Wood	Spring
Fire	Summer
Earth	Indian summer or the transition from season to season
Metal	Fall
Water	Winter

The Twelve-Stage Growth Cycle is a very important model in Chinese astrology, feng shui and numerous healing and divination arts. The Twelve-Stage Growth Cycle identifies the growth and decline stages in a cycle. The most favorable and potent stages are 4 and 5, which are adult and prime stages. The Twelve-Stage Growth Cycle is the energetic structure of the daily meridian clock.

In time-based acupuncture, or chrono acupuncture, favorable times are identified and the proper acupuncture points are selected based on nature's energy cycles. Each acupoint selected is based on multiple systems that include Twelve-Stage Growth Cycle energetics. The method identifies the prime times within cycles of time. Figure 8.4 and Table 8.7 show the Twelve-Stage Growth Cycle.

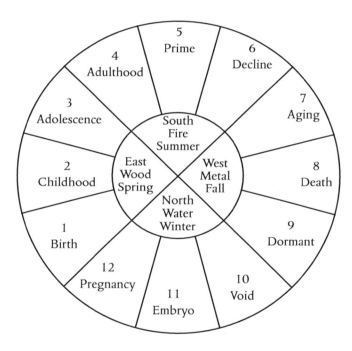

Figure 8.4 The Twelve-Stage Growth Cycle

Table 8.7 The Twelve-Stage Growth Cycle

	Cycle stage
1	Birth—*Chang Sheng* Needs energy
2	Childhood—*Mu Yu* Needs energy
3	Adolescence—*Guan Dai* Needs direction
4	Adulthood—*Lin Guan* Rising, growth
5	Prime—*Di Wang* Peak
6	Decline—*Sui* Decline
7	Aging—*Bing* Weakening
8	Death—*Si* Depletion
9	Dormancy—*Mu* Buried, storing, grave
10	Void—*Jue* Preparation
11	Embryo—*Tai* Beginning
12	Pregnancy—*Yang* New creation has begun

The Chinese Calendar

The Chinese calendar is also called the natural energy calendar or the 10,000-year calendar. According to legend it began in 2698 BC, on the first day of the first year of the reign of Huang Di, the Yellow Emperor. This calendar is the foundation for many methods in Chinese metaphysics, including calculating a Chinese astrology birth chart, which is called the "eight characters" (Ba Zi, or the Four Pillars). These are the stem and branch of the hour, day, month and year of birth. This calendar is a method of counting, using the cycle of 60 (the 60-binomial cycle). The following are the main components necessary to find correct stem and branch information:

- *Time of birth*: Use the time of the city in which you were born, do not convert your birth time to Chinese time. If you were born in New York, use the time of birth in New York.

- *Solar calendar*: The New Year begins in the month of Yang Wood, the Tiger, which is February (and not in Yin Water, the Rat, or January). The actual day of the New Year varies from year to year.

- *Day*: A new day begins after midnight. The Zi, or Rat, hour pillar spans the hours 11:00pm–1:00am, but the new day actually begins after 12:00am.

- *Hour*: The hour of birth is based on the standard double Chinese hours—for example, as already stated, the Zi (Rat) hour includes any time from 11:00pm to 1:00am.

A comprehensive Chinese calendar has 24 sections, or seasons, which are periods of 15 days. These are the 12 months, categorized into Yin–Yang: the first part of the month is Yang and the second part of the month is Yin. (The first day of the month is called *Jie*, and the first day of the second part of the month (the sixteenth day) is called *Qi*.) The daily meridian clock and the waxing and waning of the two-hour periods are also based on this energy pattern.

The solar year begins on Li Chun, or the Beginning of Spring, usually February 4 or 5, when the sun enters 15 degrees Aquarius. This is also the beginning of the month of the Tiger, or Yin Yue, and when the Big Dipper points to the East. The natural energetic flow of waxing and waning Qi for each month is applied in a micro-system to each day, and the daily meridian clock is the tool by means of which acupuncturists can utilize this cycle.

Table 8.8 shows the 24 seasons, the Chinese zodiac animals and their related monthly correspondences. The beginning day of each month is in bold type. Note the corresponding branches or Chinese animal names. The days for the months can change by a day, so please refer to the actual year calendar for exact dates and times.

There is a special form of Qi Gong called Jieqi Qi Gong, which links the 24 vertebrae of the spine and the 24 seasons. In this Qi Gong form a specific Qi Gong meditation and body posture is performed during one of the Jieqi. This practice connects, collects and energizes the human body and is an example of correspondence between the human body and cycles of time.

Table 8.8 The 24 Seasons

Date	*Jie*	*Qi*	Branch	Direction
Feb 4	*Li Chun* Beginning of Spring		*Yin* Tiger	East
Feb 19		*Yu Shui* Rain Water		
March 6	*Jing Zhu* Insects Awaken		*Mao* Rabbit	East
March 21		*Chun Fen* Spring Equinox		
April 5	*Qing Ming* Clear and Bright		*Chen* Dragon	East
April 20		*Gu Yu* Great Rain		
May 6	*Li Xia* Beginning of Summer		*Si* Snake	South
May 21		*Xiao Man* Small Surplus		

June 6	*Mang Zhong* Planting of Crops		*Wu* Horse	South
June 21		*Xia Shu* Summer Solstice		
July 7	*Xiao Shu* Lesser Heat		*Wei* Sheep	South
July 23		*Da Shu* Greater Heat		
August 7	*Li Qiu* Beginning of Autumn		*Shen* Monkey	West
August 23		*Chu Shu* Storage Heat		
September 7	*Bai Lu* White Dew		*You* Cock	West
September 23		*Qiu Fen* Autumn Equinox		
October 8	*Han Lu* Cold Dew		*Shu* Dog	West
October 23		*Shuang Jiang* Frost Falls		
November 7	*Li Dong* Beginning of Winter		*Hai* Pig	North
November 22		*Xiao Xue* Lesser Snow		
December 7	*Da Xue* Greater Snow		*Zi* Rat	North
December 22		*Dong Zhi* Winter Solstice		
January 5	*Xiao Han* Lesser Cold		*Chou* Ox	North
January 20		*Da Han* Greater Cold		

The Origin of the Daily Meridian Clock

Chapter 16 of the *Ling Shui* (Wu 2002) presents the Ying Qi cycle. Even though it does not assign time frames to the channels, their sequence has become what is commonly known as "the daily cycle" or "daily meridian clock." It is the Ying Qi, or nutritive Qi that flows through the acupuncture channels in the Ying Qi cycle sequence. This Ying Qi cycle flows from the Hand Tai Yin to Hand Yang Ming, Foot Yang Ming, Foot Tai Yin, Hand Shao Yin, Hand Tai Yang, Foot Tai Yang, Foot Shao Yin, Hand Jue Yin, Hand Shao Yang, Foot Shao Yang, and then Foot Jue Yin Channels. When one cycle of the primary channels is completed, the circulation flows up the front of the body to the vertex and down the back of the spine, and then up the front of the body to the Lungs to repeat the cycle. The flow up the front of the body and down the back comprises the Ren and Du Channels, with the pattern continuing in an endless cycle. This pattern is the path in which Ying Qi flows, and it reflects post-natal energetics. The connection to the Ren and Du is the internal channel flow, which reveals how post-natal conditions influence prenatal energetics, or how superficial influences can enter deeper, Yuan layers of the body. This cycle is the basis for a variety of clinically significant methods.

The daily meridian clock is based on several Chinese metaphysical principles, including the Nine Palaces, which is the terrain for the construction of the Ying Qi cycle. The following section presents new information and integrates it into what has already been discussed, to provide the theoretical model for the Ying Qi cycle sequence and the daily meridian clock.

The Nine Palaces

The Nine Palaces (Luo Shu) or Magic Square takes several different forms. The three diagrams in Figure 8.5 are the more common versions. The numbers include 1 through 9 in modern versions, with nine dots used in ancient versions. The first model is a dot system with no numbers, the second adds numbers to the dot system and the third uses only numbers.

The Nine Palaces has a number pattern which originates in the center, with the number 5, and then flows or flies in ascending order around the Nine Palaces from 6 through 4: 6, 7, 8, 9, 1, 2, 3, 4. Universal correspondences can be inferred from this special pattern; however, though the items placed in this pattern can change, the pattern sequence is fixed.

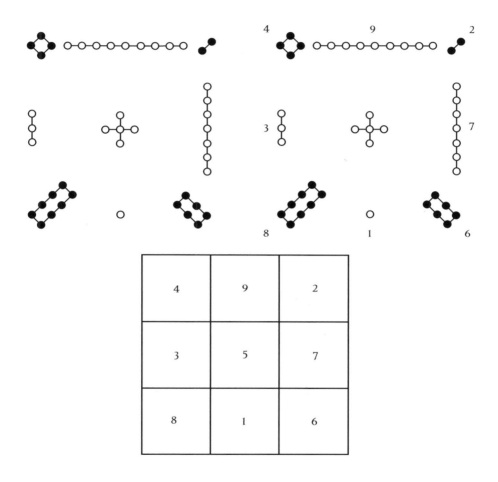

Figure 8.5 The Nine Palaces and He Tu

The Nine Palaces reflects the integration of numerous theories of Chinese metaphysics: numbers correspond to trigrams, Five Phases and their corresponding organs and channels. The Nine Palaces in Figure 8.6 contain numbers, Five Phases, trigrams and a new correspondence: the acupuncture channels.

4 *Xun* Yin Wood Liver	9 *Li* Fire Heart Small Intestine	2 *Kun* Earth-Fire Pericardium San Jiao
3 *Zhen* Yang Wood Gallbladder	5 Center Earth	7 *Dui* Yang Metal Large Intestine
8 *Gen* Mountain Earth Stomach Spleen	1 *Kan* Water Bladder Kidney	6 *Qian* Yin Metal Lung

Figure 8.6 Nine Palaces Showing Acupuncture Channel Correspondences

Each of the qualities related to trigrams and palaces can be combined with the numerical pattern inside the Nine Palaces. This is the "magic" of the Magic Square or Nine Palaces. The pattern or sequence of the numbers creates the exact order of the Ying Qi cycle, or the daily meridian clock. This pattern is also called the Dance of Yu, a movement from an ascending, or Yang, sequence of the numbers. This dance places the channels with their corresponding number, polarity, phase and trigram, revealing the Ying Qi, or daily meridian clock, order.

The Ying Qi, or daily cycle, flows in the order seen in Figure 8.6, beginning with the Lungs and flowing in an ascending or Yang pattern, revealing the complete daily cycle. The theory and logic for this exact sequence is now presented.

Ying Qi Cycle Construction Principles

Odd numbers are Yang; *even* numbers are Yin.

The center of the Nine Palaces is the beginning position and contains the Earth element. In Ba Gua theory there are eight directions, not nine, and there is no trigram for the center, and so there are eight directions and eight trigrams.

Begin in the center (5) and move palace by palace in ascending order: from 5 move to 6 then 7, 8, 9, 1, 2, 3 and 4. The first channel is placed at number 6.

- 6 is a Yin number, which is Yin Metal and relates to the Lung.

- 7 is a Yang number, Yang Metal and relates to the Large Intestine.

- 8 is Earth and relates to the Stomach/Spleen.

- 9 is Fire and relates to the Heart/Small Intestine.

- 1 is Water and relates to the Bladder/Kidney.

- 2 is Earth/Fire and relates to the Pericardium/San Jiao.

- 3 is a Yang number, Yang Wood and relates to the Gallbladder.

- 4 is a Yin number, Yin Wood and relates to the Liver.

The following Nine Palaces diagrams illustrate the eight-step numerical sequence one step at a time.

	5 Center Earth	
		6 *Qian* Yin Metal Lung ☰

6 is a Yin number, Yin Metal and relates to the Lung.

	5 Center Earth	7 *Dui* Yang Metal Large Intestine
		6 *Qian* Yin Metal Lung

7 is a Yang number, Yang Metal and relates to the Large Intestine.

		7 *Dui* Yang Metal Large Intestine ▬▬ ▬▬ ▬▬▬▬▬▬ ▬▬▬▬▬▬
	5 Center Earth	
8 *Gen* Mountain Earth Stomach Spleen ▬▬▬▬▬▬ ▬▬ ▬▬ ▬▬ ▬▬		6 *Qian* Yin Metal Lung ▬▬▬▬▬▬ ▬▬▬▬▬▬ ▬▬▬▬▬▬

8 is Earth and relates to the Stomach/Spleen.

	9 *Li* Fire Heart Small Intestine ☲	
	5 Center Earth	7 *Dui* Yang Metal Large Intestine ☱
8 *Gen* Mountain Earth Stomach Spleen ☶		6 *Qian* Yin Metal Lung ☰

9 is Fire and relates to the Heart/Small Intestine.

	9 *Li* Fire Heart Small Intestine	
	5 Center Earth	7 *Dui* Yang Metal Large Intestine
8 *Gen* Mountain Earth Stomach Spleen	1 *Kan* Water Bladder Kidney	6 *Qian* Yin Metal Lung

1 is Water and relates to the Bladder/Kidney.

	9 *Li* Fire Heart Small Intestine	2 *Kun* Fire–Earth Pericardium San Jiao
	5 Center Earth	7 *Dui* Yang Metal Large Intestine
8 *Gen* Mountain Earth Stomach Spleen	1 *Kan* Water Bladder Kidney	6 *Qian* Yin Metal Lung

2 is Earth/Fire and relates to the Pericardium/San Jiao.

	9 *Li* Fire Heart Small Intestine	2 *Kun* Earth-Fire Pericardium San Jiao
3 *Zhen* Yang Wood Gallbladder	5 Center Earth	7 *Dui* Yang Metal Large Intestine
8 *Gen* Mountain Earth Stomach Spleen	1 *Kan* Water Bladder Kidney	6 *Qian* Yin Metal Lung

3 is a Yang number, Yang Wood and relates to the Gallbladder.

4 *Xun* Yin Wood Liver	9 *Li* Fire Heart Small Intestine	2 *Kun* Earth-Fire Pericardium San Jiao
3 *Zhen* Yang Wood Gallbladder	5 Center Earth	7 *Dui* Yang Metal Large Intestine
8 *Gen* Mountain Earth Stomach Spleen	1 *Kan* Water Bladder Kidney	6 *Qian* Yin Metal Lung

4 is a Yin number, Yin Wood and relates to the Liver.

The method for deciphering the daily meridian clock within the Nine Palaces is to extract out the organ channels in sequential order. The pattern in the Nine Palaces is a Yang, or ascending pattern. The following pattern reveals the daily meridian clock:

- 6 is a Yin number, Yin Metal and relates to the Lung.

- 7 is a Yang number, Yang Metal and relates to the Large Intestine.

- 8 is Earth and relates to the Stomach/Spleen.

- 9 is Fire and relates to the Heart/Small Intestine.

- 1 is Water and relates to the Bladder/Kidney.

- 2 is Earth/Fire and relates to the Pericardium/San Jiao.

- 3 is a Yang number, Yang Wood and relates to the Gallbladder.

- 4 is a Yin number, Yin Wood and relates to the Liver.

The Nine Palaces order of primary channels is as follows, and it parallels the Ying Qi cycle sequence found in Chapter 16 of the *Nei Jing Ling Shu*.

Lung

Large Intestine

Stomach

Spleen

Heart

Small Intestine

Bladder

Kidney

Pericardium

San Jiao

Gallbladder

Liver

The Cosmological Daily Meridian Clock

The daily meridian clock is a traditional tool frequently used in the practice of Chinese medicine and is included in most books on acupuncture, but theories supporting its sequence have not been commonly presented. This section presents Chinese metaphysical principles and models that explain the theoretical basis of the Ying Qi cycle or daily meridian clock, including how the 12 channels and branches explain the channel formation on the arms and legs. For example, it explains why the Spleen, Liver and Kidneys are on the Leg Yin region.

The daily meridian clock is a multi-dimensional energetic model. It is a profound energy system integrating many principles contained in the *I Ching* and *Nei Jing*. It requires multiple Chinese metaphysical models to explain the logic for the construction of the daily meridian clock; the models include Yin–Yang, Five Phases, Twelve Branches and the Twelve-Stage Growth Cycle. This section presents classic concepts and theories explaining the building blocks of the daily meridian clock, and how it contains the origin of foundational aspects of Chinese medicine. Step by step you will come to see how the daily meridian clock model supports the groups of three Leg Yang, three Leg Yin, three Arm Yin and three Arm Yang Channels. In addition, a comprehensive daily meridian clock shows why the Lung Channel begins the clock flow between 3:00 and 5:00am.

As a cosmological imaging system, the daily meridian clock originates as a mirror image of the energetic flow of nature.

1. Yin descends and Yang ascends, reflected in the energetics of Water and Fire:

	Fire Yang	
	Water Yin	

2. Yin–Yang expands to the Five Phases and their energetic flow. Below is a traditional presentation of the elements: Water and Metal are Yin and descend, while Wood and Fire are Yang and ascend:

	Fire Yang	
Wood Yang	Earth	Metal Yin
	Water Yin	

3. The four cardinal positions are now added to their energetic flow and their corresponding elements. Notice that the Earth element is in the central palace or position, and is the only palace that touches or connects to every palace and element. Earth, then, is the transformer:

	Fire Yang South	
Wood Yang East	Earth	Metal Yin West
	Water Yin North	

4. This diagram adds major times of the day:

	Fire Yang Noon	
Wood Yang 6:00am	Earth	Metal Yin 6:00pm
	Water Yin Midnight	

The Twelve Earthly Branches reflect Earth's energy (Qi) and relate to the 12 months of the year, the 12 primary acupuncture channels and the 12 double-hours of a day. A major model used in Chinese metaphysics is the Twelve-Stage Growth Cycle, a model that integrates Yin–Yang, Five Phases and the energetic patterns of 12. The Twelve-Stage Growth Cycle numerology matches the 12 double-hours in a day and the 12 primary acupuncture channels in the body. This cycle can be viewed as an expansion of the cycle of two (Yin–Yang) and the cycle of five (the Five Phases). The Twelve-Stage Growth Cycle includes an expansion stage and a declining stage with 12 aspects, which match the 12 acupuncture channels of the body. Figure 8.4 on page 103 and Table 8.7 on page 104 contain information on the Twelve-Stage Growth Cycle.

In traditional Chinese medicine, the Twelve Branches or Chinese zodiac animals correspond to elements and directions. Figure 8.7 shows these correspondences, and Figure 8.8 adds the time of the day.

	Snake-6 Yang Fire	Horse-7 Yin Fire	Sheep-8 Yin Earth	
Dragon-5 Yang Earth		South Fire Summer		Monkey-9 Yang Metal
Rabbit-4 Yin Wood	East Wood Spring		West Metal Fall	Cock-10 Yin Metal
Tiger-3 Yang Wood		North Water Winter		Dog-11 Yang Earth
	Ox-2 Yin Earth	Rat-1 Yin Water	Pig-12 Yang Water	

Figure 8.7 The Twelve Branches, Elements and Directions

The animals and their associated acupuncture channels are presented in Figure 8.9. As mentioned earlier, a key relationship between the branches is the trinity or harmonic relationships. Select any animal and count in a pattern of four palaces or positions. The three animals in this plane have many interrelationships. For example, the Rat is located at the bottom: count four palaces, or spaces, arriving at the Dragon; and four more palaces, arriving at the Monkey. The Rat, Dragon and Monkey comprise the Water Frame, as the Rat is Water, and the other two contain a hidden element of Water. These groups are used in Chinese astrology as potential romantic partners. In acupuncture they reveal the three Leg Yang Channels or Gallbladder, Stomach and Bladder Channels.

Water, the Rat, is Yin and represents the winter solstice. Fire, the Horse, is Yang and represents the summer solstice. These opposite poles set the midnight-noon, Horse-Rat or Wu-Zi axis of a clockwise flow, with each of the Twelve Branches relating to an interval of two hours.

	Snake-6 Yang Fire 9am–11am	Horse-7 Yin Fire 11am–1pm	Sheep-8 Yin Earth 1pm–3pm	
Dragon-5 Yang Earth 7am–9am		South Fire Summer		Monkey-9 Yang Metal 3pm–5pm
Rabbit-4 Yin Wood 5am–7am	East Wood Spring		West Metal Fall	Cock-10 Yin Metal 5pm–7pm
Tiger-3 Yang Wood 3am–5am		North Water Winter		Dog-11 Yang Earth 7pm–9pm
	Ox-2 Yin Earth 1am–3am	Rat-1 Yin Water 11pm–1am	Pig-12 Yang Water 9pm–11pm	

Figure 8.8 The Twelve Branches and the Times of the Day

Notice that the Five Phases flow from Rat-Water to Rabbit-Wood to Horse-Fire and Cock-Metal: an unfolding of the Five Phases is an integral aspect of the clock. The four Earth branches or animals are in the four corners, and they transform the Qi of one Five Phase element into that of another. This clock clearly shows the key Earth function of transformation.

The Daily Meridian Clock, Channels and Internal Organs

The internal organs correspond to the Five Phases and 12 branches. When the Five Phases, Twelve Branches and time periods are matched to the internal organs, the traditional daily meridian clock is completed.

	Snake-6 Yang Fire 9am–11am Spleen	Horse-7 Yin Fire 11am–1pm Heart	Sheep-8 Yin Earth 1pm–3pm Small Intestine	
Dragon-5 Yang Earth 7am–9am Stomach		South Fire Summer ☲		Monkey-9 Yang Metal 3pm–5pm Bladder
Rabbit-4 Yin Wood 5am–7am Large Intestine	East Wood Spring ☳		West Metal Fall ☱	Cock-10 Yin Metal 5pm–7pm Kidney
Tiger-3 Yang Wood 3am–5am Lung		North Water Winter ☵		Dog-11 Yang Earth 7pm–9pm Pericardium
	Ox-2 Yin Earth 1am–3am Liver	Rat-1 Yin Water 11pm–1am Gallbladder	Pig-12 Yang Water 9pm–11pm San Jiao	

Figure 8.9 The Twelve Branches, Channels and Internal Organs

Nine Palaces theory explains the sequence of the daily meridian clock and why the Lung is the first in the sequence. The next step is to understand why the Lung begins at 3:00am. In some traditional Chinese astrology and feng shui systems, the Tiger month, February, is the beginning of the New Year. It is Yang Wood, representing the energy of ascending, growing and the beginning Qi of a new cycle. This is based on a solar calendar and solar energy patterns; however, some systems are based on the moon's patterns. According to the Nine Palaces, the Lung is the first channel in the daily meridian clock. By association with February as Yang Wood and the Tiger, the Lung is matched with the branch that begins the energy cycle; and in terms of the daily meridian clock this corresponds to 3:00 to 5:00am. Placing the remaining channels in the exact order of the Nine Palaces reveals the pattern of the daily meridian clock.

In *I Ching* theory, Heaven created the myriad things with Zhen. Zhen, the trigram Thunder, contains Yang Wood and is located in the East. The East is the direction where the sun rises and is the beginning of a new day, season and year. As shown in Figure 8.9, Yang Wood corresponds with the Tiger as the energetic beginning of a cycle. This is the theory that underpins Spring and the Earth branch Tiger as the start of a New Year or cycle.

Figures 8.10–8.13 present each of the four trinity or harmonic branch partners and their corresponding acupuncture pairs. (These pairs are also called frames.) They comprise the three-channel pairings on the arms and legs.

- The Fire trinity comprises the three Hand Yin Channels: Heart, Lung and Pericardium (Figure 8.10).

- The Wood trinity comprises the three Arm Yang Channels: Large Intestine, Small Intestine and San Jiao (Figure 8.11).

- The Metal trinity comprises the three Leg Yin Channels: Kidney, Liver and Spleen (Figure 8.12).

- The Water trinity comprises the three Leg Yang Channels: Gallbladder, Stomach and Bladder (Figure 8.13).

This presentation of the daily meridian clock provides the theoretical support for the acupuncture channel pairs and demonstrates that the clock is not just a time-based tool, but also an imaging system of the human body.

	Snake-6 Yang Fire Yang Earth Yang Metal 9am–11am Spleen	Horse-7 Yin Fire Yin Earth 11am–1pm Heart	Sheep-8 Yin Earth Ying Fire Yin Wood 1pm–3pm Small Intestine	
Dragon-5 Yang Earth Yin Wood Yin Water 7am–9am Stomach		South Fire Summer		Monkey-9 Yang Metal Yang Water Yang Earth 3pm–5pm Bladder
Rabbit-4 Yin Wood 5am–7am Large Intestine	East Wood Spring		West Metal Fall	Cock-10 Yin Metal 5pm–7pm Kidney
Tiger-3 Yang Wood Yang Fire Yang Earth 3am–5am Lung		North Water Winter		Dog-11 Yang Earth Yin Metal Yin Fire 7pm–9pm Pericardium
	Ox-2 Yin Earth Yin Water Yin Metal 1am–3am Liver	Rat-1 Yin Water 11pm–1am Gallbladder	Pig-12 Yang Water Yang Wood 9pm–11pm San Jiao	

Figure 8.10 The Fire Branch Trinity

	Snake-6 Yang Fire Yang Earth Yang Metal 9am–11am Spleen	Horse-7 Yin Fire Yin Earth 11am–1pm Heart	Sheep-8 Yin Earth Ying Fire Yin Wood 1pm–3pm Small Intestine	
Dragon-5 Yang Earth Yin Wood Yin Water 7am–9am Stomach		South Fire Summer		Monkey-9 Yang Metal Yang Water Yang Earth 3pm–5pm Bladder
Rabbit-4 Yin Wood 5am–7am Large Intestine	East Wood Spring		West Metal Fall	Cock-10 Yin Metal 5pm–7pm Kidney
Tiger-3 Yang Wood Yang Fire Yang Earth 3am–5am Lung		North Water Winter		Dog-11 Yang Earth Yin Metal Yin Fire 7pm–9pm Pericardium
	Ox-2 Yin Earth Yin Water Yin Metal 1am–3am Liver	Rat-1 Yin Water 11pm–1am Gallbladder	Pig-12 Yang Water Yang Wood 9pm–11pm San Jiao	

Figure 8.11 The Wood Branch Trinity

	Snake-6 Yang Fire Yang Earth Yang Metal 9am–11am Spleen	Horse-7 Yin Fire Yin Earth 11am–1pm Heart	Sheep-8 Yin Earth Ying Fire Yin Wood 1pm–3pm Small Intestine	
Dragon-5 Yang Earth Yin Wood Yin Water 7am–9am Stomach		South Fire Summer		Monkey-9 Yang Metal Yang Water Yang Earth 3pm–5pm Bladder
Rabbit-4 Yin Wood 5am–7am Large Intestine	East Wood Spring		West Metal Fall	Cock-10 Yin Metal 5pm–7pm Kidney
Tiger-3 Yang Wood Yang Fire Yang Earth 3am–5am Lung		North Water Winter		Dog-11 Yang Earth Yin Metal Yin Fire 7pm–9pm Pericardium
	Ox-2 Yin Earth Yin Water Yin Metal 1am–3am Liver	Rat-1 Yin Water 11pm–1am Gallbladder	Pig-12 Yang Water Yang Wood 9pm–11pm San Jiao	

Figure 8.12 The Metal Branch Trinity

	Snake-6 Yang Fire Yang Earth Yang Metal 9am–11am Spleen	Horse-7 Yin Fire Yin Earth 11am–1pm Heart	Sheep-8 Yin Earth Ying Fire Yin Wood 1pm–3pm Small Intestine	
Dragon-5 Yang Earth Yin Wood Yin Water 7am–9am Stomach		South Fire Summer		Monkey-9 Yang Metal Yang Water Yang Earth 3pm–5pm Bladder
Rabbit-4 Yin Wood 5am–7am Large Intestine	East Wood Spring		West Metal Fall	Cock-10 Yin Metal 5pm–7pm Kidney
Tiger-3 Yang Wood Yang Fire Yang Earth 3am–5am Lung		North Water Winter		Dog-11 Yang Earth Yin Metal Yin Fire 7pm–9pm Pericardium
	Ox-2 Yin Earth Yin Water Yin Metal 1am–3am Liver	Rat-1 Yin Water 11pm–1am Gallbladder	Pig-12 Yang Water Yang Wood 9pm–11pm San Jiao	

Figure 8.13 The Water Branch Trinity

Table 8.9 summarizes channel pairs for the legs and arms.

- The Rabbit/Large Intestine is Wood and the Horse/Heart is Fire; both are Yang, and their three-channel patterns are located on the Yang part of the body, the arm. The trinity pairs of these animals/ elements are located on the arm.

- The Cock/Kidney is Metal and the Rat/Gallbladder is Water; both are Yin and their three-channel patterns are located on the Yin part of the body, the leg.

This model is the basis for the location of the channels, not just their pairings.

TABLE 8.9 THE ARM AND LEG CHANNELS

Frame or trinity	Region	Channel and animal	Channel and animal	Channel and animal
Wood Frame	Three Arm Yang	Large Intestine Rabbit	Small Intestine Sheep	San Jiao Pig
Fire Frame	Three Hand Yin	Heart Horse	Pericardium Dog	Lung Tiger
Metal Frame	Three Leg Yin	Kidney Cock	Liver Ox	Spleen Snake
Water Frame	Three Leg Yang	Gallbladder Rat	Stomach Dragon	Bladder Monkey

The Chinese metaphysical models presented so far reveal in numerous ways how the ancient Chinese philosophers and practitioners evaluated their environment and constructed tools to reflect their insights. The birth of applied philosophy occurs when theories are extended to the human body and condition, and become the basis of treatment. Studying the classic Chinese metaphysical models and theories provides the opportunity to understand the unique insights of the originators of these theories and models. The remaining chapters of this book describe Chinese medical applications of the theories and models presented, which comprise the Balance Method.

PART II

CLINICAL APPLICATIONS

INTRODUCTION TO PART II

The Chinese have a unique understanding of the human body and the acupuncture channel system. The vision of the early Chinese medical practitioners and authors was that the acupuncture channels are a sequencing system, which includes levels that can be easily visualized in terms of anatomical layers. There are five major channel systems, and each layer or channel system corresponds to specific aspects of the body and their corresponding Chinese medical substances, and pathogens located there.

The pathways of the channel system provide pointers to the "sequencing" of the channels. For example, superficial channel layers deal with the exterior and the pathology related to it, and the deep channels influence the interior conditions and chronic constitutional conditions.

The Acupuncture Layering System

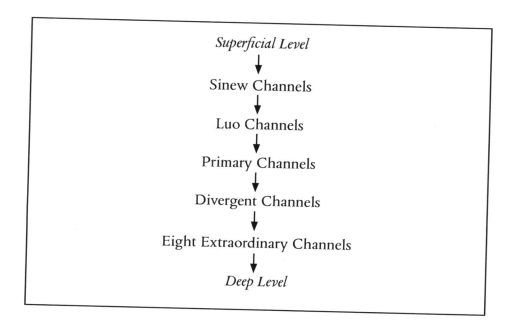

Superficial Level

↓

Sinew Channels

↓

Luo Channels

↓

Primary Channels

↓

Divergent Channels

↓

Eight Extraordinary Channels

↓

Deep Level

The following three references from the *Nei Jing Su Wen* present the sequencing or layering of channels. They also present how pathogens can be lodged in these layers, as well as that needling must be at the depth of the targeted channel system to treat the condition most effectively. These references are the basis for how to use all acupuncture channels and become a complete practitioner.

> "In general, when a pathogen invades the body, it first enters the skin level. If it lingers or is not expelled it will travel into the Micro Luo. If not expelled it travels to the regular Luo channels, if not expelled then moves to the main channels and then the internal organs... This is the progression of the pathogen from the skin level into the organs."
>
> *Nei Jing Su Wen*, Chapter 63

> "It is said the illness may be on the hair level, the skin level, the muscle level, the level of channels, tendon level, bone and marrow level. When treating the hair level do not damage the skin level. If the illness is at the skin level do not damage the muscle level, if the illness is at the muscle level needling too deeply will damage the channel level. In illness of the tendons needling too deeply will damage the bone level, in illness of the bones needling too deeply will damage the marrow."
>
> *Nei Jing Su Wen*, Chapter 50

> "When needling the bone level, take care not to needle the tendon level. When needling the tendon level do not injure the muscles. When needling the muscles, do not injure the channels and vessels. When needling the skin, do not injure the flesh or muscles."
>
> *Nei Jing Su Wen*, Chapter 51

When all the systems of acupuncture are properly applied in clinical practice, a higher degree of effectiveness can be achieved. The Balance Method offers clinical point selection strategies and methods that can be combined with all the channels of acupuncture.

One of the most important principles presented in Part I of this book is that the human body is an integrated whole, where individual aspects influence other aspects based on certain Chinese medical relationships.

Four major relationships are: Yin–Yang Primary Channel pairs, Six Channel pairs, daily meridian clock opposite pairs and Five Phases relationships. These pairings can be selected alone and/or in combinations to treat health conditions. *I Ching Acupuncture—The Balance Method* contains methods that use each of these essential channel relationships. *I Ching* acupuncture is rooted in classical Chinese medical and acupuncture theory; it contains strategies and clinical applications guided by the vision of early practitioners of the *I Ching* and Chinese medicine.

Chapter 9

BALANCE METHOD 1
BALANCING SIX CHANNEL PAIRS

- Balancing hand conditions with foot channels

- Balancing foot conditions with hand channels

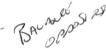

Balance Method 1 is based on anatomical relationships of the limbs, with 12 joints and six channel acupuncture pairings. These relationships include hand-to-foot and foot-to-hand connections. Needling the hand to influence the foot and needling the foot to influence the hand are examples of anatomical relationships based on the six channel acupuncture relationships. Balance Method 1 is based on Ba Gua and *Nei Jing Su Wen* theory.

> "Man corresponds with nature: In heaven, there are Yin and Yang, in man, there are 12 large joints of the limbs."

> "When one understands the principles of the 12 joints, a sage will never surpass him."
>
> *Nei Jing Su Wen*, Chapter 25

> "Diverse pricking to the right side or to the left, contra lateral insertion of pricking the upper part to cure the lower disease, and pricking the left side to cure the right."
>
> *Nei Jing Su Wen*, Chapter 27

Nei Jing Ling Shu, Chapter 7 presents the following needling method:

> "The Giant Needling method is to choose the right side for diseases on the left and choose the left side for diseases on the right."

These *Nei Jing* references are the basis for using the lower left part of the body to treat the upper right, and the upper right part of the body to treat the lower left, as well as the lower right part of the body to treat the upper left, and the upper left part of the body to treat the lower right.

A major aspect of Chinese medicine is systems of correspondences: Yin–Yang, Five Phases, Eight Trigrams, Ba Gua and the 64 Hexagrams are the major systems of correspondences. These theories and models provide the basis for *I Ching* acupuncture applications, which is to locate and needle corresponding anatomical locations.

Theory and Applications

The applications are set out in the *Nei Jing Su Wen*, Chapter 27. When an ailment is on the limbs, use the Twelve Joint theory to locate the balance area. In Balance Method 1, the acupuncture point selection method is contralateral point selection. The Twelve Joint theory includes selecting points corresponding to the ankle and wrist, the knee and elbow, and the shoulder and hip. This method requires selecting a Six Channel acupuncture pair at the anatomical and channel correspondences. This method is a one-needle acupuncture treatment.

The following are examples of Balance Method 1.

Example 1
If there is pain at right Large Intestine 11, the balancing point is left Stomach 35. This acupoint is the contralateral anatomical balance point. The Large Intestine and Stomach form the Yang Ming Six Channel pairing, and the knee is the balanced area for the elbow.

Example 2
If there is pain at right Bladder 40, select left Small Intestine 8. Bladder 40 is at the knee, and its balance point is the elbow. Bladder and Small Intestine are Tai Yang pairs, therefore, Small Intestine 8 is a balance point for Bladder 40.

Example 3
A patient has pain at the area of left Gallbladder 40. The corresponding balance point for left Gallbladder 40 is right San Jiao 4. Gallbladder 40 is located at the ankle, and its balance point is the wrist. San Jiao 4 is at the wrist, and is the Gallbladder's Shao Yang pair.

Table 9.1 presents the Twelve Joint pairings and their Six Channel partners. Locate the joint where the imbalance exists, then select the balance joint and its Six Channel location for treatment.

Six Channel pairs are presented in classic texts of Chinese medicine. In Chapter 79 of the *Nei Jing Su Wen*, these channel pairings are presented as corresponding anatomical relationships between the body and channels; they are, in effect, a body-imaging system. The following section explains how multiple theories and models, especially the Ba Gua and the Five Phases, are integrated to support Six Channel pairings.

Chinese Metaphysics and Six Channel Pairings

In texts from the Song dynasty, the 12 primary and the Ren and Du Channels were grouped together. The reason for this was that they are the only channels that have their own acupuncture points. That common link also provides a rationale for placement of these channels within Chinese metaphysical models. The integration of these channels and models discloses deep relationships within the acupuncture channel system, and supports classic pairings of the channels.

The Nine Palaces is the terrain within which to place components of Chinese models, theories and acupuncture channels. One channel sequence that is placed in the Nine Palaces is the Ying Qi or daily meridian clock cycle. Figure 9.1 shows the Nine Palaces, which is an important reference point for showing the formation of the Six Channel pairings.

TABLE 9.1 THE 12 JOINTS AND ACUPUNCTURE CHANNELS

	Ankle / Wrist	Knee / Elbow	Hip / Shoulder	Wrist / Ankle	Elbow / Knee	Shoulder / Hip
Tai Yang	Bladder / Small Intestine	Bladder / Small Intestine	Bladder / Small Intestine	Small Intestine / Bladder	Small Intestine / Bladder	Small Intestine / Bladder
Shao Yang	Gallbladder / San Jiao	Gallbladder / San Jiao	Gallbladder / San Jiao	San Jiao / Gallbladder	San Jiao / Gallbladder	San Jiao / Gallbladder
Yang Ming	Stomach / Large Intestine	Stomach / Large Intestine	Stomach / Large Intestine	Large Intestine / Stomach	Large Intestine / Stomach	Large Intestine / Stomach
Tai Yin	Spleen / Lungs	Spleen / Lungs	Spleen / Lungs	Lungs / Spleen	Lungs / Spleen	Lungs / Spleen
Shao Yin	Kidneys / Heart	Kidneys / Heart	Kidneys / Heart	Heart / Kidneys	Heart / Kidneys	Heart / Kidneys
Jue Yin	Liver / Pericardium	Liver / Pericardium	Liver / Pericardium	Pericardium / Liver	Pericardium / Liver	Pericardium / Liver

4 *Xun* Yin Wood Liver	9 *Li* Fire Heart Small Intestine	2 *Kun* Earth-Fire Pericardium San Jiao
3 *Zhen* Yang Wood Gallbladder	5 Center Earth	7 *Dui* Yang Metal Large Intestine
8 *Gen* Mountain Earth Stomach Spleen	1 *Kan* Water Bladder Kidney	6 *Qian* Yin Metal Lung

Figure 9.1 The Nine Palaces

The Nine Palaces contain trigrams and their corresponding channels. In the Nine Palaces above, each channel resides in a palace with its corresponding trigram. For example, the Lungs correspond to Yin Metal, the Liver to Yin Wood, the Heart to Fire, the Spleen to Earth, and the Kidneys to Water. The creation of the daily meridian clock was presented earlier in detail (see Chapter 8). The order of the channels in this cycle is listed below:

1. Lung (LU)

2. Large Intestine (LI)

3. Stomach (ST)

4. Spleen (SP)

5. Heart (HT)

6. Small Intestine (SI)

7. Bladder (BL)

8. Kidney (KD)

9. Pericardium (PC)

10. San Jiao (SJ)

11. Gallbladder (GB)

12. Liver (LV)

The creation of the Six Channels pairings is based on a variety of Chinese metaphysical theories, which begins with *I Ching* theory.

The *Shou Gua*, which is part of the "Ten Wings" commentary in the *I Ching*, states:

"Qian/Heaven and Kun/Earth establish the positions."

This *Shou Gua* guidance means, when placing channels in a pattern, start by placing the Qian trigram at the beginning and the Kun trigram at the end. The Early Heaven Ba Gua is the model used to identify the formation of Six Channel pairings.

The method for identifying these Six Channel relationships is a three-step process:

1. Place the Du Channel with Qian and place the Ren Channel with Kun. The Du Channel is the Sea of Yang and is matched with Qian, which is pure Yang. The Ren Channel is the Sea of Yin and is matched with Kun, which is pure Yin.

2. Arrange the Early Heaven Ba Gua horizontally, starting with Qian and ending with Kun.

3. Place the Yin–Yang channel pairs in a sequential flow from the first trigram to the last trigram—in other words, between Qian and Kun, as explained below.

Chapter 5 of the *Nei Jing Su Wen* presents the acupuncture channels as pairs, which are called liu he. The grouping of the 12 channels into two sets of six channel pairings is the guiding principle for Yin–Yang and Six Channel pairings of the acupuncture channels. These pairings include the 12 joints of the body, and are a guiding principle for selecting acupuncture points.

The Yin–Yang channel pairs are:

Lung	Large Intestine
Stomach	Spleen
Heart	Small Intestine
Bladder	Kidney
Pericardium	San Jiao
Gallbladder	Liver

Match each channel pair with its corresponding trigram, beginning with Qian, and ending with Kun. (The Du Channel is placed with Qian and the Ren Channel is placed with Kun.)

The Eight Trigrams and channel pairings are shown below.

Yang Metal	Yin Metal	Yin Fire	Yang Wood	Yin Wood	Yang Water	Yang Earth	Yin Earth
Qian	Dui	Li	Zhen	Xun	Kan	Gen	Kun
1	2	3	4	5	6	7	8
Du	LU	HT	PC	LV	KD	SP	Ren
	LI	SI	SJ	GB	BL	ST	

The process of assigning channels to trigrams is presented below in a step-by-step format.

Yang Metal	Yin Metal	Yin Fire	Yang Wood	Yin Wood	Yang Water	Yang Earth	Yin Earth

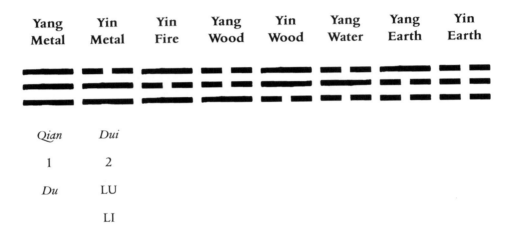

Qian

1

Du

The Lungs and Large Intestine are placed with Dui, which is Yin Metal.

Yang Metal	Yin Metal	Yin Fire	Yang Wood	Yin Wood	Yang Water	Yang Earth	Yin Earth

Qian   Dui

1   2

Du   LU

        LI

The Heart and Small Intestine are placed with Li, which is Fire.

Yang Metal	Yin Metal	Yin Fire	Yang Wood	Yin Wood	Yang Water	Yang Earth	Yin Earth

Qian   Dui   Li

1   2   3

Du   LU   HT

        LI   SI

The Pericardium and San Jiao are placed with Zhen, which is Yang Wood and close to Fire. Additionally, the Pericardium protects the Heart, and is located adjacent to it.

Yang Metal	Yin Metal	Yin Fire	Yang Wood	Yin Wood	Yang Water	Yang Earth	Yin Earth

Qian	Dui	Li	Zhen
1	2	3	4
Du	LU	HT	PC
	LI	SI	SJ

The Liver and Gallbladder are placed with Xun, which is Yin Wood.

Yang Metal	Yin Metal	Yin Fire	Yang Wood	Yin Wood	Yang Water	Yang Earth	Yin Earth

Qian	Dui	Li	Zhen	Xun
1	2	3	4	5
Du	LU	HT	PC	LV
	LI	SI	SJ	GB

The Kidneys and Bladder are placed with Kan, which is Water.

Yang Metal	Yin Metal	Yin Fire	Yang Wood	Yin Wood	Yang Water	Yang Earth	Yin Earth

Qian	Dui	Li	Zhen	Xun	Kan		
1	2	3	4	5	6		
Du	LU	HT	PC	LV	KD		
	LI	SI	SJ	GB	BL		

The Spleen and Stomach are placed with Gen, which is Yang Earth.

Yang Metal	Yin Metal	Yin Fire	Yang Wood	Yin Wood	Yang Water	Yang Earth	Yin Earth

Qian	Dui	Li	Zhen	Xun	Kan	Gen	
1	2	3	4	5	6	7	
Du	LU	HT	PC	LV	KD	SP	
	LI	SI	SJ	GB	BL	ST	

The Ren Channel is placed with Kun. This completes the principle: Qian and Kun set the positions. This finishes the process for assigning Yin–Yang paired channels to trigrams.

Yang Metal	Yin Metal	Yin Fire	Yang Wood	Yin Wood	Yang Water	Yang Earth	Yin Earth
Qian	Dui	Li	Zhen	Xun	Kan	Gen	Kun
1	2	3	4	5	6	7	8
Du	LU	HT	PC	LV	KD	SP	Ren
	LI	SI	SJ	GB	BL	ST	

A guiding principle for Yin–Yang theory and the Early Heaven Ba Gua is the relationship between trigrams in opposite positions. Figure 9.2 shows the corresponding relationships between the Six Channel pairs.

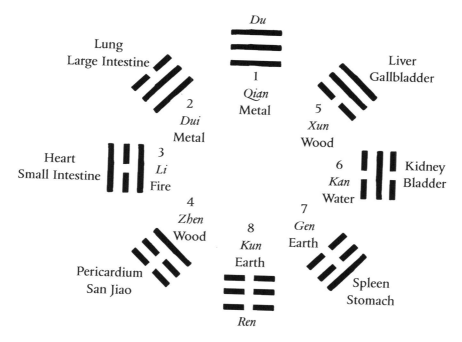

Figure 9.2 The Early Heaven Ba Gua

It can now be seen that, for example:

- Trigram 2 contains the Lung and Large Intestine, and Trigram 7 contains the Spleen and Stomach. The Stomach is opposite the Large Intestine, and they are a Yang Ming pair. The Spleen is opposite the Lung, and they are a Tai Yin pair.

- Trigram 3 contains the Heart and Trigram 6 contains the Kidney: these are a Shao Yin pair.

- Trigram 4 contains the San Jiao and Trigram 5 contains the Gallbladder: they are a Shao Yang pair.

In Balance Method I the theory of opposites, combined with Twelve Joint theory, provides the basis for an acupuncture treatment strategy. Treatment strategies include identifying the imbalanced channel, and then treating its healthy Six Channel pair. Table 9.2 lists the Six Channel pairings.

TABLE 9.2 THE SIX CHANNEL PAIRINGS

Six Stage	Foot channel	Hand channel
Tai Yang	Bladder	Small Intestine
Shao Yang	Gallbladder	San Jiao
Yang Ming	Stomach	Large Intestine
Tai Yin	Spleen	Lung
Shao Yin	Kidneys	Heart
Jue Yin	Liver	Pericardium

Chapter 10

BALANCE METHOD 2
BALANCING YIN–YANG
PAIRED CHANNELS

- Balancing hand conditions with hand channels

- Balancing foot conditions with foot channels

Balance Method 2 is based on Yin–Yang paired channels. These paired channels can be viewed as one inseparable channel, because treating one of the paired channels influences the other channel. The area to treat or influence is based on anatomical correspondences and the theory of correspondences: like treats like.

Chapter 9 of the *Nei Jing Ling Shu* presents a treatment plan for each channel, where each treatment includes Yin–Yang paired channels. From an anatomical viewpoint, this is the Twelve Joint theory in a horizontal aspect (not the contralateral method described in Balance Method 1).

The following are the anatomical relationships for this method:

- ankle and ankle

- knee and knee

- hip and hip

- wrist and wrist

- elbow and elbow

- shoulder and shoulder.

Yin–Yang paired channels connect the body in this horizontal or mirrored anatomical relationship. The method consists of choosing the same anatomical area on the opposite side, and then selecting the Yin–Yang paired channel and acupuncture point. The following are examples of Balance Method 2.

> *Example 1*
> A patient has pain on the right side of the wrist at Lung 9. In this method, select the wrist on the opposite side (the left side). Then locate the Yin–Yang channel pair of the Lung, which is the Large Intestine Channel. The balancing area for Lung 9 is Large Intestine 5. These two points have the wrist-to-wrist anatomical correspondence and they are mirror images of each other. Large Intestine 5 on the left side is therefore the acupuncture point for Balance Method 2.
>
> *Example 2*
> A patient has pain at left Spleen 9. In this method, select the opposite anatomical image, or the right knee. The acupuncture point that balances Spleen 9 is Stomach 36. The Stomach is the Spleen's Yin–Yang pair. It is also its knee-to-knee anatomical correspondence and the Balance Method 2 treatment.

Yin–Yang channels are considered inseparable because they share the same element and are linked through internal pathways. Yin–Yang acupuncture channel pairs are presented in classic texts with little or no theory to support their relationships. The following section integrates multiple theories and models to support Yin–Yang paired channels.

The Ba Gua and Yin–Yang Acupuncture Channel Pairs

Trigrams can be organized according to their Yin and Yang quality: there are four Yin trigrams and four Yang trigrams. These trigram groupings are listed below.

Straight Lines ▬▬▬ are Yang   Broken Lines ▬ ▬ are Yin

Yang Trigrams	**Yin Trigrams**
Father Pure Yang	Mother Pure Yin
First Yang Eldest Son	First Yin Eldest Daughter
Second Yang Second Son	Second Yin Second Daughter
Third Yang Youngest Son	Third Yin Youngest Daughter

All Yang trigrams have one Yang line and two Yin lines, except Qian, which is pure Yang and has three Yang lines.

All Yin Trigrams have one Yin line and two Yang lines, except Kun, which is pure Yin and has three Yin lines.

Each of the primary channels and organs are categorized according to their traditional Yin–Yang polarity. The order listed below is based on the Five Phases creation cycle.

Yin channels/organs are as follows:

- Wood and Liver

- Fire and Heart

- Earth and Spleen

- Metal and Lung

- Water and Kidney

- Wood and Pericardium.

Yang channels/organs are as follows:

- Wood and Gallbladder

- Fire and Small Intestine

- Earth and Stomach

- Metal and Large Intestine

- Water and Bladder

- Wood and San Jiao.

The acupuncture channels are matched to their corresponding trigrams, based on the Five Phases creation cycle: Wood, Fire, Earth, Metal and Water.

Yang Channels

The pattern used to assign Yang channels in this method is the Five Phases creation cycle and the Yin–Yang polarity of the channel.

As stated above, there are four Yang trigrams. The first, Qian, contains all Yang lines; the other three have one Yang line. Based on the idea that Spring and Yang Wood mark the beginning of a new year and cycle, the channels are placed in the following pattern, which is based on the creation cycle:

- Gallbladder is Yang Wood and is placed with the first trigram, Qian.

- Small Intestine is Yang Fire and is placed with Gen.

- Stomach is Yang Earth and is placed with Kan.

- Large Intestine is Yang Metal and is placed with Zhen.

When those four trigrams have been matched, the pattern repeats from Qian to accommodate six channels matching to four trigrams. The pattern of channel placement is Wood, Fire, Earth, Metal and Water, and then repeats Wood and Fire to accommodate all six Yang channels, as shown below.

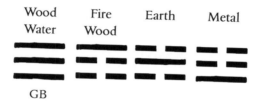

	Qian	Gen	Kan	Zhen
	Wood	Fire	Earth	Metal
	Water	Wood		
	1	2	3	4
	5	6		
	GB	SI	ST	LI
	BL	SJ		

The following is a step-by-step presentation of this assignment process:

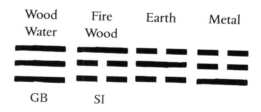

Wood   Fire   Earth   Metal
Water Wood

GB

Wood   Fire   Earth   Metal
Water Wood

GB   SI

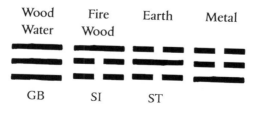

Wood   Fire   Earth   Metal
Water Wood

GB   SI   ST

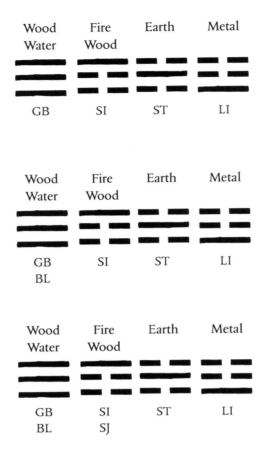

Yin Channels

For Yin channels and trigrams, the same theory and process applies as for the Yang channels and trigrams, producing the pattern shown below.

The following is a step-by-step presentation of this assignment process:

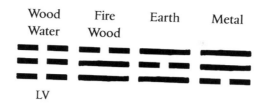

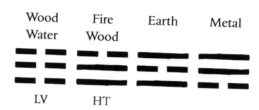

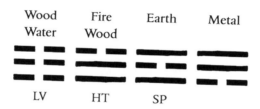

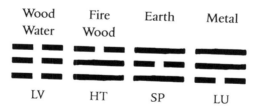

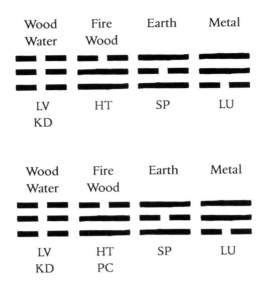

The Ba Gua and Opposite Channel Pairs

When channel and trigram correspondences are placed on the Early Heaven Ba Gua, it shows opposite trigrams to be Yin–Yang pairs; this is Ba Gua theory supporting Yin–Yang acupuncture channel pairings. Figure 10.1 is the Ba Gua for Balance Method 2, and Table 10.1 lists the anatomical relationships. Combining Ba Gua, *Su Wen* and *Ling Shu* theory, a strategy using Yin–Yang paired acupuncture channels is formed for clinical point selection.

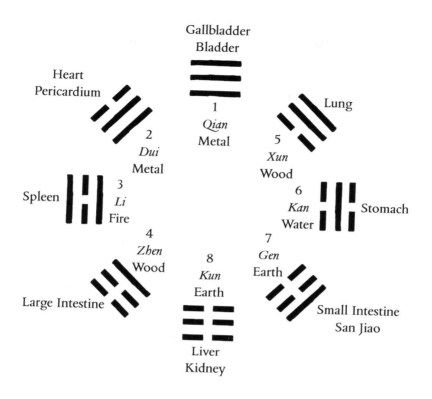

Figure 10.1 The Ba Gua with the 12 Acupuncture Channels

TABLE 10.1 THE BODY AND THE YIN– YANG ACUPUNCTURE CHANNELS

Yin–Yang channels	Anatomical relationship
Gallbladder and Liver	Foot to foot
Bladder and Kidneys	Foot to foot
Heart and Small Intestine	Hand to hand
Pericardium and San Jiao	Hand to hand
Spleen and Stomach	Foot to foot
Large Intestine and Lungs	Hand to hand

Applying Balance Method 2

The application for this method is based on anatomical imaging, Twelve Joint theory and Yin–Yang acupuncture channel pairs; the three are combined to locate the balance area.

Example 1

When a patient has pain at right Bladder 60, select the Yin–Yang paired channel of the Bladder at the ankle. The channel is the Kidneys and the point is left Kidney 3. This method combines ankle treating ankle, Yin–Yang channel pairs, and treating the opposite side of the condition. These three aspects are based on *Nei Jing* and Ba Gua theory.

Example 2

A patient has pain at right Large Intestine 5. In this method, treat the corresponding opposite area, which is left Lung 9. This example combines Yin–Yang channel pairs (in this case the Large Intestine and Lungs), anatomical correspondence of wrist and wrist, and opposite balance theory.

Example 3

A patient has pain at Heart 3 on the left hand. The acupoint for Balance Method 2 is Small Intestine 8, on the right hand. This example combines Yin–Yang paired channels: The Heart and Small Intestine. The anatomical correspondences are the ankle and wrist; combining these two correspondences is an application of contralateral and opposite balance theory.

Chapter 11

BALANCE METHOD 3
BALANCING WITH STREAM AND SEA ACUPOINTS—THE 3–6 BALANCE METHOD

The *Su Wen* and *Ling Shu* present Antique or Transporting points as a primary category of acupoints for treating channel and organ conditions. The five Antique points influence the entire channel and organs that they relate to. They can be used to balance conditions in their own channel and organs, and also to influence channels to which they are connected, based on acupuncture theory, and especially channel theory. The Ying Qi daily meridian clock cycle contains 12 channels, and these can be grouped into three sets of four channels. The grouping of the channels is based primarily on Yin–Yang and Six Channel pairings. When a set of four channels is viewed as a unit or circuit, it can be seen that the four support each other because they are connected by two of the strongest channel theory relationships: Yin–Yang and Six Channel pairs.

The following are the three circuits:

- Lungs—Large Intestine—Stomach—Spleen

- Heart—Small Intestine—Bladder—Kidneys

- Pericardium—San Jiao—Gallbladder—Liver

The Lungs and Large Intestine and the Stomach and Spleen are Yin–Yang pairs, and support each other. The Spleen and Lungs are Tai Yin Pairs, and the Large Intestine and Stomach are Yang Ming pairs, and they support each other. The Lungs and Large Intestine are Metal and the Stomach and

Spleen are Earth. The Five Phases relationship between the channels is the parent–child Five Phase relationship. These four channels, then, are related according to three of the strongest Chinese medical theories: Yin–Yang and Six Channel pairs, and the Five Phases.

The Heart and Small Intestine are Yin–Yang paired channels, as are the Bladder and Kidneys. The Heart and Kidneys are Shao Yin pairs and the Small Intestine and Bladder are Tai Yang pairs.

The Pericardium and San Jiao are Yin–Yang paired channels, as are the Gallbladder and Liver. Pericardium and Liver are Jue Yin pairs and San Jiao and Gallbladder are Shao Yang pairs.

These three four-channel circuits all contain Yin–Yang and Six Channel pairs, which can be combined in treatments to utilize four channels to influence a condition. The channels in each four-channel set influence and support each other; they can be combined to obtain a synergy in treating an imbalance within the four-channel circuit.

Assigning Acupuncture Points to Hexagrams

The *Nei Jing* presents the Five Antique (Transporting), Connecting and Source points for each of the 12 primary channels. When those points are matched to the six lines of a hexagram, each line contains one acupuncture point. Tables 11.1 and 11.2 list the acupuncture points and the lines of a hexagram.

Table 11.1 The Yang Channels: Hexagram Lines and Acupuncture Points

Line of hexagram	GB	SI	ST	LI	BL	SJ
6-Sea	34	8	36	11	40	10
5-River	38	5	41	5	60	6
4-Source	40	4	42	4	64	4
3-Stream	41	3	43	3	65	3
2-Spring	43	2	44	2	66	2
1-Well	44	1	45	1	67	1

For Yang channels, the Source points are not the Stream point, and are placed at the fourth line. The Connecting points are not added to the Yang channels.

TABLE 11.2 THE YIN CHANNELS: HEXAGRAM LINES AND ACUPUNCTURE POINTS

Line of hexagram	LV	HT	SP	LU	KD	PC
6-Sea	8	3	9	5	10	3
5	5-Luo	4-River	5-River	7-Luo	7-River	5-River
4	4-River	5-Luo	4-Luo	8-River	4-Luo	6-Luo
3-Stream	3	7	3	9	3	7
2-Spring	2	8	2	10	2	8
1-Well	1	9	1	11	1	9

For Yin channels, Source points are Stream points, which requires adding Luo (Connecting) points to the six lines to match a point for each line in the hexagram.

Applying Balance Method 3

The basics of a hexagram line structure and how to assign acupoints to each line in the hexagram will now be explained by presenting the hexagram Qian, showing the acupoints that correspond with each line. This method is applied to all channels.

This hexagram is Qian, and it contains all Yang lines:

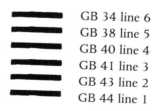

GB 34 line 6
GB 38 line 5
GB 40 line 4
GB 41 line 3
GB 43 line 2
GB 44 line 1

Balance Method 3 works with the five Antique points, and the Connecting and Source points; and there are several applications for this method. The first method is to select two points that can balance the channel.

From a numerical and positional perspective, lines 3 and 6 are balanced positions in a hexagram. These points are the Stream and Sea points, or the third and sixth points in a hexagram—respectively, points at the middle and top of a hexagram. They are the third and sixth points on Yin–Yang paired channels; they are also the acupoints around the middle and top of the upper and lower limbs. The hexagram and limbs, then, mirror each other; they are, in effect, holograms.

The Antique points have a powerful influence on moving and balancing Qi and Blood, and they can treat channel and organ conditions.

Applications for Balance Method 3 include treating a single channel, the two Yin–Yang channel pairs, the two Six Channel pairs, or all four channels as a complete circuit (outlined at the beginning of this chapter). Table 11.3 contains a list of all the Stream and Sea point combinations.

TABLE 11.3 THE STREAM AND SEA POINTS

Channel	Stream (third)	Sea (sixth)
Lungs	9	5
Large Intestine	3	11
Stomach	43	36
Spleen	3	9
Heart	7	3
Small Intestine	3	8
Bladder	65	40
Kidneys	3	10
Pericardium	7	3
San Jiao	3	10
Gallbladder	41	34
Liver	3	8

The Stream and Sea points can be treated on each channel. For example, if there is an imbalance on the Lung Channel, needle the third and sixth points: Lung 9 and Lung 5.

Two channels can be combined, using the Stream and Sea points. For example, if there is an imbalance in the Spleen, the strategy is to combine Stomach and Spleen Channels and points: needle Spleen 3 and 9 and Stomach 43 and 36.

Example 1

A patient has sciatica on the left side of the body. Select Gallbladder 41 and 34. If your style treats the same side, needle the left side. If you prefer Ba Gua theory, select the opposite side, or right Gallbladder 41 and 34.

Example 2

A patient has chronic diarrhea. In this case, select the Stream and Sea points on the Large Intestine and Lungs. Insert the points on the root channel of the condition first. If it is the Large Intestine, needle Large Intestine 3, then 11. After needling the Large Intestine points, needle Lung 9 and Lung 5. This method combines Yin–Yang pairs to provide support to a paired channel. This is a bilateral and four-needle treatment.

Example 3

A patient has suffered a stroke. The treatment plan is to treat Yang Ming Channels to build Qi and Blood. The method is to treat Stomach 43 and 36. After completing the Stomach Channel, treat Large Intestine 3 and 11. This application treats two channels (the Six Channel pairs) and includes four needles in the treatment.

Combining Yin–Yang and Six-Channel Pairs

Balance Method 3 includes combining Yin–Yang and Six-Channel pairs. This is the acupuncture channel circuit that includes all four channels. Acupuncture channel combinations for the four-channel circuit are as follows.

Tai Yang: Bladder Condition

First set of needles: Bladder 65 then 40.
Second set of needles: Kidney 3 then 10.
Third set of needles: Small Intestine 3 then 8.
Fourth set of needles: Heart 7 then 3.

Tai Yang: Small Intestine Condition

First set of needles: Small Intestine 3 then 8.
Second set of needles: Heart 7 then 3.
Third set of needles: Bladder 65 then 40.
Fourth set of needles: Kidney 3 then 10.

Yang Ming: Stomach Condition

First set of needles: Stomach 43 then 36.
Second set of needles: Spleen 3 then 9.
Third set of needles: Large Intestine 3 then 11.
Fourth set of needles: Lung 9 then 5.

Yang Ming: Large Intestine Condition

First set of needles: Large Intestine 3 then 9.
Second set of needles: Lung 9 then 5.
Third set of needles: Stomach 43 then 36.
Fourth set of needles: Spleen 3 then 9.

Shao Yang: Gallbladder Condition

First set of needles: Gallbladder 41 then 34.
Second set of needles: Liver 3 then 8.
Third set of needles: San Jiao 3 then 10.
Fourth set of needles: Pericardium 7 then 3.

Shao Yang: San Jiao Condition

First set of needles: San Jiao 3 then 10.
Second set of needles: Pericardium 7 then 3.
Third set of needles: Gallbladder 41 then 34.
Fourth set of needles: Liver 3 then 8.

TAI YIN: SPLEEN CONDITION

First set of needles: Spleen 3 then 9.
Second set of needles: Stomach 43 then 36.
Third set of needles: Lung 9 then 5.
Fourth set of needles: Large Intestine 3 then 11.

TAI YIN: LUNG CONDITION

First set of needles: Lung 9 then 5.
Second set of needles: Large Intestine 3 then 11.
Third set of needles: Spleen 3 then 9.
Fourth set of needles: Stomach 43 then 36.

SHAO YIN: KIDNEY CONDITION

First set of needles: Kidney 3 then 10.
Second set of needles: Bladder 65 then 40.
Third set of needles: Heart 7 then 3.
Fourth set of needles: Small Intestine 3 then 11.

SHAO YIN: HEART CONDITION

First set of needles: Heart 7 then 3.
Second set of needles: Small Intestine 3 then 8.
Third set of needles: Kidney 3 then 10.
Fourth set of needles: Bladder 65 then 40.

JUE YIN: LIVER CONDITION

First set of needles: Liver 3 then 8.
Second set of needles: Gallbladder 41 then 34.
Third set of needles: Pericardium 7 then 3.
Fourth set of needles: San Jiao 3 then 10.

JUE YIN: PERICARDIUM CONDITION

First set of needles: Pericardium 7 then 3.
Second set of needles: San Jiao 3 then 10.
Third set of needles: Liver 3 then 8.
Fourth set of needles: Gallbladder 41 then 34.

Balance Method 3 Guidance

There is a variety of acupuncture needling insertion methods based on varying theories. The following method is common in clinical practice. Females are Yin and males are Yang; Yin is the right side and Yang is the left side. When conditions are bilateral or organ-related, needle the right side first for females, and the left side first for males. For one-sided conditions, contralateral or same-sided treatments can be selected. Base the needling method on your preference.

Balance Method 3 includes a four-step treatment method. This method is presented here, followed by an example.

1. The first needle is on the problem channel. Treat the third point, and then the sixth point on the channel. (These are the Stream and Sea points respectively.)

2. The second needle is on the Yin–Yang paired channel of the problem channel. Treat the side of the body *opposite* to that treated in step 1. Treat the third (Stream), and then the sixth (Sea) point on the channel.

3. The third set of needles is the Six Channel pair of the problem channel. Treat the side *opposite* to the side needled in step 1, and then insert needles at the third (Stream) and sixth (Sea) points on the channel.

4. The fourth channel treated is the Yin–Yang pair of the Six Channel pair used in Step 3. Treat the side of the channel *opposite* to the side needled in Step 3, and needle the third (Stream) and sixth (Sea) points.

Example

The patient is a female and the diagnosis is Liver Blood deficiency.
The following points and sequence are the acupuncture plan:

1. Right side Liver 3 and 8.

2. Left side Gallbladder 41 and 34.

3. Left side Pericardium 7 and 3.

4. Right side San Jiao 3 and 10.

Chapter 12

Balance Method 4
Balancing the Daily Meridian Clock

A primary principle of the Ba Gua is that opposites balance each other, and this is the basis of distal point selection. This application of the Ba Gua can be applied to the Ying Qi cycle or the daily meridian clock. In this method, ignore the time aspect of the clock and just treat the opposite channel. This application is based on Yin–Yang theory and the relationship between opposite channels.

Applying Balance Method 4

The process for Balance Method 4 is as follows:

1. Identify the problem channel.

2. Identify the channel at the opposite end of the daily meridian clock, and needle this channel to treat the problem channel.

3. A variety of points can be selected in this method. For example, for pain, select Cleft points or an anatomical image point from Balance Method 1 and 2.

Examples
Liver and Small Intestine Treat Each Other

1. If there is pain in the scapula or at Small Intestine 11, select Liver 6, the Cleft acupoint.

2. If there is pain on the Liver Channel, select Small Intestine 6, the Cleft point.

Lung and Bladder Treat Each Other

1. If there is pain at the lower back, select Lung 5, which is a corresponding anatomical location.

2. If there is pain on the forearm at Lung 6, select Bladder 57, which is a corresponding anatomical location.

Large Intestine and Kidney Treat Each Other

1. If there is pain around Bladder 23 or in the spine, select Large Intestine 3. This is a Stream point, which treats pain. Large Intestine 3 is at the second metacarpal bone, which images and treats the spine.

2. If there is pain at Large Intestine 5, select Kidney 3.

Stomach and Pericardium Treat Each Other

1. If there is pain on the Stomach Channel, select Pericardium 6 or Pericardium 4.

2. If there is pain at Pericardium 3, select Stomach 36.

Spleen and San Jiao Treat Each Other

1. If there is pain at San Jiao 3, select Spleen 8, the Cleft point.

2. If there is pain at Spleen 3, select San Jiao 3. Both of these points are the third points and Stream points on each channel.

Heart and Gallbladder Treat Each Other

1. If there is pain at Gallbladder 30, select Heart 6. This point is the Cleft point and treats pain.

2. If there is pain at Heart 7, select Gallbladder 40 or Gallbladder 36.

Figure 12.1 shows the daily meridian clock in a circular format. The corresponding times are not listed for each channel; in Balance Method 4, simply identify the problem channel and treat the opposite channel.

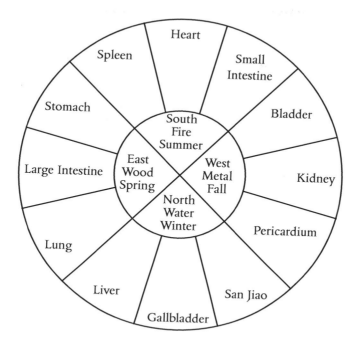

Figure 12.1 The Daily Meridian Clock in a Circular Format

Figure 12.2 shows the times for each of the 12 acupuncture channels. The way to use this table is to select the acupuncture channel opposite the problem channel to treat the latter, as follows; refer back to the examples provided at the beginning of this chapter.

1. Liver and Small Intestine treat each other.

2. Lung and Bladder treat each other.

3. Large Intestine and Kidney treat each other.

4. Stomach and Pericardium treat each other.

5. Spleen and San Jiao treat each other.

6. Heart and Gallbladder treat each other.

	9–11am Spleen	11am–1pm Heart	1–3pm Small Intestine	
7–9am Stomach				3–5pm Bladder
5–7am Large Intestine				5–7pm Kidney
3–5am Lung				7–9pm Pericardium
	1–3am Liver	11pm–1am Gallbladder	9–11pm San Jiao	

Figure 12.2 The Daily Meridian Clock in a Grid

Chapter 13

BALANCE METHOD 5
BALANCING CHANNEL CORRESPONDING NAMES AND POSITIONS

The Balance Method is based on the relationship between anatomical areas and the acupuncture channels on the body. In Balance Method 5, the position of the acupuncture channels in a trigram is the guiding theory for the clinical application of this method.

When two trigrams are placed side by side, there is correspondence between their lines, i.e. between lines 1 and 1, 2 and 2 and 3 and 3, as shown here.

Figure 13.1 Two Trigrams and their Corresponding Lines

Hexagrams are composed of two trigrams, as shown in Figure 13.2. The lines of a hexagram can be labeled by their location in the trigram or hexagram, as shown in Figure 13.2.

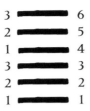

Figure 13.2 Hexagram Composed of Two Trigrams

Correspondences can treat each other. Balancing the Six Channels with Balance Method 5 begins by assigning one of the Six Channel pairings to each line of a hexagram.

Figure 13.3 shows a hexagram with the Six Stages. These correspondences are the basis of acupuncture treatments.

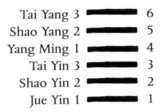

Figure 13.3 Hexagram with the Six Stages

The Six Channel pairs can be explained as follows.

1. Jue Yin and Yang Ming are lines 1 and 1 within their separate trigrams. They are also lines 1 and 4 respectively within a hexagram.

2. Shao Yin and Shao Yang are lines 2 and 2 within their separate trigrams. They are also lines 2 and 5 respectively within a hexagram.

3. Tai Yin and Tai Yang are lines 3 and 3 within their separate trigrams. They are also lines 3 and 6 respectively within a hexagram.

These channel–line correspondences can be represented as shown below.

- 1–4   1-Jue Yin corresponds to 4-Yang Ming.

- 2–5   2-Shao Yin corresponds to 5-Shao Yang.

- 3–6   3-Tai Yin corresponds to 6-Tai Yang.

Applying Balance Method 5

The principle underlying treatment application is that these pairs treat each other.

- Jue Yin and Yang Ming treat each other.

- Shao Yin and Shao Yang treat each other.

- Tai Yin and Tai Yang treat each other.

Tables 13.1 and 13.2 show the hexagram lines and acupuncture points for Yang and Yin channels respectively.

TABLE 13.1 THE YANG CHANNELS: HEXAGRAM LINES AND ACUPUNCTURE POINTS

Line of hexagram	GB	SI	ST	LI	BL	SJ
6-Sea	34	8	36	11	40	10
5-River	38	5	41	5	60	6
4-Source	40	4	42	4	64	4
3-Stream	41	3	43	3	65	3
2-Spring	43	2	44	2	66	2
1-Well	44	1	45	1	67	1

TABLE 13.2 THE YIN CHANNELS: HEXAGRAM LINES AND ACUPUNCTURE POINTS

Line of hexagram	LV	HT	SP	LU	KD	PC
6-Sea	8	3	9	5	10	3
5	5-Luo	4-River	5-River	7-Luo	7-River	5-River
4	4-River	5-Luo	4-Luo	8-River	4-Luo	6-Luo
3-Stream	3	7	3	9	3	7
2-Spring	2	8	2	10	2	8
1-Well	1	9	1	11	1	9

Application 1

Balancing channel names and positions is based on the names shared by Six Channel paired channels and their positions in trigrams and hexagrams. For example, if the diagnosis is a Yang Ming condition, needle the lines that correspond to Yang Ming and its pair Jue Yin, i.e. lines 4 and 1 respectively—for example, if applicable, Pericardium 9 and Large Intestine 4. All channel and point combinations for this application are listed in Table 13.3.

Table 13.3 Hexagrams and the Six Channels: Application 1

Hexagram relationships	Lines	Channel	Channel
Jue Yin–Yang Ming	1–4	Pericardium 9	Large Intestine 4
Jue Yin–Yang Ming	1–4	Pericardium 9	Stomach 42
Jue Yin–Yang Ming	1–4	Liver 1	Large Intestine 4
Jue Yin–Yang Ming	1–4	Liver 1	Stomach 42
Shao Yin–Shao Yang	2–5	Heart 8	Gallbladder 38
Shao Yin–Shao Yang	2–5	Heart 8	San Jiao 6
Shao Yin–Shao Yang	2–5	Kidney 2	Gallbladder 38
Shao Yin–Shao Yang	2–5	Kidney 2	San Jiao 6
Tai Yin–Tai Yang	3–6	Spleen 3	Bladder 40
Tai Yin–Tai Yang	3–6	Spleen 3	Small Intestine 8
Tai Yin–Tai Yang	3–6	Lung 9	Bladder 40
Tai Yin–Tai Yang	3–6	Lung 9	Small Intestine 8

Example

A male patient complains of a migraine headache, and the location is the temporal area. The channel where the pain is located is the Gallbladder and is Shao Yang, and its channel pair is Shao Yin. When there is pain on the Shao Yang Gallbladder Channel there are four options:

1. Gallbladder 38 and Heart 8. These channels are Shao Yang and Shao Yin, and hexagram lines 5 and 2.

2. Gallbladder 38 and Kidney 2. These channels are Shao Yang and Shao Yin, and hexagram lines 5 and 2.

3. San Jiao 6 and Heart 8. These channels are Shao Yang and Shao Yin, and hexagram lines 5 and 2.

4. San Jiao 6 and Kidney 2. These channels are Shao Yang and Shao Yin, and hexagram lines 5 and 2.

Application 2

This application includes selecting the numerical corresponding channels and allows any appropriate point selection (unlike Application 1, which has specific points to treat). The key to this application is to select the appropriate channel. For example, if there is pain, select Cleft or Stream points. If there is a deficiency, select source or Sea points to treat the deficiency. Select the appropriate points based on your preference and clinical experience.

Jue Yin and Yang Ming treat each other: 1–4.

1. Liver treats the Stomach and Large Intestine.

2. Pericardium treats the Stomach and Large Intestine.

3. Stomach treats the Liver and Pericardium.

4. Large Intestine treats the Liver and Pericardium.

Shao Yin and Shao Yang treat each other: 2–5.

1. Kidneys treat the Gallbladder and San Jiao.

2. Heart treats the Gallbladder and San Jiao.

3. Gallbladder treats the Kidneys and Heart.

4. San Jiao treats the Kidneys and Heart.

Tai Yin and Tai Yang treat each other: 3–6.

1. Lungs treat the Bladder and Small Intestine.

2. Spleen treats the Bladder and Small Intestine.

3. Bladder treats the Lungs and Spleen.

4. Small Intestine treats the Lungs and Spleen.

Example 1

A female has nausea. Select lines 1–4, which are Jue Yin and Yang Ming Channels. Both these channels treat the Stomach and Spleen, the organs related to nausea in this case. Pick the points on these channels based on your experience.

Example 2

A male has low back pain, and the pain is centralized at the Bladder Channel. Select lines 3–6, which are Tai Yin and Tai Yang Channels. Select the Tai Yin Lung Channel to treat the Tai Yang Bladder Channel. Pick the points on this channel based on your experience.

Chapter 14

BALANCE METHOD 6
BALANCING HEXAGRAMS

A major theory within Chinese medicine concerns systems of correspondences and relationships between two or more aspects of life. Balance Method 6 is based on the relationships between two hexagrams and their corresponding acupuncture channels.

The first step in this method is to make a diagnosis and select the corresponding channel to treat the condition. Once the correct channel is selected, a favorable hexagram for that channel and diagnosis is chosen. The selection of a favorable hexagram is based on numerous qualities. The key criteria for selecting a favorable hexagram include the way the Five Phases for the trigrams within a hexagram influence the channels or organs treated. For example, if there is a deficiency, the treatment plan is to supplement the organ or channel. Selecting a hexagram containing trigrams that are the parent phase or the same phase as the problem channel or organ supplements; and so the hexagram's Five Phases energies will balance the condition.

There are a few ways to evaluate hexagrams and trigrams. If the hexagram has a favorable outcome we can use it, regardless of the trigram relationships. If the trigrams have favorable aspects, we can use them without considering the hexagram outcome.

Balance Method 6 contains aspects of the healing methods of ancient Chinese healers. Systems of correspondences include the principle of like treating like. In this method we determine the hexagram for the imbalanced or diseased channel or organ, and then a favorable hexagram is selected for it. These two hexagrams are placed side by side, so that all six lines of each hexagram are next to each other. These lines represent their channels and conditions, as well as their acupuncture points. In this method, lines that differ in polarity are identified—for example, a Yin and a Yang line. The acupuncture points at these lines are needled because they are the locations of stagnations in the channels, and these stagnations can be cleared by needling them. The treatment changes the Qi in the channel, removing the imbalance in the channel so that the condition is balanced. When a line is the same in both hexagrams, no needling is required at those acupuncture points. This method matches the imbalanced channel and its hexagram to a healthy hexagram: the imbalanced lines are identified and their acupuncture points are needled to transform to the healthy condition. Balance Method 6 changes or transforms the Qi in a channel by attuning one hexagram to another, changing the quality of Qi in the channel and body.

The 64 Hexagrams are contained in the *Book of Changes* or *I Ching*, and it can be interpreted in a variety of ways. Two major ways to evaluate hexagrams are the symbolism and numbers methods. Both of these methods are applied to Balance Method 6 (balancing hexagrams).

The treatment plan for this method is a five-step process:

1. Make a diagnosis.

2. Select the channels for treatment.

3. Identify the channel's corresponding hexagram.

4. Select a balancing hexagram for the condition and channel.

5. Needle the correct lines and points.

This chapter presents how to perform Steps 4 and 5. The process for Step 5 starts with placing the problem channel's hexagram next to a favorable hexagram. (Selecting a favorable hexagram is discussed later in this chapter.) By comparing the two hexagrams we can identify the differing lines, and when we needle their points we can change the Qi in the body (channel or organ). The hexagrams identify which points to needle. We only change the condition in the problem channel. The change from Yin to Yang happens when we needle an acupuncture point; the needling causes the change. The goal of this method is to switch the imbalanced channel or organ to the favorable hexagram. This is done by needling the differing lines on the problem channel.

The hexagrams and their corresponding primary channels are listed in Table 14.1.

TABLE 14.1 HEXAGRAMS AND PRIMARY CHANNELS

Qian	Dui	Li	Zhen	Xun	Kan	Gen	Kun
Bladder Gall-bladder	Heart Pericardium	Spleen	Large Intestine	Lungs	Stomach	Small Intestine San Jiao	Liver Kidneys

Tables 14.2 and 14.3 show the acupuncture points for each channel, which are needled in treatments.

TABLE 14.2 THE YANG CHANNELS: HEXAGRAM LINES AND ACUPUNCTURE POINTS

Line of hexagram	GB	SI	ST	LI	BL	SJ
6-Sea	34	8	36	11	40	10
5-River	38	5	41	5	60	6
4-Source	40	4	42	4	64	4
3-Stream	41	3	43	3	65	3
2-Spring	43	2	44	2	66	2
1-Well	44	1	45	1	67	1

TABLE 14.3 THE YIN CHANNELS: HEXAGRAM LINES AND ACUPUNCTURE POINTS

Line of hexagram	LV	HT	SP	LU	KD	PC
6-Sea	8	3	9	5	10	3
5	5-Luo	4-River	5-River	7-Luo	7-River	5-River
4	4-River	5-Luo	4-Luo	8-River	4-Luo	6-Luo
3-Stream	3	7	3	9	3	7
2-Spring	2	8	2	10	2	8
1-Well	1	9	1	11	1	9

The following is an example of this method.

1. Begin by making a diagnosis.

2. Identify the problem organ or channel and its associated hexagram. For example, if the condition is bitter taste in the mouth due to Shao Yang excess, indicating a Gallbladder condition, select the Gallbladder hexagram. Qian is the trigram for the Gallbladder.

Gallbladder

Qian

3. Double the trigram, which creates the Gallbladder hexagram with six Yang lines:

Gallbladder

Qian

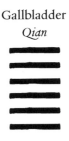

4. Select a favorable hexagram for this condition. A good hexagram for this condition is Zhong Fu, Hexagram 61. All of the favorable hexagrams for the purposes of this method are presented on pages 195–254.

Evaluating Zhong Fu includes the Five Phases for both trigrams and the list of qualities below the hexagram. In this example, the Gallbladder Channel is imbalanced, and it is also Wood. Zhong Fu is composed of two trigrams: Xun above, which is Wood, and Dui below, which is Metal. Wood treats Wood and Metal controls Wood; these Five Phases elements directly relate to the Gallbladder and can treat it. The Five Phases is the reason why this hexagram is selected.

Hexagram 61

Zhong Fu
Faithfulness
Inner sincerity
Central sincerity
Centering and connecting to the spirits

XUN-4-WOOD

DUI-7-METAL

1. Core, center.

2. Hit the mark.

3. Site of initiation.

4. Drive out evil spirits.

5. Creative transformation.

6. Connection to the spirit.

7. It is a time of perseverance.

8. Connect the heart to the spirit.

9. Connect your inner and outer lives.

10. Return to the center to find health and happiness.

11. Focus on your body and emotions; they may reveal the root of the health condition.

Zhong Fu contains the trigram Dui at the bottom and the trigram Xun at the top.

Zhong Fu
Hexagram 61

```
6  ━━━━━
5  ━━━━━
4  ━━  ━━
3  ━━  ━━
2  ━━━━━
1  ━━━━━
```

Place the Gallbladder hexagram alongside Hexagram 61, and compare the lines.

Note the lines that are not the same polarity—i.e. Yang to Yin or Yin to Yang.

In this example, lines 3 and 4 are not the same polarity, these lines and their corresponding acupoints are needled.

Gallbladder   *Zhong Fu*
Qian   Hexagram 61

```
━━━━━   6   ━━━━━
━━━━━   5   ━━━━━
━━━━━   4 *  ━━  ━━
━━━━━   3 *  ━━  ━━
━━━━━   2   ━━━━━
━━━━━   1   ━━━━━
```

Note that the third and fourth points on the Gallbladder Hexagram are Gallbladder 41 and 40.

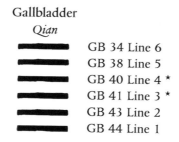

Gallbladder

Qian

GB 34 Line 6
GB 38 Line 5
GB 40 Line 4 *
GB 41 Line 3 *
GB 43 Line 2
GB 44 Line 1

If the patient is female, needle Gallbladder 41 and 40 on the right side and then Liver 3 and 4 on the left side. The Liver is the Yin–Yang paired channel and supports the treatment. (See Tables 14.2 and 14.3 on pages 183 and 184.)

Selecting Favorable Hexagrams

The *I Ching* is a profound system that reveals correspondences between a hexagram and related universal correspondences, including the human body. The 64 Hexagrams can be evaluated in a variety of ways. The most common method is the Symbol or Image method, where trigrams and hexagrams are metaphors for aspects of life such as family members or seasons, and it is found in all *I Ching* books. Imaging is the oldest method of evaluation; it is an aspect of the original work of King Wen and his son, King Wu.

In Table 14.4 the favorable hexagrams are identified with shading; Figure 14.1 lists only the favorable hexagrams. The quality of each hexagram is based on the Symbol or Image viewpoint. It is a good exercise to review a hexagram in several *I Ching* books and identify the nature of the outcome, whether it is favorable, or will become favorable, for health.

TABLE 14.4 THE 64 HEXAGRAMS

	Qian-1	Dui-2	Li-3	Zhen-4	Xun-5	Kan-6	Gen-7	Kun-8
Qián	1	43	14	34	9	5	26	11
Dui	10	58	38	54	61	60	41	19
Li	13	49	30	55	37	63	22	36
Zhen	25	17	21	51	42	3	27	24

46	7	15	2
18	4	52	23
48	29	39	8
57	59	53	20
32	40	62	16
50	64	56	35
28	47	31	45
44	6	33	12
Xun	*Kan*	*Gen*	*Kun*

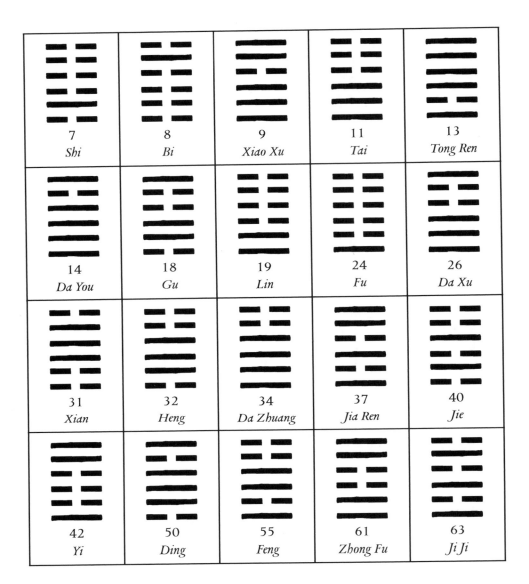

Figure 14.1 The Favorable Hexagrams

A Step-by-Step Explanation for Balancing Hexagrams

The following steps summarize how to apply Balance Method 6:

1. Make a diagnosis that can be converted to the 12 primary channels.

2. Select the correct hexagram for the primary channel being treated.

3. Select a favorable hexagram from the table of favorable hexagrams, and place it alongside the problem channel.

4. Note the lines that have a different Yin or Yang polarity.

5. Refer to the acupuncture point charts (see Tables 14.2 and 14.3 on pages 183 and 184) and locate the points that are highlighted in Step 4. Needle the points on the problem channel that were found in Step 1.

6. Needle the corresponding point(s) on the primary channel's Yin–Yang paired channel. Review the selection of case studies at the end of the book for examples.

A Synopsis of the Favorable Hexagrams

This section presents basic information for each of the 20 favorable hexagrams, following the sequence in which they appear in Figure 14.1. This information is derived from many sources and from the author's experience, and it focuses on health and transformation. Balance Method 6 requires an understanding of the image and elemental quality of hexagrams. Please review the "Ten Wings" section in the *I Ching*, which provides theory for the meanings of the trigrams.

Example

Each hexagram in this section is presented according to the following example.

Number: **7**

Name: **Shi**

Qualities: Leader
              Multitude
              Group action

Upper trigram: KUN-2-EARTH

Lower triagram: KAN-1-WATER

In Hexagram Shi-7, Kun-2 is the top trigram and Kan-1 is the lower trigram. The numbers for trigrams are from the Later Heaven (Hou Tian) Ba Gua (see Figure 14.2).

Note the element of each trigram and how the two interact with each other: whether it is the promoting, controlling or reduction cycle (see pages 49–53). Also, evaluate how each trigram's element phase interacts with the element phase of the hexagram of the problem channel.

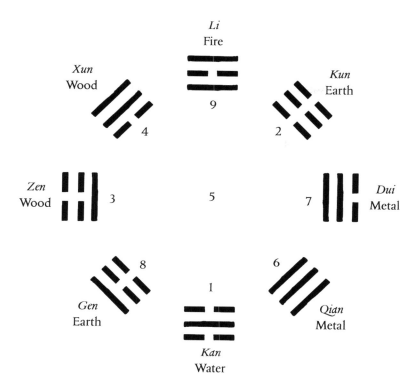

Figure 14.2 The Later Heaven Ba Gua

In the tables on pages 195–254 the hexagrams for the 12 primary channels are shown in the second column. In the third column are the favorable hexagrams. In the fourth column the differing lines are noted, along with the acupoints that should be needled. The table on the following page shows the first two rows for the example hexagram, Shi-7.

Hexagram	Problem channel	Favorable hexagram: *Shi*	Acupoints to needle
Qian Heaven	BL or GB	*Shi*-7	Lines 1, 2, 4, 5, 6
Dui Lake	HT or PC	*Shi*-7	Lines 1, 4, 5 Heart 9, 5, 4 or Pericardium 9, 6, 5

7
SHI

Leader
Multitude
Group action

KUN-2-EARTH

KAN-1-WATER

1. Sage.

2. A good omen.

3. A symbol of hidden power.

4. A mandate from heaven to take action.

5. Master of martial arts.

6. Organized, functional, order.

7. Organizing disorder to become order.

8. Organizing for the release of transformative energy.

9. The gentle energy of Earth controls the unknown and ambiguous energy of Water.

10. Guidance by an experienced leader with constancy brings good fortune.

11. Be aware of external health influences—for example, family, friends, school.

12. Follow an organized and specific health plan.

13. Avoid external emotional and psychological influences.

14. Cultivate your higher self.

15. Primordial/Yuan/original changes false patterns.

Hexagram	Problem channel	Favorable hexagram: *Shi*	Acupoints to needle
Qian Heaven	BL or GB	*Shi*-7	Lines 1, 3, 4, 5, 6 Bladder 67, 65, 64, 60, 40 or Gallbladder 44, 41, 40, 38, 34
Dui Lake	HT or PC	*Shi*-7	Lines 1, 4, 5 Heart 9, 5, 4 or Pericardium 9, 6, 5
Li Fire	SP	*Shi*-7	Lines 1, 2, 3, 4, 6 Spleen 1, 2, 3, 4, 9
Zhen Thunder	LI	*Shi*-7	Lines 1, 2, 4 Large Intestine 1, 2, 4
Xun Wind	LU	*Shi*-7	Lines 3, 5, 6 Lung 9, 7, 5

Kan Water	ST	*Shi*-7	Line 5 Stomach 41
Gen Mountain	SI, SJ	*Shi*-7	Lines 2, 3, 6 Small Intestine 2, 3, 8 or San Jiao 2, 3, 10
Kun Earth	LV or KD	*Shi*-7	Line 2 Liver 2 or Kidney 2

8
BI

Union
Accord
Loyalty
Closeness
Fellowship
Gathering the spirits

KAN-1-WATER

KUN-2-EARTH

1. Good fortune.

2. Mutual support, spirit kinship.

3. Site of creative transformation.

4. A ritual of gathering energies.

5. Intimacy, closeness.

6. Correct any imbalances.

7. A group setting provides favorable energy.

8. Support brings a favorable result.

9. You receive assistance from others.

10. Image includes bright stars encircling the North Star.

11. View things in a holistic way, not in a narrow or limited way.

12. An image is "Yu the Great" bringing spirits together to tame flooding.

13. King Yu called an assembly of Shen, lords and spirits on Mao Shan, the sacred mountain to help people.

14. The waters were transformed to become an ever-flowing source to nourish all.

15. The jar used for medicines is put on the top shelf, health is good.

16. A withered tree produces beautiful flowers, good fortune after a spell of difficulties.

Hexagram	Problem channel	Favorable hexagram: *Bi*	Acupoints to needle
Qian Heaven	▬▬▬ ▬▬▬ ▬▬▬ ▬▬▬ ▬▬▬ ▬▬▬ BL or GB	▬ ▬ ▬▬▬ ▬ ▬ ▬ ▬ ▬ ▬ ▬ ▬ *Bi*-8	Lines 1, 2, 3, 4, 6 Bladder 67, 66, 65, 64, 40 or Gallbladder 44, 43, 41, 40, 34
Dui Lake	▬ ▬ ▬▬▬ ▬▬▬ ▬ ▬ ▬▬▬ ▬▬▬ HT or PC	▬▬▬ ▬▬▬ ▬ ▬ ▬ ▬ ▬ ▬ ▬ ▬ *Bi*-8	Lines 1, 2, 4 Heart 9, 8, 5 or Pericardium 9, 8, 6
Li Fire	▬▬▬ ▬ ▬ ▬▬▬ ▬▬▬ ▬ ▬ ▬▬▬ SP	▬ ▬ ▬▬▬ ▬ ▬ ▬ ▬ ▬ ▬ ▬ ▬ *Bi*-8	Lines 1, 3, 4, 5, 6 Spleen 1, 3, 4, 5, 9
Zhen Thunder	▬ ▬ ▬ ▬ ▬ ▬ ▬ ▬ ▬▬▬ LI	▬ ▬ ▬ ▬ ▬ ▬ ▬ ▬ ▬ ▬ *Bi*-8	Lines 1, 4, 5 Large Intestine 1, 4, 5

Xun Wind	LU	*Bi-8*	Lines 2, 3, 6 Lung 10, 9, 5
Kan Water	ST	*Bi-8*	Line 2 Stomach 44
Gen Mountain	SI or SJ	*Bi-8*	Lines 3, 5, 6 Small Intestine 3, 5, 8 or San Jiao 3, 6, 10
Kun Earth	LV or KD	*Bi-8*	Line 5 Liver 4 or Kidney 7

9
XIAO XU

Taming force
Small accumulates
Gathering the ghosts

XUN-4-WOOD

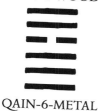

QAIN-6-METAL

1. Progress and success.

2. It is a time of a proactive covering, shell or womb.

3. Men and women dance to bring spirits and souls into the world.

4. It is the cultivation or nurturing of the smallest thing that causes change.

5. It is an aspect of the Tao, barely visible, but will lead to illumination.

6. Take time to regenerate setting the seeds for growth.

7. Channel and control your emotions and energies.

8. Good for transforming psychological conditions.

9. A gentle approach is the way to success and harmony.

10. Be humble to grow.

11. Submitting to external truth develops inner strength.

12. A new group must have a place to accumulate and gather souls; accept this and use the energy of Xiao Xu.

13. Represents the timing and location for harvesting, particularly providing the environment for receiving incoming spirits.

Hexagram	Problem channel	Favorable hexagram: *Xiao Xu*	Acupoints to needle
Qian Heaven	BL or GB	*Xiao Xu*-9	Line 4 Bladder 64 or Gallbladder 40
Dui Lake	HT or PC	*Xiao Xu*-9	Lines 3, 4, 6 Heart 7, 5, 3 or Pericardium 7, 6, 3
Li Fire	SP	*Xiao Xu*-9	Lines 2, 4, 5 Spleen 2, 4, 5
Zhen Thunder	LI	*Xiao Xu*-9	Lines 2, 3, 4, 5, 6 Large Intestine 2, 3, 4, 5, 11
Xun Wind	LU	*Xiao Xu*-9	Line 1 Lung 11
Kan Water	ST	*Xiao Xu*-9	Lines 1, 3, 6 Stomach 45, 43, 36

Gen Mountain SI or SJ	*(hexagram)*	*(hexagram)* *Xiao Xu*-9	Lines 1, 2, 5 Small Intestine 1, 2, 5 or San Jiao 1, 2, 6
Kun Earth LV or KD	*(hexagram)*	*(hexagram)* *Xiao Xu*-9	Lines 1, 2, 3, 5, 6 Liver 1, 2, 3, 5, 8 or Kidney 1, 2, 3, 4, 10

11
TAI

Peace
Advance
Harmony
Pervading
Great rituals
Good opportunity

KUN-2-EARTH

QIAN-6-METAL

1. Union of heaven and earth.

2. Good health.

3. Flexibility leads to success.

4. Activity brings good fortune.

5. Favorable for all situations.

6. A time for growth and prosperity.

7. Insights will appear, act on these insights.

8. Perfect balance of Yin–Yang, male–female.

9. Represents the integration and harmony of heaven and earth.

10. The King offered sacrifices and made direct communication to Di (heaven); the goal was to open communication of heaven and humanity.

11. Tai represents the stars of the Big Dipper, which is the place of the High Lord who directs the fates of people.

12. Its root is water, hidden wealth and fertility.

13. Yang energy ascends and Yin energy descends, the natural integration of Yin–Yang.

14. Address your weaknesses at this time in an honest way and you will transform them.

15. Seek a specialist for unusual conditions.

Hexagram	Problem channel	Favorable hexagram: *Tai*	Acupoints to needle
Qian Heaven	BL or GB	*Tai*-11	Lines 4, 5, 6 Bladder 64, 60, 40 or Gallbladder 40, 38, 34
Dui Lake	HT or PC	*Tai*-11	Lines 3, 4, 5 Heart 7, 5, 4 or Pericardium 7, 6, 5
Li Fire	SP	*Tai*-11	Lines 2, 4, 6 Spleen 2, 4, 9
Zhen Thunder	LI	*Tai*-11	Lines 2, 3, 4 Large Intestine 2, 3, 4

Xun Wind LU		*Tai*-11	Lines 1, 5, 6 Lung 11, 7, 5
Kan Water ST		*Tai*-11	Lines 1, 3, 5 Stomach 45, 43, 41
Gen Mountain SI or SJ		*Tai*-11	Lines 1, 2, 6 Small Intestine 1, 2, 8 or San Jiao 1, 2, 10
Kun Earth LV or KD		*Tai*-11	Lines 1, 2, 3 Liver 1, 2, 3 or Kidney 1, 2, 3

13
TONG REN

Union
Fellowship of people
Harmonizing people
Seeking harmony among people

QIAN-6-METAL

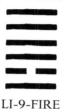

LI-9-FIRE

1. Advancement.

2. Seek harmony.

3. Progress and success.

4. Perseverance brings success.

5. Look to qualified people for advice.

6. Begin a health or exercise program, it will be very favorable.

7. People unite to celebrate the Zhou victory over the Shang.

8. The ancient Wu, who were practitioners of divination, healing, magic, talisman and *I Ching*.

9. Great sacrifices on the sacred Tai Shan Mountain, where people danced and celebrated together in the original unity of Tao.

10. Do not be too preoccupied with conditions, as they will become the cause of new problems.

11. Do not allow unfavorable thoughts and feelings to prevent your actions for health and success.

Hexagram	Problem channel	Favorable hexagram: *Tong Ren*	Acupoints to needle
Qian Heaven	BL or GB	13-*Tong Ren*	Line 2 Bladder 66 or Gallbladder 43
Dui Lake	HT or PC	13-*Tong Ren*	Lines 2, 3, 6 Heart 8, 7, 3 or Pericardium 8, 7, 3
Li Fire	SP	13-*Tong Ren*	Line 5 Spleen 5
Zhen Thunder	LI	13-*Tong Ren*	Lines 3, 5, 6 Large Intestine 3, 5, 11
Xun Wind	LU	13-*Tong Ren*	Lines 1, 2, 4 Lung 11, 10, 8
Kan Water	ST	13-*Tong Ren*	Lines 1, 2, 3, 4, 6 Stomach 45, 44, 43, 42, 36

Gen Mountain	 SI or SJ	 13-*Tong Ren*	Lines 1, 4, 5 Small Intestine 1, 4, 5 or San Jiao 1, 4, 6
Kun Earth	 LV or KD	 13-*Tong Ren*	Lines 1, 3, 4, 5, 6 Liver 1, 3, 4, 5, 8 or Kidney 1, 3, 4, 7, 10

14
Da You

Great being
Great possessions
Great harvest

LI-9-FIRE

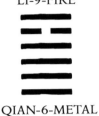

QIAN-6-METAL

1. Things respond to you.

2. Sunlight provides for all of life.

3. Look deep for the root of the condition.

4. Represents the moon and favorable changes.

5. A medicine giving off light, very effective remedy.

6. A woman accepting medicine, it is good for her.

7. A woman releasing Qi from the abdomen, a joyful time.

8. Clarity of mind, actions driven by spirit are expressions of health.

9. A sign of people being full of power and virtue and the power to become a fully realized person.

10. Sages, diviners, Wu, leaders are connected to the nature and in the flow of Tao and they can protect people.

Hexagram	Problem channel	Favorable hexagram: *Da You*	Acupoints to needle
Qian Heaven	BL or GB	14-*Da You*	Line 5 Bladder 60 or Gallbladder 38
Dui Lake	HT or PC	14-*Da You*	Lines 3, 5, 6 Heart 7, 4, 3 or Pericardium 7, 5, 3
Li Fire	SP	14-*Da You*	Line 2 Spleen 2
Zhen Thunder	LI	14-*Da You*	Lines 2, 3, 6 Large Intestine 2, 3, 11
Xun Wind	LU	14-*Da You*	Lines 1, 4, 5 Lung 11, 8, 7
Kan Water	ST	14-*Da You*	Lines 1, 3, 4, 5, 6 Stomach 45, 43, 42, 41, 36

Gen Mountain SI or SJ		14-*Da You*	Lines 1, 2, 4 Small Intestine 1, 2, 4 or San Jiao 1, 2, 4
Kun Earth LV or KD		14-*Da You*	Lines 1, 2, 3, 4, 6 Liver 1, 2, 3, 4, 8 or Kidney 1, 2, 3, 4, 10

18
GU

Renovating
Remedying
Arresting decay
Correcting the corruption

GEN-8-EARTH

XUN-4-WOOD

1. Offering service to the ancestors.

2. Allow things to rot so that new beginning will occur.

3. Unfavorable situation cannot last, it must change.

4. Handle the situation properly and great success will manifest.

5. The source of new growth, follow a plan for health and there will be success.

6. Image includes a vase containing five poisonous creatures: snake, scorpion, centipede, gecko and toad. These five are put in a jar until one eats the others, it kills all poisons.

7. Image includes a container with worms in it: this is an environment for them to thrive. Make a clear diagnosis, this is the key and takes action for a favorable result.

8. Image includes three vampires sucking blood; unfavorable situation cannot last, the time is for change.

9. Evaluate your condition in depth; peruse deep levels to begin the process of change.

Hexagram	Problem channel	Favorable hexagram: *Gu*	Acupoints to needle
Qian Heaven	BL or GB	18-*Gu*	Lines 1, 4, 5 Bladder 67, 64, 60 or Gallbladder 44, 40, 38
Dui Lake	HT or PC	18-*Gu*	Lines 1, 3, 4, 5, 6 Heart 9, 7, 5, 4, 3 or Pericardium 9, 7, 6, 5, 3
Li Fire	SP	18-*Gu*	Lines 1, 2, 4 Spleen 1, 2, 4
Zhen Thunder	LI	18-*Gu*	Lines 1, 2, 3, 4, 6 Large Intestine 1, 2, 3, 4, 11
Xun Wind	LU	18-*Gu*	Line 5 Lung 7
Kan Water	ST	18-*Gu*	Lines 3, 5, 6 Stomach 43, 41, 36

Gen Mountain	SI or SJ	18-*Gu*	Line 2 Small Intestine 2 or San Jiao 2
Kun Earth	LV or KD	18-*Gu*	Lines 2, 3, 6 Liver 2, 3, 8 or Kidney 2, 3, 10

19
LIN

Nearing
Advancing
Approaching
Releasing the spirit

KUN-2-EARTH

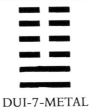

DUI-7-METAL

1. Take action.

2. Very favorable hexagram.

3. Begin a new health program.

4. Know the cyclical nature of life.

5. Be determined and focused for success.

6. Cooperate with advisors for success.

7. Utilize the body's self-healing processes.

8. It is a doorway or connection to heaven.

9. Deal promptly with conditions that make it difficult for a seed to grow.

10. A time to plant seeds of your highest qualities.

11. A calling to heaven above for protection of all the people.

12. Great accomplishments can manifest with proper sacrifice.

13. Cultivate Yuan energy and transform patterns and conditioning.

14. Represents ceremonies of the transformation of a person to a soul.

Hexagram	Problem channel	Favorable hexagram: *Lin*	Acupoints to needle
Qian Heaven	BL or GB	19-*Lin*	Lines 3, 4, 5, 6 Bladder 65, 64, 60, 40 or Gallbladder 41, 40, 38, 34
Dui Lake	HT or PC	19-*Lin*	Lines 4, 5 Heart 4, 5 or Pericardium 5, 6
Li Fire	SP	19-*Lin*	Lines 2, 3, 4, 6 Spleen 2, 3, 4, 9
Zhen Thunder	LI	19-*Lin*	Lines 2, 4 Large Intestine 2, 4
Xun Wind	LU	19-*Lin*	Lines 1, 3, 5, 6 Lung 11, 9, 8, 5
Kan Water	ST	19-*Lin*	Lines 1, 5 Stomach 45, 41

| Gen
Mountain |

SI or SJ |

19-*Lin* | Lines 1, 2, 3, 6
Small Intestine 1, 2, 3, 8
or
San Jiao 1, 2, 3, 10 |
| Kun
Earth |

LV or KD |

19-*Lin* | Lines 1, 2
Liver 1, 2
or
Kidney 1, 2 |

24
FU

Renewal
Returning
Turning back

KUN-2-EARTH

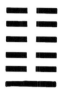

ZHEN-3-WOOD

1. Yang.

2. Return to the source.

3. Return of life.

4. Quick success.

5. New beginnings.

6. Put the past behind you.

7. The path brings progress.

8. The seventh day brings a new cycle.

9. Cultivate and gather your energy.

10. Rebirth, renewal, re-establishment.

11. It is the root of power and virtue.

12. Unfavorable energy surrenders to the light.

13. Change occurs based on nature's patterns.

14. Restore your energy and health step by step.

Hexagram	Problem channel	Favorable hexagram: *Fu*	Acupoints to needle
Qian Heaven	BL or GB	24-*Fu*	Lines 2, 3, 4, 5, 6 Bladder 66, 65, 64, 60, 40 or Gallbladder 43, 41, 40, 38, 34
Dui Lake	HT or PC	24-*Fu*	Lines 2, 4, 5 Heart 8, 5, 4 or Pericardium 8, 6, 5
Li Fire	SP	24-*Fu*	Lines 3, 4, 6 Spleen 3, 4, 9
Zhen Thunder	LI	24-*Fu*	Line 4 Large Intestine 4
Xun Wind	LU	24-*Fu*	Lines 1, 2, 3, 5, 6 Lung 11, 10, 9, 7, 5
Kan Water	ST	24-*Fu*	Lines 1, 2, 5 Stomach 45, 44, 41

Gen Mountain	䷳ SI or SJ	䷖ 24-*Fu*	Lines 1, 3, 6 Small Intestine 1, 3, 8 or San Jiao 1, 3, 10
Kun Earth	䷁ LV or KD	䷖ 24-*Fu*	Line 1 Liver 1 or Kidney 1

26
Da Xu

Great saving
Great accumulation
Great taming force
Gathering the spirits

GEN-8-EARTH

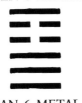

QIAN-6-METAL

1. Support.

2. Nourishment.

3. Gather spirit.

4. Harvesting.

5. Be active.

6. Success.

7. Great achievement.

8. Bringing things together.

9. Avoid spreading yourself too thinly.

10. Rely on professional guidance.

11. Be focused on the goal for a favorable result.

12. Manage the gathering of numerous energies.

13. Focus your energy in positive and favorable areas.

Hexagram	Problem channel	Favorable hexagram: *Da Xu*	Acupoints to needle
Qian Heaven	BL or GB	26-*Da Xu*	Lines 4, 5 Bladder 64, 60 or Gallbladder 40, 38
Dui Lake	HT or PC	26-*Da Xu*	Lines 3, 4, 5, 6 Heart 7, 5, 4, 3 or Pericardium 7, 6, 5, 3
Li Fire	SP	26-*Da Xu*	Lines 2, 4 Spleen 2, 4
Zhen Thunder	LI	26-*Da Xu*	Lines 2, 3, 4, 6 Large Intestine 2, 3, 4, 11
Xun Wind	LU	26-*Da Xu*	Lines 1, 5 Lung 11, 7
Kan Water	ST	26-*Da Xu*	Lines 1, 3, 5, 6 Stomach 45, 43, 41, 36

Gen Mountain	䷳ SI or SJ	䷙ 26-*Da Xu*	Lines 1, 2 Small Intestine 1, 2 or San Jiao 1, 2
Kun Earth	䷁ LV or KD	䷙ 26-*Da Xu*	Lines 1, 2, 3, 6 Liver 1, 2, 3, 8 or Kidney 1, 2, 3, 10

31
XIAN

Influence
Uniting in spirit
Mutual attraction

DUI-7-METAL

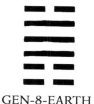

GEN-8-EARTH

1. Strong attraction.

2. Place of transformation.

3. Bringing together what belongs together.

4. Ancient Wu contacted "Shen" in these locations.

5. The Heart-Shen is filled and moved with spirit.

6. Is the sensing of spirit moving inside.

7. Avoid the influence of others.

8. Heaven and earth; celestial and terrestrial are harmonized.

9. Sensing the Tao within and moving us.

10. Embrace the Yin; be open to receiving and following.

11. Someone will assist you in a way you never thought possible.

12. Energetic health systems can be effective.

13. Location of the Xian Qi, location of the sun as it begins its new journey each day.

Hexagram	Problem channel	Favorable hexagram: *Xian*	Acupoints to needle
Qian Heaven	BL or GB	31-*Xian*	Lines 1, 2, 6 Bladder 67, 66, 40 or Gallbladder 44, 43, 34
Dui Lake	HT or PC	31-*Xian*	Lines 1, 2, 3 Heart 9, 8, 7 or Pericardium 9, 8, 7
Li Fire	SP	31-*Xian*	Lines 1, 5, 6 Spleen 1, 5, 9
Zhen Thunder	LI	31-*Xian*	Lines 1, 3, 5 Large Intestine 1, 3, 5
Xun Wind	LU	31-*Xian*	Lines 2, 4, 6 Lung 10, 8, 5
Kan Water	ST	31-*Xian*	Lines 2, 3, 4 Stomach 44, 43, 42

Gen Mountain	[hexagram] SI or SJ	[hexagram] 31-*Xian*	Lines 4, 5, 6 Small Intestine 4, 5, 8 or San Jiao 4, 6, 10
Kun Earth	[hexagram] LV or KD	[hexagram] 31-*Xian*	Lines 3, 4, 5 Liver 3, 4, 5 or Kidney 3, 4, 7

32
Heng

Constancy
Conjoining
Uniting in spirit

ZHEN-3-WOOD

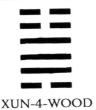

XUN-4-WOOD

1. Image of sacred sites where spirits live.

2. Places where the Wu communicate with Shen.

3. Feeling in the bones.

4. Sensation of spirit moving in the body.

5. Heaven and earth are integrating in the body.

6. Sun and moon shine bright, auspicious.

7. A Taoist priest provides guidance.

8. Be firm and correct for a favorable result.

9. Evaluate old patterns as the possible root.

Hexagram	Problem channel	Favorable hexagram: *Heng*	Acupoints to needle
Qian Heaven	BL or GB	32-*Heng*	Lines 1, 5, 6 Bladder 67, 60, 40 or Gallbladder 44, 38, 34
Dui Lake	HT or PC	32-*Heng*	Lines 1, 3, 5 Heart 9, 7, 4 or Pericardium 9, 7, 5
Li Fire	SP	32-*Heng*	Lines 1, 2, 6 Spleen 1, 2, 9
Zhen Thunder	LI	32-*Heng*	Lines 1, 2, 3 Large Intestine 1, 2, 3
Xun Wind	LU	32-*Heng*	Lines 4, 5, 6 Lung 8, 7, 5
Kan Water	ST	32-*Heng*	Lines 3, 4, 5 Stomach 43, 42, 41

Gen Mountain	SI or SJ	32-*Heng*	Lines 2, 4, 6 Small Intestine 2, 4, 8 or San Jiao 2, 4, 10
Kun Earth	LV or KD	32-*Heng*	Lines 2, 3, 4 Liver 2, 3, 4 or Kidney 2, 3, 4

34
DA ZHUANG

Power of the great
Great strength
Invigorating strength

ZHEN-3-WOOD

QIAN-6-METAL

1. Advance.

2. Full vitality.

3. Listen to advice.

4. Great invigoration.

5. Persevere for success.

6. Time to move forward.

7. Avoid extreme emotions, seek balance.

8. Manage your energy in a favorable direction.

9. A powerful hexagram; focus your energy with sensitivity for a favorable result.

Hexagram	Problem channel	Favorable hexagram: *Da Zhuang*	Acupoints to needle
Qian Heaven	BL or GB	34-*Da Zhuang*	Lines 5, 6 Bladder 60, 40 or Gallbladder 38, 34
Dui Lake	HT or PC	34-*Da Zhuang*	Lines 3, 5 Heart 7, 4 or Pericardium 7, 5
Li Fire	SP	34-*Da Zhuang*	Lines 2, 6 Spleen 2, 9
Zhen Thunder	LI	34-*Da Zhuang*	Lines 2, 3 Large Intestine 2, 3
Xun Wind	LU	34-*Da Zhuang*	Lines 1, 4, 5, 6 Lung 11, 8, 7, 5
Kan Water	ST	34-*Da Zhuang*	Lines 1, 3, 4, 5 Stomach 45, 43, 42, 41

Gen Mountain			
	SI or SJ	34-*Da Zhuang*	Lines 1, 2, 4, 6 Small Intestine 1, 2, 4, 8 or San Jiao 1, 2, 4, 10
Kun Earth	LV or KD	34-*Da Zhuang*	Lines 1, 2, 3, 4 Liver 1, 2, 3, 4 or Kidney 1, 2, 3, 4

37
Jia Ren

Family
Dwelling people

XUN-4-WOOD

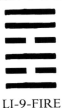

LI-9-FIRE

1. Support.

2. Nourishment.

3. A time for fruition.

4. Support at the dwelling.

5. Cultivate the inner.

6. Turn inward, "know thyself."

7. Join with others, avoid isolation.

8. Nurture one's energy for the situation.

9. Symbol of flowers turning to fruit; favorable.

10. Cultivate your health with good diet and exercise.

11. Spirit blessings from ancestors and the mothers.

Hexagram	Problem channel	Favorable hexagram: *Jia Ren*	Acupoints to needle
Qian Heaven	BL or GB	37-*Jia Ren*	Lines 2, 4 Bladder 66, 64 or Gallbladder 43, 40
Dui Lake	HT or PC	37-*Jia Ren*	Lines 2, 3, 4, 6 Heart 8, 7, 5, 3 or Pericardium 8, 7, 6, 3
Li Fire	SP	37-*Jia Ren*	Lines 4, 5 Spleen 4, 5
Zhen Thunder	LI	37-*Jia Ren*	Lines 3, 4, 5, 6 Large Intestine 3, 4, 5, 11
Xun Wind	LU	37-*Jia Ren*	Lines 1, 2 Lung 11, 10
Kan Water	ST	37-*Jia Ren*	Lines 1, 2, 3, 6 Stomach 45, 44, 43, 36

Gen Mountain	䷳ SI or SJ	䷤ 37-*Jia Ren*	Lines 1, 5 Small Intestine 1, 5 or San Jiao 1, 6
Kun Earth	䷁ LV or KD	䷤ 37-*Jia Ren*	Lines 1, 3, 5, 6 Liver 1, 3, 5, 8 or Kidney 1, 3, 7, 10

40
JIE

Relief
Loosening
Deliverance
Removing obstacles
Dissolution of the problem

ZHEN-3-WOOD

KAN-1-WATER

1. Letting go.

2. Untie knots.

3. Relieve pain.

4. Advice is good.

5. Solving problems.

6. Freed from suffering.

7. New cycle is beginning.

8. Difficulties come to an end.

9. Release of blocked energy.

10. Remedy has intended effect.

11. Let go of old emotional patterns.

12. Evaluate your habits and actions as the potential root of the condition.

Hexagram	Problem channel	Favorable hexagram: *Jie*	Acupoints to needle
Qian Heaven	BL or GB	40-*Jie*	Lines 1, 3, 5, 6 Bladder 67, 65, 60, 40 or Gallbladder 44, 41, 38, 34
Dui Lake	HT or PC	40-*Jie*	Lines 1, 5 Heart 9, 4 or Pericardium 9, 5
Li Fire	SP	40-*Jie*	Lines 1, 2, 3, 6 Spleen 1, 2, 3, 9
Zhen Thunder	LI	40-*Jie*	Lines 1, 2 Large Intestine 1, 2
Xun Wind	LU	40-*Jie*	Lines 3, 4, 5 Lung 9, 8, 7
Kan Water	ST	40-*Jie*	Lines 4, 5 Stomach 42, 41

Gen Mountain			Lines 2, 3, 4, 6 Small Intestine 2, 3, 4, 8 or San Jiao 2, 3, 4, 10
	SI or SJ	40-*Jie*	
Kun Earth			Lines 2, 4 Liver 2, 4 or Kidney 2, 4
	LV or KD	40-*Jie*	

42
YI

Benefit
Increasing
Augmenting
The blessing

XUN-4-WOOD

ZHEN-3-WOOD

1. Developing.

2. Expanding.

3. Focus on inner healing.

4. Site of transformations.

5. Empty bowl ready to be filled.

6. The connection of heaven and earth.

7. Hexagram invokes growth and springtime.

8. Favorable for taking initiative and action.

9. Generosity and compassion are keys to transformation.

Hexagram	Problem channel	Favorable hexagram: *Yi*	Acupoints to needle
Qian Heaven	BL or GB	42-*Yi*	Lines 2, 3, 4 Bladder 66, 65, 64 or Gallbladder 43, 41, 40
Dui Lake	HT or PC	42-*Yi*	Lines 2, 4, 6 Heart 8, 5, 3 or Pericardium 8, 6, 3
Li Fire	SP	42-*Yi*	Lines 3, 4, 5 Spleen 3, 4, 5
Zhen Thunder	LI	42-*Yi*	Lines 4, 5, 6 Large Intestine 4, 5, 11
Xun Wind	LU	42-*Yi*	Lines 1, 2, 3 Lung 11, 10, 9
Kan Water	ST	42-*Yi*	Lines 1, 2, 6 Stomach 45, 44, 36

Gen Mountain SI or SJ	(hexagram) 42-*Yi*		Lines 1, 3, 5 Small Intestine 1, 3, 5 or San Jiao 1, 3, 6
Kun Earth LV or KD	(hexagram) 42-*Yi*		Lines 1, 5, 6 Liver 1, 5, 8 or Kidney 1, 7, 10

50
DING

Cauldron
Stability
The vessel
Harmonization
Transformation
Establishing the new

LI-9-FIRE

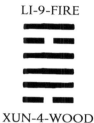

XUN-4-WOOD

1. Hold.

2. Found.

3. Established.

4. Sacred vessel.

5. Progress and success.

6. Contain and transform.

7. Highest good fortune.

8. Stability after revolution.

9. New order after disorder.

10. Structure in your life brings success.

11. Review possible misunderstandings.

12. Develop favorable lifestyle behavior to develop health and vitality.

Hexagram	Problem channel	Favorable hexagram: *Ding*	Acupoints to needle
Qian Heaven	BL or GB	50-*Ding*	Lines 1, 5 Bladder 67, 60 or Gallbladder 44, 38
Dui Lake	HT or PC	50-*Ding*	Lines 1, 3, 5, 6 Heart 9, 7, 4, 3 or Pericardium 9, 7, 5, 3
Li Fire	SP	50-*Ding*	Lines 1, 2 Spleen 1, 2
Zhen Thunder	LI	50-*Ding*	Lines 1, 2, 3, 6 Large Intestine 1, 2, 3, 11
Xun Wind	LU	50-*Ding*	Lines 4, 5 Lung 8, 7
Kan Water	ST	50-*Ding*	Lines 3, 4, 5, 6 Stomach 43, 42, 41, 36

Gen Mountain	䷠ SI or SJ	50-*Ding*	Lines 2, 4 Small Intestine 2, 4 or San Jiao 2, 4
Kun Earth	䷁ LV or KD	50-*Ding*	Lines 2, 3, 4, 6 Liver 2, 3, 4, 8 or Kidney 2, 3, 4, 10

55
FENG

Prosperity
Abounding
Abundance
Receiving the mandate

ZHEN-3-WOOD

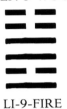

LI-9-FIRE

1. Full.

2. Fertility.

3. Plentiful.

4. Expansion.

5. Great change.

6. Harmony.

7. A sign of change.

8. Embrace change.

9. Action, success.

10. Inner creative energy.

11. Abundant, harvest, plentiful.

12. Attention prevents problems.

13. Step into the brightness of the present.

14. Use your energy to develop long-term health.

Hexagram	Problem channel	Favorable hexagram: *Feng*	Acupoints to needle
Qian Heaven	BL or GB	55-*Feng*	Lines 2, 5, 6 Bladder 66, 60, 40 or Gallbladder 43, 38, 34
Dui Lake	HT or PC	55-*Feng*	Lines 2, 3, 5 Heart 8, 7, 4 or Pericardium 8, 7, 5
Li Fire	SP	55-*Feng*	Line 6 Spleen 9
Zhen Thunder	LI	55-*Feng*	Line 3 Large Intestine 3
Xun Wind	LU	55-*Feng*	Lines 1, 2, 4, 5, 6 Lung 11, 10, 8, 7, 5
Kan Water	ST	55-*Feng*	Lines 1, 2, 3, 4, 5 Stomach 45, 44, 43, 42, 41

Gen Mountain SI or SJ	☶ SI or SJ	55-*Feng*	Lines 1, 4, 6 Small Intestine 1, 4, 8 or San Jiao 1, 4, 10
Kun Earth LV or KD	☷ LV or KD	55-*Feng*	Lines 1, 3, 4 Liver 1, 3, 4 or Kidney 1, 3, 4

61
ZHONG FU

Faithfulness
Inner sincerity
Central sincerity
Centering and connecting to the spirits

XUN-4-WOOD

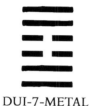

DUI-7-METAL

1. Core, center.

2. Hit the mark.

3. Site of initiation.

4. Drive out evil spirits.

5. Creative transformation.

6. Connection to the spirit.

7. It is a time of perseverance.

8. Connect the heart to the spirit.

9. Connect your inner and outer lives.

10. Return to the center to find health and happiness.

11. Focus on your body and emotions, they may reveal the root of the health condition.

Hexagram	Problem channel	Favorable hexagram: *Zhong Fu*	Acupoints to needle
Qian Heaven	BL or GB	61-*Zhong Fu*	Lines 3, 4 Bladder 65, 64 or Gallbladder 41, 40
Dui Lake	HT or PC	61-*Zhong Fu*	Lines 4, 6 Heart 5, 3 or Pericardium 6, 3
Li Fire	SP	61-*Zhong Fu*	Lines 2, 3, 4, 5 Spleen 2, 3, 4, 5
Zhen Thunder	LI	61-*Zhong Fu*	Lines 2, 4, 5, 6 Large Intestine 2, 4, 5, 11
Xun Wind	LU	61-*Zhong Fu*	Lines 1, 3 Lung 11, 9
Kan Water	ST	61-*Zhong Fu*	Lines 1, 6 Stomach 45, 36

Gen Mountain	SI or SJ	61-*Zhong Fu*	Lines 1, 2, 3, 5 Small Intestine 1, 2, 3, 5 or San Jiao 1, 2, 3, 6
Kun Earth	LV or KD	61-*Zhong Fu*	Lines 1, 2, 5, 6 Liver 1, 2, 5, 8 or Kidney 1, 2, 7, 10

63
Ji Ji

Finished
Fulfilled
Completion
Already crossing
After crossing the water

KAN-1-WATER

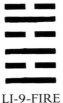

LI-9-FIRE

1. Proceed.

2. Underway.

3. Stable vessel.

4. In progress.

5. Correct alignment.

6. Focus on preventive health.

7. Symbol is Yin matching Yang.

8. Avoid overextending yourself.

9. Maintain a daily health regimen.

10. Souls and spirits entering the great Stream.

11. Maintain health and prepare for the future.

12. Manage your accomplishments and prepare for the future.

13. Water and Fire are balanced, very favorable; transformation is favorable.

Hexagram	Problem channel	Favorable hexagram: *Ji Ji*	Acupoints to needle
Qian Heaven	BL or GB	63-*Ji Ji*	Lines 2, 4, 6 Bladder 66, 64, 40 or Gallbladder 43, 40, 34
Dui Lake	HT or PC	63-*Ji Ji*	Lines 2, 3, 4 Heart 8, 7, 5 or Pericardium 8, 7, 6
Li Fire	SP	63-*Ji Ji*	Lines 4, 5, 6 Spleen 4, 5, 9
Zhen Thunder	LI	63-*Ji Ji*	Lines 3, 4, 5 Large Intestine 3, 4, 5
Xun Wind	LU	63-*Ji Ji*	Lines 1, 2, 6 Lung 11, 10, 5
Kan Water	ST	63-*Ji Ji*	Lines 1, 2, 3 Stomach 45, 44, 43

Gen Mountain SI or SJ	(hexagram)	(hexagram) 63-*Ji Ji*	Lines 1, 5, 6 Small Intestine 1, 5, 8 or San Jiao 1, 6, 10
Kun Earth LV or KD	(hexagram)	(hexagram) 63-*Ji Ji*	Lines 1, 3, 5 Liver 1, 3, 5 or Kidney 1, 3, 7

Guidance for Acupuncture Needling

1. If the condition is one-sided, select points on the contralateral side.

2. If the condition is bilateral, insert needles on the right side first for females, and the left side first for males; then needle the opposite side.

3. Needling technique includes choices: one-sided or bilateral needling are options, and it is up to you to select your preference.

4. The Yin–Yang paired channel can always be added to the treatment by selecting the corresponding points of the problem channel. For example, if you needled Spleen 3 and 9, select its Yin–Yang pair channel and needle Stomach 43 and 36; both are Stream and Sea points or 3–6 acupoint combinations.

Appendix I

Six Clinical Cases for Balance Method 6

Case 1

1. Your patient suffers from an occipital headache. The channel in this case is the Bladder and the hexagram is Qian, which has six Yang lines. The favorable hexagram selected is Tai-11.

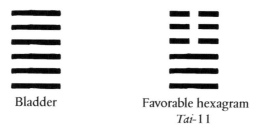

Bladder   Favorable hexagram
Tai-11

2. Compare the two hexagrams. Count hexagram lines from the bottom to the top and note lines that are different, which in this case are lines 4, 5 and 6. These are the lines to needle, and they correspond to lines 4, 5 and 6 on the Bladder Channel.

3. The acupoints that correspond to lines 4, 5 and 6 are Bladder 64, 60 and 40 (marked with an asterisk in the table below).

Line	Bladder
6-Sea	40 *
5-River	60 *
4-Source	64 *
3-Stream	65
2-Spring	66
1-Well	67

4. Treat the contralateral side if it is a one-sided condition. Treat bilaterally if the condition is on both sides.

Case 2

1. A patient has chest pain along the right side of the Stomach Channel. The hexagram that corresponds with the Stomach Channel is Kan. The time of year for the treatment is spring.

2. Select a favorable hexagram. Yi-42 is the hexagram selected for this condition. Yi is comprised of trigrams Zhen-Wood and Xun-Wood. These two trigrams and the season of treatment contain the Wood element, and all of them support Wood and the treatment. Wood is the child of the hexagram Kan, which is the Water element; this hexagram reduces the condition. Wood also controls Earth, which is the Stomach Channel.

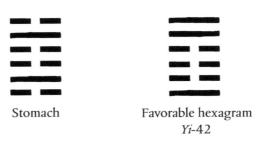

Stomach   Favorable hexagram
                        Yi-42

3. Note the lines that are different: 1, 2 and 6.

4. Needle Stomach 45, 44 and 36 on the left (contralateral) side. In the treatment of pain, treat the contralateral side; this is Yang treating Yin or Yin treating Yang, and contralateral acupuncture.

Line	Stomach
6-Sea	36 *
5-River	41
4-Source	42
3-Stream	43
2-Spring	44 *
1-Well	45 *

Case 3

1. A patient has back pain during the spring, and the pain is located on the Bladder Channel.

2. Hexagram Heng-32 is selected. Heng is a spring hexagram and it contains two Wood trigrams, which also correspond to spring. The seasonal phase is Wood and reinforces the hexagram Heng, which contains Wood.

3. Note the lines that are different: 1, 5 and 6, corresponding to Bladder 67, 60 and 40; needle these acupoints.

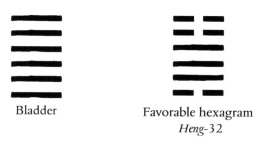

Bladder

Favorable hexagram
Heng-32

Line	Bladder
6-Sea	40 *
5-River	60 *
4-Source	64
3-Stream	65
2-Spring	66
1-Well	67 *

Case 4

1. A female patient suffers from long-term emotional disharmony. The emotions are sadness and grief, which are related to the Lungs and the Metal element.

2. The Pericardium Channel is selected to treat the Shen for this condition. The corresponding hexagram is Dui, which is the Metal element.

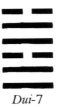

Dui-7

3. The favorable hexagram selected is Lin-19. Lin contains the Earth and Metal elements, which are favorable to the Metal hexagram for the Pericardium. The image includes *Releasing the spirit*, a Shen-related quality.

Kun-2-Earth

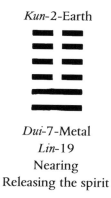

Dui-7-Metal
Lin-19
Nearing
Releasing the spirit

4. Comparing the two hexagrams, the lines that differ are 4 and 5, and they relate to Pericardium 5 and 6. Needle those acupoints on the right side for a female, and balance the treatment by needling the Yin–Yang paired channel: needle San Jiao 4 and 6.

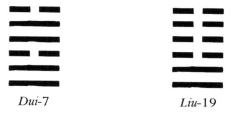

Dui-7   *Liu*-19

Line	Pericardium
6-Sea	3
5-River	5 *
4-Luo	6 *
3-Stream	7
2-Spring	8
1-Well	9

The Liver could have been selected as the balance channel instead of San Jiao. (It is the Jue Yin pair of the Pericardium.)

Case 5

1. A female patient has been unable to become pregnant. The diagnosis for this patient is Kidney Yang deficiency.

2. The hexagram for the Kidney is Kun, and it contains all Yin lines. The favorable hexagram selected is Feng-55. Feng contains the following qualities: full, fertility, plentiful, expansion, harmony, sign of change, abundant, harvest and plentiful.

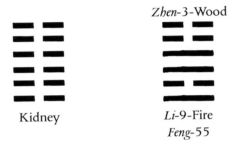

Zhen-3-Wood

Kidney

Li-9-Fire
Feng-55

3. The lines that are different between the two hexagrams are 1, 3 and 4, corresponding to Kidney 1, 3 and 4.

4. Treat Kidney 1, 3, and 4 on the right side. Bladder is the Yin–Yang pair of Kidney, so treat Bladder 67, 65 and 64 on the left side.

Line	Kidney
6-Sea	10
5-River	7
4-Luo	4 *
3-Stream	3 *
2-Spring	2
1-Well	1 *

Case 6

1. A 45-year old male complained of anger, irritability and asthma. The diagnosis included Wood insulting Metal or Liver insulting the Lungs.

    The favorable hexagram selected is Heng.

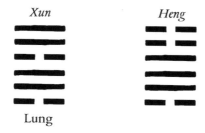

2. Note that lines 4, 5 and 6 are opposite polarities, and these lines correspond to Lung 8, 7 and 5.

3. The Lung's Yin–Yang partner, the Large Intestine Channel, can be needled to balance the treatment. The Large Intestine points to needle are at lines 4, 5 and 6, or Large Intestine 4, 5 and 11.

Line	Lung
6-Sea	5 *
5-River	7 *
4-Source	8 *
3-Stream	9
2-Spring	10
1-Well	11

Line	Lung	Large Intestine
6-Sea	5	11
5-River	7-Luo	5
4-Source	8-River	4
3-Stream	9	3
2-Spring	10	2
1-Well	11	1

SUMMARY OF I CHING ACUPUNCTURE—THE BALANCE METHOD

Balance Method 1

- Balancing Six Channel pairs.

- Balancing hand conditions with foot channels.

- Balancing foot conditions with hand channels.

Needling method for pain: Opposite side of the condition.

Balance Method 2

- Balancing Yin–Yang paired channels.

- Balancing hand conditions with hand channels.

- Balancing foot conditions with foot channels.

Needling method for pain: Opposite side of the condition.

Balance Method 3

- Balancing with Stream and Sea acupoints: the 3–6 Balance Method.

Needling method:

- For pain, needle the same or opposite side of the pain.

- Needle bilaterally for organ conditions and to balance the entire channel.

Balance Method 4

- Balancing the daily meridian clock.

Needling method for pain: Same side or opposite side of the condition.

Balance Method 5

- Balancing channel corresponding names and positions: 1-Jue Yin and 4-Yang Ming; 2-Shao Yin and 5-Shao Yang; 3-Tai Yin and 6-Tai Yang.

Needling method:

- For pain, needle the same or opposite side of the pain.

- Needle bilaterally for organ conditions.

Balance Method 6

- Balancing hexagrams.

Needling method:

- For pain, needle the same or opposite side of the pain.

- When treating organ conditions select the insertion method based on gender, or any method you prefer, and then select the Yin–Yang paired channel on the opposite side.

Summary Table

Balance Method	Conditions
Balance Method 1 *Balancing Six Channel pairs*	*Treats pain.* The hand treats the foot, and the foot treats the hand: 12 Joint theory. Select the problem channel's Six Channel paired channel. Opposite side needling.
Balance Method 2 *Balancing Yin–Yang paired channels*	*Treats pain.* The hand treats the other hand and the foot treats the other foot: 12 Joint theory. Select the problem channel's Yin–Yang pair. Opposite side needling.
Balance Method 3 *Balancing with Stream and Sea acupoints: the 3–6 Balance Method*	*Treats pain or any imbalance on the channel.* *Treats internal organ conditions.* One-channel treatments. Combine Yin–Yang channel pairs. Combine Six Channel pairs. Select the Stream and Sea points on the channel. (This is the 3–6 Balance Method.) For pain, select the same side or opposite side. For organ conditions needle bilaterally.
Balance Method 4 *Balancing the daily meridian clock*	*Treats pain.* Select the opposite channel on the daily meridian clock. Same or opposite side needling.
Balance Method 5 *Balancing channel corresponding names and positions*	*Treats pain or any imbalance on the channel.* *Treats internal organ conditions.* Balancing channels with the same name: Jue Yin–Yang Ming; Shao Yin–Shao Yang; Tai Yin–Tai Yang, 1–4; 2–5; 3–6. For pain, select the same side or opposite side. For organ conditions needle bilaterally.
Balance Method 6 *Balancing hexagrams*	*Treats pain.* *Treats internal organ conditions.* For pain, select the same side or opposite side. When treating organ conditions, select the insertion method based on gender, or any method you prefer, and then select the Yin–Yang paired channel on the opposite side.

CONCLUSION

The ancient Chinese had a unique understanding of their world and the human body, and they created equally unique theories, principles and models to express their insights. Their ways of expressing their insights permeate every aspect of Chinese culture, including the healing arts.

It is very interesting that the classics of Chinese medicine do not always include the theories that clinical methods are based upon. The first part of this book is my attempt to explain important Chinese philosophical theories that guide acupuncture applications. The second part of this book integrates theory and clinical practice. The clinical methods presented can be practiced alone as a complete method, or combined with other acupuncture methods.

The theories, models and methods in this book are a key to unlock many of the mysteries of Chinese healing arts. Additionally, a grasp of these Chinese philosophies and methods allows entry into many of the Chinese divination and prediction arts, including feng shui, Chinese astrology, *I Ching*, qi men dun jia and inner alchemy (nei dan). I hope this book inspires you to continue your studies of these fascinating arts. I welcome any feedback and comments about this book, and your experience applying them in clinical practice.

David Twicken, DOM, LAc
1 April 2011
Year of the Metal Rabbit

BIBLIOGRAPHY

Bertschinger, R. (2011) *The Secret of Everlasting Life*. London: Singing Dragon.

Chang, S. (1985) *The Great Tao*. Reno, NV: Tao Longevity.

Clearly, T. (trans) (2001) *The Inner Teachings of Taoism*. Boston, MA: Shambhala Publications.

Hsi, C. and Adler, J. (2002) *Introduction to the Study of the Classic of Change*. New York, NY: Global Scholarly Publications.

Huang, A. (2000) *The Numerology of the I Ching: A Sourcebook of Symbols, Structures, and Traditional Wisdom*. Rochester, VT: Inner Traditions.

Huang, A. (2004) *Complete I Ching: The Definitive Translation*. Rochester, VT: Inner Traditions.

Hwa, J. (1989) *The Tao of I Ching*. Rutland, VT: Tuttle Publishing.

Karcher, S. (2009) *Total I Ching*. New York, NY: Piatkus Books.

Liu, D. (1979) *I Ching Numerology*. New York, NY: Routledge & Kegan Paul Limited.

Lynn, J. (2004) *The Classic of Changes: A New Translation of the I Ching as Interpreted by Wang Bi*. New York, NY: Columbia University Press.

Moran, E. and Yu, J. (2001) *The Complete Idiot's Guide to I Ching*. New York: Alpha Books.

Schipper, K. (1994) *The Taoist Body*. Berkeley, CA: University of California Press.

Twicken, D. (2002) *Treasures of Tao*. Bloomington, IN: iUniverse.

Twicken, D. (2011) *Chinese Astrology*. Los Angeles, CA: Healing Qi Publishing.

Veith, I. (1966) *The Yellow Emperor's Classic of Internal Medicine*. Berkeley, CA: University of California Press.

Wilhelm, R. and Baynes, C. (1967) *The I Ching (Book of Changes)*. Princeton, NJ: Princeton University Press.

Wu, J. (2002) *Ling Shu: Or The Spiritual Pivot*. Hawaii: University of Hawaii Press.

Wu, N. and Wu, A. (2002) *Yellow Emperor's Canon of Internal Medicine*. China Science and Technology Press.

Wu, Z. (2009) *Seeking the Spirit of the Book of Change: 8 Days to Mastering a Shamanic Yijing (I Ching) Prediction System.* London: Singing Dragon.

Yoke, H. (1985) *Li, Qi and Shu: An Introduction to Science and Civilization of China.* Hong Kong: Hong Kong Unversity Press.

Printed in Great Britain
by Amazon

Thadd Presley Presents

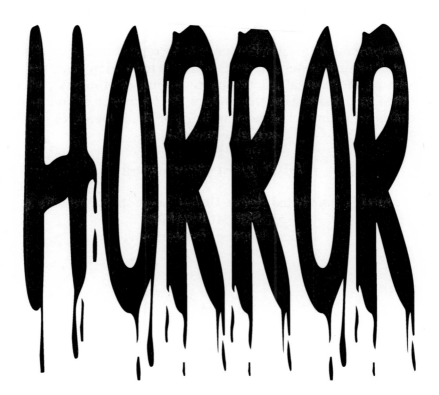

C000165300

HORROR

STATIC MOVEMENT

short stories to make you scream

Table of Contents

Thadd Presley Presents: Horror..1
The Pit by Nate Burleigh...3
Shadow Man by Charlotte Emma Gledson.......................18
Lady Killers by Todd Martin..32
Alena's Piece by Stacy Bolli...39
Adrift by Michael Dortmundt..44
Birds of a Feather by Charlotte Emma Gledson................57
Heart of an Angel by Jonathan Moon.................................72
Closed Caption by Nate D. Burleigh..................................75
It's Up to You, New York by JD Stone...............................85
The Conscience of Janice Clovell by S. Wayne Roberts...103
The Old Fishin' Hole by Todd Martin.............................120
Allie, Advantageous by S. Wayne Roberts......................128
Rain of Terror by Todd Martin...140
The Rock Garden by Stacy Bolli.......................................147
Grind by JD Stone...157
You'd Better Learn by Thadd Presley..............................173
Fallow Ground by Thadd Presley.....................................176
Born to Fight... Commanded to Kill by Jason Hughes...183
Poisoned Meat by Jonathan Moon....................................206
AuthorPages..217

Thadd Presley Presents

Horrors

WHEN I BEGAN WRITING short stories and novellas, it was my dream to have them published in magazines alongside great writers. As the stories began to be accepted, I noticed that I wrote more stories than I could ever have published. So, I began to compile my stories by genre and plan out short story books. My first short story book was published in 2008, entitled *Full Spectrum*, and it was very satisfying to have a book that I could send friends and hold in my hands.

Then in 2009, stories began to fade and I began to write poetry. When my inspiration for writing longer pieces fades, I filled the void with poetry, music, and editing for other writers. And surprisingly, in 2011, by accumulating poetry over 2009 and 2010, I published my first poetry book, entitled *Poetry Principia*. During those years I edited for many writers and learned of new places to have the stories I'd written before published. These places were not magazines but instead anthologies. It opened me up to many writers who I would later come to work with many times.

During the years of 2011, I was published in seven anthologies, including *Sins and Tragedies*, and edited for a very satisfying e-zine called *The Dark Fiction Spotlight*, where I met three good friend and great writers by the

1

name of S. Wayne Roberts, Stacy Bolli, and Daniel Fabiani. These writers each have stories in this book and along with the other authors were invited especially by me. I wanted this book to showcase some of the people who had helped me out along my way.

And now for the first time in my career, I join the ranks of Alfred Hitchcock and Rod Serling by presenting my own set of stories and the authors who wrote them. Get ready to sink into your most comfortable chair and spent the night reading what Thadd Presley Presents.

Thadd Presley Presents

The Pit
Nate D. Burleigh

I'M IN A CLOSET. It's not much wider than the one back home, but it's deeper and I'm safe. I hope.

Their screams echo through my mind as I huddle tight in the back corner of this man-made cave. It's dark, dismal, and silent. I'm alone. Knowing that my wife and three children are safe at home helps me focus. They probably think I'm having the time of my life. This morning when I called them, I was. But now I'm afraid. Frightened that I may never see them again, hold them in my arms, or tell them how much I love them. What scares the hell out of me is that they'll never find out what happened and I'll end up like so many other tourists that go hiking in the outback — lost forever. I reminisce of the events that took place today leading me to this cabin in the middle of nowhere, hoping to survive this hellish nightmare.

***

MY YOUNGER BROTHER DAVID had started his own restaurant. He'd saved up some money and flew me, our older brother, and his two best friends down to Australia for a two week vacation at his home on Bondi Beach. Hiking hadn't been in the itinerary, at least not in mine. Mine consisted of lying around on the beach, bikini scoping, and getting a tan. Things my psychiatrist said would be therapeutic.

"We have to go," Jamon said, eying the brochure like a child ogling another kid's Oreo.

"I hate hiking," I said and the other four looked at me like I was the biggest wuss on the planet. "You know I get wicked shin splints." Which was a feeble attempt to justify my cowardice.

In truth, I just didn't like doing anything that involved exercise, the outdoors, or being in public. Since turning thirty-eight I hadn't done so much as take a Sunday stroll with my family. My doctor calls it "anhedonia". Basically, it's the loss of will to do anything pleasurable. Manic depression and chronic anxiety will do that to you. Like impious succubi, they can drain your very essence, and if you're not careful, the essences of those closest to you.

Stress from my work as a Disability Claim's Manager in an insurance company, failures at church, and strained family relations were like plates of rock being piled on my chest, crushing my will and my soul. Evidenced by the medicine wheel on my bedside table, now almost completely full of antidepressant, antianxiety, and antipsychotic prescriptions. Although without them, I'd most likely be in a padded cell somewhere, singing to children that don't exist.

***

THE INCESSANT SCREAMS ARE getting louder. I hear other sounds: grinding, crunching, and gasping. The shrieks of terror subside for a moment and my thoughts revert back through the day's events.

***

"I've never been on this particular hike before; looks pretty fun," my brother David said. He swept the brochure out of Jamon's hands and plopped onto the couch. David was my younger brother.

***

THE *WAS* HITS ME HARD. He's gone and nothing can be done about that now. Tears well up in my eyes and erupt, spilling down both cheeks. The blood on my left ankle seems to have congealed. Double checking the bandage makes me wince. A sudden jolt of pain shoots up my calf and thigh as I tighten the cloth. I have to focus. The need for self-preservation kicks in and I know I have to survive — for them.

***

OUR OLDER BROTHER, CHARLES, and David's friend, Ryan, both agreed with Jamon. They outvoted me four-to-one. We were going on the hike and I could either stay in the condo and wallow in self-pity, or go with.

I reached over and snatched the brochure from Ryan. "I'll take a look, but I'm not promising anything."

"Great," Jamon said with a wide smile. He'd always been like that with everything. Even as the only boy out of eight and the youngest of the lot, his optimism about life soared above the norm; this was one of the many reasons he'd been given command of his own nuclear submarine.

Ryan had been David's best friend since grade-school. His unmotivated nature directly contrasted David's strive for success and Jamon's sanguine outlook on life.

Jamon had great book smarts, but I'd never met a person with more raw intelligence than my older brother.

Charles could pick up any how-to book and become an overnight expert on the topic. I guess that's why he never went to college, yet still did fairly well for himself with his own computer consulting firm.

***

I REACH INTO MY pocket to find the crumpled brochure. It's too dark to read. I imagine what it will say:

> **Bush walk of a lifetime.**
> **Take a walk in the beautiful outback.**

Yeah right, I think.

> **On this nature trail you will be able to enjoy the plethora of life that resides in the outback. You'll see Kangaroos, Koala bears, and so on...**

I toss the useless paper into the dark space ahead of me. There's no need for it now.

***

DAVID SLAMMED ON THE breaks, bringing the car to a stop at the trail-head with an explosion of red dust. When the dust settled, I got out, dug into my backpack and pulled out the sunscreen. My bald-head, neck, ears, and face would burn for certain if I didn't rub gobs of the thick white lotion onto them.

The narrow path leading away from the car looked like a ribbon of red dirt. It snaked up the hill toward an endless horizon. I tossed my pack over my shoulders and hurried to catch up.

Jamon had taken the lead. With brochure in hand, he pointed out lizards, kangaroos, wild orchids, and a snake of some sort. The sun started to scorch through the sunscreen and I felt a burn developing.

"I'm too hot, we need to stop for a bit," I said, using the front of my t-shirt to wipe the stinging sweat out of my eyes.

"Look, just up the way a bit should be a *'beautiful pond for our swimming, drinking, and viewing pleasure'*." Jamon pointed at a spot on the brochure.

"I say we keep going," David said.

"Yeah, maybe there's some chicks skinny dipping," Ryan chimed in.

"I'm with Nathan, let's take a break," Charles said. He, like me, wasn't the most adept at outdoor adventures.

Jamon took a swig of water and hoisted his pack back to his shoulders. "Fine, Ryan and I will scout up ahead and see if we can't find him a girlfriend."

"Sweet," Ryan said. "You brothers have a nice rest. We'll try and save some of the girls for you." He sniggered.

A stump under a rather shady tree looked very inviting. I sat down and furiously rubbed at my shin splints. At that moment my head started to spin, my vision blurred, and everything went black. It felt as if something had pushed me off of the stump. Even though I only fell a few feet, it felt like I fell for hours. A sharp pain twinged up my backside.

Blinking helped bring the world back into focus. I was on my back, staring at the weeping tree above. It mocked me for falling. Cursing under my breath, I got up, smacked the dust off my backside, and picked up in the middle of a conversation my brothers were having.

We were discussing David's restaurant business plans when we heard Ryan yelling from up the trail, "Help!

Guys! Come quick!" He didn't have his pack on and looked like he'd seen a ghost.

"What is it?" David asked, jumping up with his pack in hand.

"Does anyone have a rope?" Ryan managed to say between heavy breaths.

"Yeah..." David said, "... Jamon."

"Holy shit!" Ryan grabbed his head. "Jamon fell into some sort of pit."

"What?" I inquired, having joined my brothers at Ryan's side.

Ryan rambled on, "We were walking up a small embankment. I turned to look at a Koala when I heard him scream. It echoed for some time and then just stopped. I got to the top of the hill and in front of me was a..."

"Well," I said impatiently.

"... a pit."

"A pit?" Charles pulled off his baseball cap and rubbed the bald spot on his head.

"Yeah, a fetching hole as big as my VW bus, right in the middle of the damn trail. I leaned in and yelled and when he didn't answer, I ran here as fast as I could."

We sprinted up the trail behind him. When we reached the top of Ryan's hill, he shrieked. "What the hell?"

We stood next to him, eying an empty trail.

"It was right here. I swear to God."

"I don't see anything," David said. He crouched down and stared into the distance, squinting as if that would bring Jamon into view.

Charles had gone off the trail looking for clues. "Nothing over here," he bellowed from behind some brush.

I too couldn't find any sign of a pit, crevice, drop off or anything of that nature.

Ryan looked dumbfounded. He'd gotten on his knees and dug into the dirt. "It had to have been a sink hole. Maybe it caved in on him."

"Jamon... Jamon!" David shouted. He'd abandoned his pack and took off into a grove of trees.

Panic had been replaced by exhaustion. We gave up our search and gathered at the site where Ryan first saw the *pit*.

"Maybe you were further than you thought?" Charles said.

"Yeah, let's hike up a ways and see what we can find." David turned and started walking back up the trail.

I donned my gear and followed. Movement adjacent to us in the bushes, a shadow on the ground, caught my eye. Chalking it up to tricks of the light, I trudged on with the rest of the group.

***

THE CLOSET QUAKES VIOLENTLY and I'm ripped from my reminiscent daydream. Or had I fallen asleep and dreamed the whole thing? I don't think so. I brace my arms against the cold walls in a vain effort to stop the tremors. A large crash makes me jump. It's just a matter of time before it tears its way through the cabin and finds me.

Silence again.

Scooting toward the closet door, I reach up. Do I dare open it? What if "*It*" is waiting for me and I'm swallowed whole, like the rest of them? Then what? I make a hasty retreat for the back of the closet and resume my fetal position. Wracking my mind, trying to make some sense of the situation, I continue backtracking through the events of the day.

***

"WE'VE BEEN WALKING FOR forty-five minutes. I think

we need to head back and get local law enforcement," David said.

"I'll second that motion," Charles said.

"Alright, but I have to take a leak first." Ryan dropped his pack and climbed over some rocks to get behind a nearby tree. "Guys, come quick!" he yelled.

The Sandalwood and outcropping of large boulders skewed my view. Then we heard a gut wrenching scream.

Charles, David and I ran as fast as we could to the tree. We couldn't believe our eyes. A large cavernous, rocky crevice sat deep in the earth behind the tree. Like Ryan said, it looked about the length and width of his VW bus. A blood curdling scream echoed from the depths of the pit.

"Ryan!" David hollered down the hole.

"Help me!" Ryan's scream was followed by a loud chomping sound, like a tractor had opened and closed its metal teeth. The snap echoed. Ryan shrieked. Then a grinding sound, as if someone were eating chips into a microphone, filled the darkness.

"Ryan!" Charles and I yelled at the same time.

"Jamon," David added weakly. "I'm going down there." He turned and started to climb down the side of the chasm.

"Are you out of your frickin' mind?" I grabbed him by the shoulder and pulled. "Didn't you hear what just happened down there?"

"It's just the sounds playing tricks on us. He probably landed on a ledge and slipped. We were just hearing the sound of him falling further down the hole. I'm going." David brushed my hand off of his shoulder and continued his descent.

"Don't do it," Charles pleaded. "Something's not right."

"I have to." The pain in David's eyes let us both

know we couldn't stop him.

I reached into my pack and pulled out my lighter and an extra t-shirt. On the other side of the trail I saw a fallen tree. The limbs were dry. I snapped one from the trunk and wrapped the shirt around it. "I'm going to drop this down there and see if we can find the bottom, or your ledge." I lit the shirt with my lighter.

David had already climbed down a good fifteen feet. "Just don't hit me," he said, looking up at me.

I moved to the far end of the pit and dropped my torch. The flame roared as it plummeted into darkness. It came to a halt and I could barely see the flickering light. "Can you see where it landed?" I yelled. He'd stalled his descent as he watched the torch fall.

"Not yet," he called to us while continuing down the rock face.

"This is crazy," Charles whispered.

"I know." I concurred. "What I don't understand is… is where the hell did it come from? And how could Jamon have fallen in when it was way up here, behind a tree?"

"Doesn't make any sense," Charles answered.

I dumped the contents of my pack on the ground and started making a rope with my jeans and t-shirts. Charles followed suit and added the contents of David and Ryan's packs. When we finished, we had a fifteen-foot homemade rope.

"Lot of good this will do," Charles said.

I concentrated on finding David in the darkness. While we had worked on the rope, he'd climbed down further into the pit, out of our sight.

"Dave!" I yelled.

"Yeah!"

"Just checking to see if you're still with us. Can you see anything yet?"

"Yeah, your torch is starting to burn out."

The glow from the torch had dulled.

"Let's make another one." Charles untied one of the shirts from the end of our rope. He located a suitable branch, lit the torch and let it fall close to mine.

For a faint second I saw David clinging to the side of the pit, searching for the next foot and hand holds. Charles' torch landed several feet away from mine. It had to be the bottom, because the flame seemed closer to the center.

"I see it," David yelled. "The bottom's right here."

One of my anxiety attacks hit. It hit hard, taking me over as if I'd been crushed by a sneaker wave. My breaths came faster and harder. I gulped, sucking for air that I couldn't find. My chest felt like someone had kicked it. Faculties and focus were lost. The world went dark.

Charles ran to my side and sat me down next to a tree. He retrieved one of the water bottles from his pack and sprayed me in the face.

"Snap out of it," he said, handing me the bottle. "We really don't have time for your shit right now."

He never did understand my chemical imbalance. I started regulating my breathing and took a drink.

"I'm... okay. Check on Dave."

He turned and went back to the crevice. "You see anything, Dave?"

I heard a murmuring echo, but couldn't make out what David had hollered up to Charles.

"What did he say?" I managed to ask.

"He said he thinks he found Jamon's backpack, but didn't see anyone."

I crawled back to the edge of the precipice. The torch moved back and forth in the depths.

"I think I see something else!" The torch slowly moved to the other side of the pit and then flickered out.

"Dave!" Charles screamed.

The torch reappeared.

"There's a cave. It smells disgusting. I'm not sure how far back it goes, but there's some sort of water source. The walls are covered in slime. I'm going further in to see what I can find."

"Be careful," Charles said.

The torch disappeared. I focused on the darkness, willing myself to see where my brother had gone. We heard a terrible screeching echo that chilled me to the core.

"Dave!" Charles yelled again, panic riddled his voice.

The torch came into sight. It moved fast, bobbing up and down as it headed for the other end of the pit.

"Heeeelp!" David screamed. The torch stopped and seemed to drop. Then the chomping sound came again. He let out another blood curdling, banshee like wail and gasped. The torch moved rapidly back toward the cave entrance. We heard two more chomping sounds and the torch disappeared.

"David!" Charles cried.

I couldn't find my voice. The ground trembled around us.

"Earthquake!" Charles leapt up.

"I don't think so." I pointed at the pit.

"Is that damn thing alive?" Charles asked, terror stricken.

It inched toward us. A faint grinding sound echoed from within. The pungent smell wafting through the air reminded me of a dead cat I once found in our woodshed.

"Run!" I didn't even think about grabbing my pack, but for some reason I'd gathered the man-made rope into my arms. We ran down the trail toward the car. I caught the shadow of something moving parallel to us.

Charles rounded a bend some thirty yards ahead of me and went over a small embankment, out of site. His scream sent chills up my spine. I stopped, waiting for the awful crunching and grinding to start.

Charles came barreling over the hill straight at me as fast as his forty-year-old legs could carry him. "Run! It's right behind me!"

I saw the knoll behind him disappear in blackness as the pit came through in its pursuit. Still with a sizable lead, I ran back toward the area where the other three had disappeared, passed the recognizable tree, and down through a grove of brush. Charles' feet pattered the dirt trail behind me, his pants for breath almost as loud as his footsteps. Then I heard a faint grunt, looked back and he was gone. The pit looked like a mirage rippling across the path as it closed the gap between us with every step I took.

I rounded a bend blocked by several large rocks on either side. The pit veered off the path. I assumed it had to go around the rocks, but it seemed to devour trees and shrubs for a second and then they would reappear behind it as if they had never left. In front of me I saw the oasis from the brochure. I figured if it couldn't go through rocks, maybe water had the same effect. I wrapped the man-made rope around my waist and dove head first into the large pond.

The cold water soothed my burning skin. I burst to the surface, treading water as I scanned every direction, searching for my assailant. The water in front of me started to churn like a toilet bowl flushing. It hadn't deterred the pit. I swam as fast as I could for shore on the other side.

A dirt trail came into view and became my new destination. The land started creeping further away as the pit slowly moved through the shallows, slurping water, dragging me backwards.

The shore stood just out of reach. My strength had almost completely given out. I needed balance. I thrust my legs down and my feet found deep mud. I stood. The evil undertow pulled at my ankles. I trudged through the slime and mud, but every second the pit got closer.

A rather large stump jutted up from the shore. The idea came fast. I untied the soaking wet clothing rope from around my waist. Using it like a jump rope, I flung it around the stump. My right ankle slipped into the mouth of the pit. When I yanked on the rope, I felt flesh being torn from my shin. My plan worked and I broke free of its evil will.

Warm dirt clung to my wet skin as I crawled onto the dry land. The water behind me gurgled and splashed inside the mouth of the pit as it ascended. I abandoned my rope and limped up the path.

That's when I saw the cabin. I bashed the door in with my shoulder and found my hiding spot in this closet.

***

THE GROUND TREMORS AGAIN and I brace myself. The next one will probably destroy the door. While I await my grinding death and pray to my God for forgiveness of my sins, the walls of the closet cave in, crashing around me in wooden splinters. I clench my eyes tight, anticipating the plummet into unending darkness. But I don't fall. I hear an unfamiliar voice.

"Oy! I found 'em."

I open my eyes slowly. Blinding light from high above skews my vision. There's a man dangling in the shadow of the light by a rope. Jolts of pain shoot through my head and throughout all my body, most of it coming from my ankle. I don't understand.

"Mate, you're bloody lucky to be alive, eh," the man says.

He has a safety helmet on with one of those lights on his head, something you'd wear spelunking. I realize

I'm lying on a piece of wood. I look up and see the pit's walls; they've been shored up with timber. Half of one of the sides looks like it caved in. I look down and my ankle is crushed under a large boulder.

"Don't move, yeah. We'll have you out in a jiff," the man says. "Oy!" he yells up.

Another man is repelling my direction.

"Pass down the basket," the second guy hollers to the crew waiting above.

"You could've died easy from that fall, mate," the first man says.

I still don't understand.

Then I'm falling. It's pitch black and I can't see. My head smashes against the side of the pit as I plummet. I reach out, clawing my fingers into the rocks. My wedding ring gets caught and the skin is torn from my finger, completely de-gloving it. Blood and parts of the bone are the only thing left. Reaching forward, I try to brace myself from the impact coming. When I hit, my arms snap like toothpicks; the right one at the wrist, the left one up by my shoulder. My head bounces off a moss covered boulder. My skull is crushed. I have no idea how I'm still alive. Wood from parts of the cabin kept my legs from breaking, but I can't move. I think I broke my neck.

A large spotlight looms over me. Someone is lying next to me. The rope wrapped around his waist had snapped. He's not breathing. His safety helmet is crushed. I try to say something, but I vomit blood. Lucky I landed with my head turned or I would have drowned in my own puke. I hear the chomping sound again. The man's body starts to move away from me and disappears into a hole in the side of the pit. The crunch sends chills through my mind. I'd probably have gooseflesh if I could feel anything. The cave opening in the side of the pit had closed when it took the rescuer. The grinding sound echoes through the cavern as it opens again, ready to partake of another meal. There's no stopping it now. It's over. My eyes won't close.

The light high above flickers out as I'm dragged by something toward the pits grotesque mouth. I see stalactites and stalagmites in rows, dripping with bloody entrails of its past victims. I hear, "chomp, crunch," and glance down. Its teeth are deep inside my legs. The mouth opens and chunks of my own flesh and bone slide off the rocky incisors leaving two mangled, bloody stumps.

It draws me in up to my chest. I still can't feel anything. I'm turned and get one last glance at the claw of a crane dangling back and forth high overhead. A huddled group of four familiar men are standing on the ledge, anxiously awaiting my rescue from the depths of the pit.

It closes on me.

The world goes dark.

I'm gone forever.

"Think he'll ever snap out of it, Doctor?" I hear.

Thadd Presley Presents

SHADOW MAN
Charlotte Emma Gledson

FLUSTERED, EMMA STUFFED HER four year old son's arm into the sleeve of his thick padded coat. Threads of pain wormed around within her head, along with a creeping sense of malaise.

"Off we go now, darlin'. Here's your beaker. And remember, Shelly Danvers is picking you up because you are having lunch with Liam today." She handed her son his drink, who in return nodded sullenly. "Come on now, you will have fun sweetie!"

"But you won't be there mum…" Alfie whimpered, a tear falling from his eye.

Emma was determined for her son not to dwell on his anxieties, so changed the subject swiftly. "… And when I am in town I will buy you a pressie and we can have spaghetti for tea! How about that?"

"What you gonna get me? A toy gun?" A glimmer of joy crossed his young searching face.

"Maybe, sweetie, we'll see." Emma winked at Alfie, then surveyed the gloomy winter skies from the kitchen window. In spite of her weary state, she was reveling in the notion that she would be able to spend a few hours alone. Shopping, a visit to the library and a cup of tea or two were on her agenda for the first time in months. She loved Alfie dearly, but as a single mother, times were hard. Alfie was a needy child, constantly draining Emma with his continuing demands; but she knew it was all part and parcel of being a mother. Without him however, Emma would have no one, so she rarely complained. *She wouldn't have it any other way.* Her only living relation was her self-sufficient mother, who lived up in the crags of the Scottish Highlands. After her father dying suddenly when she was fifteen, she took care of her mother until she moved down to Portsmouth University where she studied English, fell in love, and had a baby. But the 'ideal' was short lived; her partner left her in the lurch. Now living as a single parent, she coped with the strains of everyday life by doting on her young son, finding solace by walking the Solent cliffs and writing for a local community magazine.

Emma bundled Alfie into the buggy and strapped him securely. Walking hastily to the Nursery, she chatted reassuringly to her son who had become disgruntled due to a restless night. He had kept her awake with worries about how he was scared that he wouldn't see her again. "Mum, you'll never leave me will you…" he had sobbed in the early hours of the morning. "You will be home when I come back from play school won't you?"

"Honey, I am not going anywhere. Now that *is* a promise!" Emma had calmed him with loving caresses and consoling words, leaving herself exhausted. Alfie had finally fallen asleep, but she had lain awake tending to a blinding headache that lasted throughout the rest of the night. Emma put his insecurities down to the new start of his Nursery Education. This was only his fourth day. The first day was a nightmare; the staff noted his nervous behavior, but comforted Emma that some children do have anxieties about leaving their mums at this age. The two of them were exceptionally close, sharing every day, every hour together. Having no family around her, and only a few select friends, Alfie and Emma faced the world together, in their own precious and untainted universe.

Arriving at the Nursery, a flurry of mums dropping off their kids reassured her that Alfie was in good hands, and he would feed upon the excitement from the other children. Once in the classroom, she kissed Alfie lightly on the lips and ruffled his snowy blonde hair. "Love you little man," she whispered into his ear, then watched her son run straight to the sandpit area.

"Love you Mummy…" Alfie replied over his shoulder giving her a shy smile as he dug a digger deep into the sand.

Feeling reassured, but still with that maternal tug in her heart, she made her way down the looming corridor towards the exit. Feeling brighter after seeing Alfie more at ease, Emma felt optimistic, in spite of the monotonous ache that remained embedded within her head. *No tears this time. My brave little soldier.*

As she neared the door, she noticed a tall man walking with a slight gait coming towards her. Feeling unsettled, she looked down for a few seconds, then looked up again. She had not recognized him before at the start of the week, but that was not the cause of her unease. A shadow passed her eyes briefly obscuring her vision, but once she re-focused; she was alarmed at the way the intimidating man held her stare. A speck of sunlight from the hallway's dusty window caught the nasty scar that ran down the left side of his eye. She noticed as he came closer, a long black fingernail on his little finger, starkly clashing with the stained grey duffel coat that hung from his gangly frame. He passed glaring sinisterly at her and for a second Emma felt as if she was about to fall with a sudden dizziness so strong she felt immediately sick. A child scuttled behind him, studying Emma with bitter ashen eyes. Composing herself, the strange feeling soon evaporated, once she saw her friend hovering outside the entrance.

"Hiya, hon! You look a bit peaky. You OK?"

"Yes, fine thanks Shelly. Just had a rough night, that's all." Emma forced a meek smile, trying to look relaxed.

"Ah, bless you, I'm sorry. So, I will drop Alfie off at yours about two then, that OK with you?" Shelly asked with a hint of stress coloring her tone.

Emma noticed her harassed mood. "Yes, that's fine, but *only* if you are sure it's no trouble," she insisted.

"Not at all Emma. My boy loves having new friends over for lunch, and they are going to watch Fireman Sam, so I can put my feet up for a second or two!"

"Thanks so much, Shel," Emma responded. "I know Alfie will be a bit shy, but the more he mixes in with new people, the less clingy he will be."

"Absolutely, so no worries hon, you can have the time that you deserve. Mine will be next week. Have my sister and her little one coming down so Liam will have a playmate for a week, and that will take some of the load off me!" Shelly laughed rather too loudly, and gave Emma a cheeky smile before she chased her young son down the long hallway. "See you at two," she called back over her shoulder. Her voice diminishing as she and her youngster disappeared down the corridor.

After a brisk walk to the bus stop, Emma stood calmly waiting for the number 84. It came into view as she looked down at her watch.

Searching for her purse she was excited about the pending time alone. The threatening rain eventfully started to patter on the back of her Macintosh, bouncing off the material like small plastic BB gun pellets. Finally after a final fumble, she found her money and boarded the bus. The smell of ash and fumes filled her nostrils causing her to gag. Handing the correct fare over to the uniformed driver, an icy awareness swept over her, along with a déjà vu sensation, rippling within her head. The driver examined her with an air of knowing, looking at her with a sneer, yet a twinkle in his eye, leaving Emma feeling unsteady once more. She felt a clench of disorientation when she noticed the serrated scar down his eye, and the black fingernail gripping the steering wheel of the double decker bus. Darting her eyes to the ground, she hurriedly walked through to the middle of the bus. Sitting down, Emma attempted to scrutinize the driver behind the bobbing heads in front of her. Though the bus was busy, she did manage to see his face in the rear view mirror. He returned her gaze with an analytical eye. Feeling nervy, she trembled as she fiddled with her bus ticket. His stare was intent. With her pulse quickening, her face flushing with prickly heat, beads of icy moisture started to bubble across her hairline. A relentless headache hammered hard within her skull like a constant drumming from a slave's galley.

It can't be HIM. He was walking in, as I was walking out!

With these thoughts, Emma looked down at the cigarette stubs littering the floor, kicking a few out of her way with the tip of her boot. She tried desperately to ignore the pain in her head. Turning her head to the window she noticed her stop was next. *Thank God.* The rain continued to splatter blotches of water onto the window, reminding her of bullet holes that had blasted through glass. Walking towards the exit doors, she watched them swish and hiss nosily as they opened. Stepping down onto the pavement she gave a quick glance over her shoulder at the driver, who was now staring ahead looking through the windscreen, his finger nail tapping against the steering wheel rhythmically. *Thank God he's not watching me.* The bus, with its sooty diesel fumes and droning engine, drove off into the distance, leaving Emma standing in the pouring rain, baffled and stressed.

Trying hard to fathom how a man could be in two

places at once, disturbed Emma. *There couldn't possibly be two men with a scar and a hideous nail like that around here!* There was no way he could have been driving a bus when only ten minutes earlier he was walking into the Nursery with a child at his heel. What troubled her more was the way he was watching her through the mirror, with a mean cunning grin.

Rain continued to batter against her coat as the library finally came into view. Entering the heavy doors she relished the blast of warm air engulfing her face. Wet strands of auburn hair were plastered against her glowing cheeks like long sucking leeches. Using her pale index finger she placed the limp hair behind her ears. *Warm and dry, thank God.* In her youth the library was her comfort zone, her haven. She loved to submerge herself in biographies and history books, feeding upon all the things that interested her. Fingering the books in a carefree manner, she searched for the biography of Grace Kelly. She had always admired this fairytale film star, who had a fairytale lifestyle, and also the inevitable tragic 'not so fairytale' ending. Emma finally found the book she was searching for. As she was about to pull the book away from its shelf, she heard a noise coming from behind the bookcase. *A muffled whispering.* The library was relatively quiet at this time of day, hence her desire to be there first thing in the morning. The whispering continued in sibilant waves, invading her ears disturbingly. Emma made her way towards the area of sound, but was only faced with a hovering shadow that suddenly fleeted past her. Perplexed, she looked around. *Nothing.* The whispering then stopped. All the aisles were empty. A stark yet distance snigger caused her to jump, the pain in her head abruptly intensifying. "Just kids..." she reassured herself and swallowed hard, eradicating her growing apprehension and panic. She retrieved the book she wanted, pulled it out and walked purposely to the withdrawal desk for it to be scanned.

Approaching the counter, Emma stopped in her tracks. The man with the ugly scar and black fingernail was waiting to receive her, and her book. Wearing a cream Arran jumper, he smiled maliciously and stooped forward, with a fixed hard stare. His gaze never wavered from hers. Black greasy hair with a bluish tinge, flat and smooth against his scalp, reminded Emma of a bowling ball. His skin was pallid, colorless, verging on translucent. The peculiar man fondled his black nail, stroking the vile talon tenderly, and then put it to his lips and licked the inky cuticle, wrapping his red thin tongue around the sharp hideous tip.

Emma's heart hammered, the recurring feeling of foreboding tumbled inside her once more. Panic clutched at her chest, spasms of white eclectic heat immersed within her head. Almost keeling over, she dropped the book, ran outside into the cold rain that mercifully saturated her flushed face. Once outside, her heart finally steadied and she knew this kind of stress was making her ill.

Emma had to face the fact that certain types of anxiety could be dangerous and because she had dangerously high blood pressure, she felt extremely vulnerable. But she religiously took her pills and the doctors had reassured her that she was fighting fit, providing she underwent the six month check-ups and tried to avoid high levels of stress. However, the prospect of a stroke hovered over her like a colossal vulture, ready to consume the entirety of her life, as it did her father.

God, how she missed him.

His death was a constant tragic reminder how precarious life was, and how she must value each second she shared with Alfie.

In order to calm her nerves, she turned to the nearest café, sat down and ordered a strong cup of tea. She sat pensively at her table, breathing deeply to steady her nerves. Had she known any one that wanted to frighten her? Did someone hold a grudge against her?

Emma recalled the day, months ago; when she had a mild altercation with a neighbor in her street over the fact that she hadn't brought her bins off from the street on the day of collection. Her thin weedy husband had leered and grinned at her from behind a grimy net curtain. It was petty and trivial, but the man skulking behind the nets had spooked her. *Could it be him?*

Her mind wandered to her ex-boyfriend Andy, Alfie's father. He was madly possessive over her at first, but as soon as she fell pregnant he had the temerity to deny that the baby was even his and his obsession miraculously disappeared, as did he. Maybe he wanted to creep her out because he wanted her back? *But it didn't explain how the man appeared out from nowhere after having seen him only moments earlier somewhere else.*

With a painful head full of rattling queries, Emma reached for her bag and pulled out some tablets for the headache. She popped out two painkillers from their plastic seal and swigged them down with the cooling tea.

"Everything alright? You look worried." The tall blonde waiter hovered over Emma, interrupting her troubled thoughts. He had an angelic face, captivating.

"Yes, fine, just a little shaky. Awful headache, but I'll be alright, thanks."

"Can I get you anything else?" His smile was wide, sensual. Emma felt the stirrings of desire trickle within her.

"No, it's OK, I'm fine, honestly. Nothing a strong brandy couldn't fix. But hey, it's still early so I'll just have to finish my tea and painkillers instead." Emma was feeble at small talk, especially if it was to a handsome young man, but she gave it her best shot under the circumstances.

The waiter smiled. "I hope to see you here again sometime, and maybe I could buy you a drink?" He took her cup away and she blushed shyly then nodded eagerly in agreement. Emma felt giddy by the waiter's attention, her mood lightening as she studied the slender physique of the gorgeous man. Giving her a wink, he then smiled and disappeared amongst the mass of occupied tables that cluttered the bustling café. Her thoughts of the sinister man were now only on the cusp of her mind, not consuming as it was before. *Oh to have someone look at me that way...* Emma stood up to leave the café, scanning the busy room as she did so. The tall calming stranger watched her from afar, smiling genuinely. He raised his arm to wave, and then he was gone.

The bus journey home was uneventful. The rain had eased, and a sliver of light was trying its best to cut through the membrane of the darkened clouds. The driver was a woman this time; she had a merry face with a reddish complexion that reminded Emma of a stereotypical farmer's wife. With her headache finally subsiding, she pondered on the chores that would greet her once she arrived home. Resting against the smeary window, she nursed a small plastic gun in her lap. Thinking of the waiter once more, she smiled to herself contentedly. The fear that beheld her earlier that morning was now a distant memory.

Ramming the key into the lock, Emma walked into her narrow hallway. Thin ribbons of sunlight from the front door could not penetrate the dinginess. Once inside the kitchen, she took off her coat, placed her handbag and the toy gun onto the table. Checking the kettle was full, Emma slammed the switch down hard.

Sitting at the small oval breakfast table she waited for the kettle to boil by flicking through the pages of a magazine, kicking off her boots in the process. A sharp knock at the door interrupted her. Feeling annoyed Emma rooted herself into her seat in protest. "Go away, I want this time alone," she uttered under her breath irritably.

After a long pause and thinking that the person had gone, she let out a relieved sigh. A second knock more urgent and louder, boomed into the hallway. Grumpily Emma heaved herself up from the table, only due to the slim possibility that her friend Shelly was arriving early with Alfie. She knew it wasn't the postman; he had already delivered her mail earlier during the morning. Yet another insistent knock pummeled the door. Reluctantly she went through to the front room and peered out from her curtain to see who the unrelenting knocker was. From her concealed view, she made out a figure in a blue uniform, holding a clip board. Tufts of black wiry hair hung loosely around the collar, but she couldn't see the face. Looking to her left up towards the path, she saw a gas board van outside her house.

Oh No, not the bloody Gas Man. Smoothing the curtain back into place, she walked into the hallway. Begrudgingly, Emma reached out to open the front door, but as she did so, the knocking returned with a vengeance. The booming thud was so pressing; she flattened her palms against her ears. The banging continued unremittingly, her heartbeat accelerating with every thump. She stepped back, terrified. A strong sense of vagueness swamped her brain, dizzy flourishes washed over her exhausted body. Emma connected her fingertips with the wall for balance. A sudden gush of pain peaked behind her eyes, seeping into the rest of her skull. Nausea swelled inside her, rising and falling like a surging angry sea. Taking a few deep breaths, Emma leaned her back against the wall to try and compose herself. The banging unexpectedly stopped, leaving a dull buzzing ringing within her ears. Only then did she tentatively open the door.

Narrowing her eyes in pain and panic, she let the tall man in, leaving the door ajar. Ushering him inside impatiently, Emma pointed to the staircase clutching her head with both hands. "Go, there, under the stairs, you will find the meter in the cupboard." Incensed with the pain she eventually turned to look at the man, who in return inquired, "Miss Williams is it? 27 Grove Avenue?" Emma in her debilitating pain nodded intolerantly. Only then did she notice the black fingernail jutting out like a poisonous viper's tongue from the spindly little finger that clutched the clip board. In spite of the grueling pain in her head, she locked eyes with the man as he stood opposite her, smirking. Shock entrenched her to the spot. His eyes began to bugle with enthusiasm as he finally spoke to her in a sickly slithery voice. "So, you have let me in. That's good. Now, you may well be aware why I am here?"

Emma's insides sloshed around like a spin dryer as she stood stunned, racked in excruciating pain. He came closer. The stranger's arms seemed unnaturally long, unfolding from under his sleeves. He stretched them towards Emma, pointing at her with his long black fingernail. Forcefully he pushed her body against the wall, causing the mirror that hung above her to smash to the ground. Shards of glass scattered to the floor like falling icy stalactites. Emma felt the sharp splinters cut into her feet, feeling tiny particles of glass slice between her toes. The man clutched Emma's head at both sides squeezing the already inflamed cranium with extreme vigour. Unable to scream, Emma could only focus on the stranger's eyes that blared with lunacy as he penetrated and invaded her vision with his manic eyes and sallow leathery skin. Blood veined and yellowing, his eyes pierced her soul with a look of such malice, Emma threw up, spilling the contents of her stomach onto the lapels of his uniform, splattering his mouth with chunks of vomit. He licked his lips in pleasure.

"Don't mind me Emma, this happens a lot," he sneered and then carefully slid his blackened fingernail into Emma's nostril penetrating deep down into the septum, severing the Spheroid sinus behind her eye. The soft tissue popped deep within her head. Blood oozed from the nostrils and spread into her hair, her left eye drooping within the socket. The pain was so huge, Emma's legs and body shook. She convulsed in pain, throwing her into a chasm of blinding bright heat, her head and body burning from the inside out. Managing a meager whimper, Emma mustered only a few words, *"Who are you? Why?"*

"Why, you know me, Emma. Have you not noticed me? Your time is up! It comes to us all eventually, my sweet!" He hissed, licking his nail clean, like a cat cleaning its paw. The nail was stained, tangled with fibrous matter. Emma's head hung weakly as he continued to hold her up against the wall with his right arm, his strength unwavering as her body shuddered and drooped loosely.

Panting and in complete agony, from the corner of her right eye Emma saw the front door push fully open. Standing in the doorway was Shelly and Alfie. Her son screamed. Shelly's face whitened. Reaching into the crevices of her dwindling conscious mind, she found the strength to utter a few final words as the stranger let go, her body slumping to the ground like a rag doll.

"Help me Shelly, Get this man off me… don't let Alfie see this…"

Shelly steered Alfie aside and directed him to stand in the front room. He didn't listen, but stood in the doorway gaping in horror. She knelt down and cradled Emma's head within her arms. "Sweetheart, I will call an ambulance, hang in there, you will be fine."

"Keep that man… away… from Alfie!" Emma spluttered, blood curdling in her throat.

"Honey, there is no man. There is no-one here. You are having a seizure of some kind. You are going to be just fine, just hold still." Shelly delved into her coat pocket for her mobile phone and called the emergency services, Alfie stood at his mother's feet, weeping weakly, wringing his hands.

"Mum...?"

Looking on, the evil caller inspected the scene, folding his arms. Only Emma was aware of his presence. "Your friend can't see me, my sweet. You see, I am your *FEAR*. This is what I look like. I am the one that comes for you before you die. Your grim reaper. I am the shadow that you see, the perpetual warning that life comes to an end. Go on, you have one last look at your son and say goodbye."

Emma turned her head shakily, her neck twisting rigidly in the desperate endeavor to see her last vision of her son. Alfie stood alone harboring such a pained expression of sadness, it left Emma reeling in helplessness and utter despair. The physical pain she experienced was nothing compared to the tortuous pain of losing her son, along with the notion that he will be alone in this world, without her. *"Mum, you'll never leave me will you..."*

Emma could only manage a pathetic moan in the vain attempt for Alfie to know she would be OK and not to worry. "Al... fieee..."

"Shhh, it's going to be fine, shhh..." Shelly soothed as she continued to support Emma's head nervously, waiting for the ambulance.

The Shadow Man knelt down to Emma's heaving body, and with one final deed, plunged his dark claw deep into Emma's ear canal. In spite of the unspeakable pain, she could hear the grinding and scraping of the long spiky nail burrowing into her ear drum. It probed deep into her middle ear cavity and pierced right through to the cochlea, resulting in her final pain, her final breath and the final unbearable truth that she was about to die and leave Alfie without a mother.

Who will look after Alfie now? With this final thought

Emma then observed, for the last time, the image of her weeping son, fizzling out rapidly like a burning photograph.

Thadd Presley Presents

Lady Killers
Todd Martin

DANIEL WOKE UP LONG before the sun came up on Christmas morning. After several failed attempts to make Olivia get out of bed he gave up and headed downstairs alone, leaving her on the bed snoring blissfully. He loved Christmas and just couldn't understand why anyone would want to sleep in since there was so much excitement in the air.

He went into the kitchen and put on a pot of coffee, fighting the urge to try at least one more time to wake Olivia up. He noticed a box of glazed doughnuts on the counter and briefly considered snagging one before he realized that he was too excited to eat anything. So he ended up leaving them behind and making his way into the living room.

The living room was basically a shrine to Christmas. A huge tree loaded with ornaments sat in the corner with roughly a ton of wrapped gifts under it. There were decorations all over the walls and mistletoe hanging over the door. It was hard to walk across the room without bumping into a Santa Claus or snowman figurine. Olivia had complained that it was too much (her exact words had been "It looks like the holiday section of Target threw up in here,") but Daniel didn't agree in the least. If anything he thought that they didn't have enough decorations and wished he'd bought a few more.

The outside of their house was equally decorative. There were several blow up Santas, snowmen, and penguins stationed in the front yard as well as an assortment of reindeer and elves. There were enough Christmas lights on the house that it could probably be seen from outer space. Olivia said that she hoped an airplane didn't land in their yard because there were so many lights the pilot could confused it for an airport. Daniel didn't care what she said though; he loved Christmas and wanted everyone to know it. If he had it his way there would be a lot more lights on the house.

He glanced over at the clock on the wall and saw that it was just a little after 7:00 A.M. He found some holiday music on the radio and then started building a fire in the fireplace as he listened to "I Saw Mommy Kissing Santa Claus," humming along with it as he lit some newspaper. Once he got the fire going he went back into the kitchen and poured himself a cup of coffee before returning to the living room where he sat down in his recliner and enjoyed the Christmas music.

Olivia came stumbling into the room about fifteen minutes later wearing her robe, looking like she was still mostly asleep. She scowled at him before mumbling something about the music being too loud and continuing into the kitchen to get a cup of coffee (she was always unbearable in the morning until she had her first cup.)

Daniel got up and warmed his hands by the fire for a moment before he walked over to the tree and stood there looking at all the gifts. He started counting them and saw that at least seven of them belonged to him. He got down on his hands and knees and picked some of them up, shaking them in turn, no longer able to resist the urge to know what might be inside. Olivia came back into the room with her cup of coffee and shook her head when she saw what he was doing.

"Jesus, you're worse than a little kid," she said before taking a sip from her cup with a grimace. She always complained that the coffee that Daniel made tasted like mud.

"Hey, Christmas is my favorite holiday, what can I say?"

"No shit. I would've never guessed."

"Can we open the presents," he asked, ignoring her smart ass comment.

"Not right now, you know we have to wait for Teresa and the girls to get here."

"What time are they coming?"

"When I talked to her last she said that they'd be here around noon or so."

He frowned and set his attention back to the fire so she wouldn't see the exasperated expression on his face. He loved Olivia's sister Teresa, but he hated that fact that she was never, ever on time. No matter what she was always guaranteed to be late and as he pushed around on the logs in the fire place with the poker he figured that since she claimed that they would be there at noon or so they wouldn't actually show up until somewhere around the neighborhood of 2:00 or even 3:00.

He glanced back over at all the gifts under the tree again and he realized that there was no way on God's green earth that he could wait that long to open them.

"Come on, let's at least open some of them," he whined.

"No Daniel. What did I just say?"

"Can we just open one a piece then?"

"Daniel!"

"Please?"

"No! We have to wait for Teresa and the girls," she snapped. "It would be rude to open one without them!"

"Oh come on, it's just one! How are they going to know that we just opened one of them?!

She took a long drink of her coffee and sat there for a moment, silently debating with herself if she should let him open a gift or not. He knew her well enough to know that she would most likely give in and let him have one just so he would shut up and leave her alone.

"OK, fine, open one," she exclaimed, throwing her arms up in defeat. "I swear to God, it's like I'm married to a ten-year-old sometimes."

Daniel put the poker down and made his way over to the tree with the same enthusiasm as a cat approaching an unsuspecting bird. He looked over all the gifts that he knew were his and tried to decide which one to grab. There was a huge one toward the back pressed up against the wall that he assumed was the big screen TV that he wanted, (Lord knew he'd dropped enough hints about it around Olivia,) so he made his way toward it when she stopped him.

"Not so fast, kiddo, I forgot to tell you about the stipulation." She said this with a smile that he didn't much care for because it was the one that she only used when she was about to screw him out of doing something he wanted.

"What stipulation?" He dreaded her response.

"I get to pick the one that you open."

"Then pick this one," he replied, pointing at the large one that he'd already set his mind on opening.

"I don't think so; I think that's the one we should save for the grand finale. Let's find another one for you."

He started to argue with her about it but changed his mind. He knew if he pushed it he would end up getting pissed off and then she wouldn't let him open anything. He kept his mouth shut and just nodded instead, as he watched her rummage around through the gifts. He suspected that she would pick up the smallest one that even a blind person could see was a bottle of cologne.

"Here you go, knock yourself out," she said as she handed it to him.

"Hold on and I'll get one for you too," he replied, planning on giving her either something that she'd picked out herself or the red blouse that he wasn't too sure that she was going to like. It was a present he'd grabbed at the store at the last minute.

"That's okay, I don't want to open one now."

"Why not?"

"Because unlike you I can wait and open them together like we're supposed to do."

"Whatever," he mumbled, not really caring if she opened one or not.

He ripped the wrapping paper off of his gift and as he suspected it was a bottle of cologne. It was in a black box with "Lady Killer" written across the front in bold, blood red letters. He'd never even heard of it, but that didn't surprise him since he really wasn't a fan of cologne. The only kind that he ever wore was Old Spice but for some reason Olivia always gave him a different bottle of cologne every year for Christmas. He supposed that one day he would have to just break down and tell her to stop buying them for him. He thought that the fact that he had six bottles in the bathroom that had only been used once or twice each would have been a pretty good clue, but so far she hadn't managed to catch on.

"Try it, it's supposed to smell really good," she said. "The woman at the store said that people had been buying the hell out of it and they were having a hard time keeping it in stock."

"Really," he asked, trying to feign an interest even though he really didn't give a shit about what she was saying. He opened the box and took out the bottle. As he sprayed some on himself, he immediately decided that he didn't like it. It had a weird musty smell that made his nostrils burn and his eyes water. It wasn't like anything he'd ever smelled before in his life and it made him actually feel a bit queasy.

"So, do you like it?" She ask this, obviously not aware of the fact that he was fighting the urge to vomit. But, before he could lie and tell her that he loved it as he always did every year he felt a rage overcome him and all he wanted to do was to rip her to pieces. He'd never felt so filled with raged before and it was then and there that he realized that he despised Olivia.

He reached over and grabbed the poker from the fireplace then hit her across the face with it. She cried out in pain and fell to her knees holding her face. When he saw the blood pouring out of the huge gash on her forehead it seemed to make him angrier so he hit her with the poker again, this time striking her right in the temple.

She fell back and hit the back of her head on the floor. He saw that her nose was broken and several of her teeth had been knocked out. He leaned down and struck her once again.

She screamed at first but he barely even heard her. All he wanted to do was to kill her so he blocked everything else out and focused on hitting her again and again. It wasn't too long until her once beautiful face was reduced to a bloody pulp that looked like a special effect from a horror film that only Tom Savini could have created.

He didn't stop hitting her until he knew for certain that she was dead. Once he was sure he'd succeeded in beating the life out of her he felt the rage inside him subside and he walked back over to the recliner. He threw the poker across the room, bent down, and picked up the bottle of the cologne again. He sprayed himself with it again and took a moment to enjoy the way it smelled before he took a seat.

He liked the scent of it a little better the second time

around. Something about it just made him feel warm and happy like he didn't have a care in the world. He didn't know why he didn't care for it when he first used it but he was starting to really like it.

He flipped on the television and watched several Rankin Bass Christmas specials as he waited for Teresa and his nieces to arrive. As the hours passed they kept showing commercials for a new perfume from the makers of "Ladykiller" called "Maneater" and he couldn't help but smile when he saw them.

Next door Mrs. Tanner sprayed herself with the very perfume her husband had given her and a few seconds later Daniel heard Mr. Tanner screaming.

Thadd Presley Presents

Alena's Piece
Stacy Bolli

ALENA WRAPPED THE JACKET tightly around her shoulders and kept her head bent against the relentless drizzle. Tears tinged with blood dripped down from Alena's battered face and stained the front of her white vinyl windbreaker. Alena did not care to reach up and wipe away these soiled tears from her eyes; she just kept trudging down the darkened country road with one thing consuming her thoughts: revenge.

Alena kept her zombie like pace until she reached her front doorstep. She slowly opened the door so not to disturb her sleeping Grandmother on the couch. Grammy always slept on the couch during her date nights. She did not like her boyfriend Jason, in fact she hated him. Grammy warned Alena multiple times that she saw hostility hiding in his dark brown eyes. Alena always laughed it off with a kiss to Grammy's cheek.

"Jason is the gentlest creature on this planet; he would never hurt a fly!" Alena would assure Grammy.

Grammy would always grumble in response and take her usual post on the couch.

That night when Alena attempted to slip by Grammy unnoticed, the old lady reached out and grabbed Alena's arm and Alena was forced to look into the old lady's matronly eyes.

Grammy sat up and turned on the lamp beside the couch. "Look at me, LeLe!" Grammy ordered.

Alena slowly turned her damaged face and saw Grammy turn sheet white.

"My LeLe, he did this to you?" Grammy reached up to touch Alena's cheek and Alena flinched.

"He hurt you! I told you this boy was no good; I saw the devil in his eyes!"

"Grammy, he was angry with me. I flirted with another boy and he saw me, it's my fault," Alena tried to explain but her words ended in a pathetic whimper. Alena gathered her thoughts and recanted the horrible evening to her Grammy.

"Jason saw me talking with another boy and he touched my hand. Jason became so angry he stormed from the party. I followed him to his car so we could talk. I wanted to assure Jason I did not instigate this other boy! Jason started the car and we drove to Old Dixie's Crossing so he could cool off. Well, the more we drove the angrier he became and we started shouting at each other. He pulled to the side of the road and slapped me hard across the cheek. I tried to fight back Grammy, but he is so big!" Alena bowed her head and wept.

Grammy pulled Alena next to her and wrapped her arms around the small, trembling teenager. Alena let her head fall against Grammy's warm bosom and her hand fell open to reveal what she was holding. Nestled in the center of her palm was a bloody, gold ring with a small shred of tissue hanging from the clasp.

"LeLe, what is this?" Grammy asked.

"It is Jason's nipple ring. I ripped it from his chest as he pushed me out of the moving car."

"Oh LeLe, this is very good! I am going to show you what to do."

Alena gave her Grammy a puzzled look and dropped the bloody ring into her grandmother's outstretched hand. Grammy recited a few unrecognizable words and blew onto the ring. She then gingerly removed the small piece of flesh from the ring and handed it to Alena.

"Swallow it."

"What? Grammy, I will throw up!"

"Swallow it, LeLe. You must do what I tell you to make the magic work."

Alena got a glass of water and the flesh easily slid down her throat.

"Now go to bed, LeLe. I cannot explain any further, but the magic will reveal itself to you in the next couple days."

The next morning Jason's younger sister had called Alena in hysterics. Jason had been in a car accident last night and died instantly when his car skidded off the road and hit a massive Oak tree.

Alena hung up the phone numb with emotion, not with sorrow but anger. Anger that Grammy's magic did not have time to exact its revenge on Jason.

That weekend was Jason's funeral. Alena and her Grandmother attended the burial out of respect for his family. A large crowd had gathered under the heavy blanket of the Florida summer and said their good byes. Night came quickly after the funeral and Alena fell into a deep sleep as Herbie, her Teddy Bear hamster, ran frantically in his squeaky exercise wheel.

Late in the night Alena woke with a start as a loud crash erupted from the front porch. Alena jumped to her feet and frantically ran to the front room to check on Grammy.

Grammy was already awake and opening the dead bolt on the front door.

"Grammy, who is here?" Alena asked.

Grammy flung open the door and turned to Alena with a wide smile crumpling her triumphant face.

"Your old Grammy still has it in her! I have not used the Magic in so long I was afraid it would not work, but like a true friend it never left."

Alena gasped as the broken and filthy body of Jason lurched through the front door. His head flopped unnaturally onto his right shoulder and his right leg was bent to a distorted angle. Alena could still see his dark eyes roll in their sockets, like loose marbles. The most eerie fact was that his eyes still held complete comprehension and terror.

"Grammy!" Alena screamed and ran behind the couch. "What is this?"

"Shh," Grammy whispered. "Don't be afraid, he is yours now! His soul will forever be trapped within this lifeless and broken body. He will feel the pain of his death until the last vestige of his bone and flesh dissipate from this Earth. Get the ax, LeLe."

Alena and Grammy quartered up Jason's embalmed body and wrapped the wriggling pieces into plastic and tucked them into the freezer chest in the corner of the garage, all but one piece.

"This special and intimate piece is for you to deal with right now, Alena."

Alena barely made it to her room, she could feel the cool chunk twitching in her palm and a couple times she almost threw it to the floor in disgust. When Alena made it to her bedroom she closed the door. Her gaze settled on Herbie's cage. She hurried to the cage as Herbie looked at her with curiosity in his beady black eyes. Alena threw the wrinkled male reproductive organ into the cage and watched it undulate through the wood shavings like an obese earthworm. Herbie squealed at the bald intruder in anger but cautiously approached it. He sniffed his new companion with his quivering little nose and then began to nibble...

Thadd Presley Presents

Adrift
Michael Dortmundt

WE WATCHED HORRIFIED AS our ship gave up the ghost and sank silently into the hungry sea to forever rest upon her forgotten and murky, unknown fathoms below. Ship and crew alike vanished into the cold dark beneath the endless expanse of the still night sea, and we four alone survived in the tiniest of lifeboats without the faintest hint of supplies to keep us alive.

The strange assortment of half castes and sinister looking specimens that made up the crew of the offending ship sailed on without hesitation as our ship disappeared from sight to join the ranks of debris forever lost on the bottom of the ocean. We had at first supposed them to be pirates, as pirates were rumored to frequent this stretch of ocean as of late. But the hostile way in which they opened fire upon our ship without so much as a warning or threat and then continued on their way without even casting a glance in our direction or even the slightest indication of a desire to plunder our sinking vessel soon dispelled any reason to continue in this line of thought. These were no pirates. They were madmen. They were murderers on the high seas.

We four knew our chances of survival out here in this minuscule raft were virtually nonexistent and this unspoken horror hung between us without being voiced by a single survivor. We drifted along in silence. Stunned. The reality of the dreadful situation affecting each man in his own way, and on his own time. That first night was passed in silence and I'm not wholly sure when the sun made its first appearance, nor do I care to recall the event, for my thoughts were elsewhere as I'm sure were the thoughts of every man on that craft. My first and primary concern was with rescue, and as the pirates had already run most of the ships away from this general area, I slowly came to the unavoidable realization that we would surely die out here. I attempted to dispel any delusions of a possible rescue and calmly accept what deemed to be my approaching fate.

In retrospect I'd lived a full and accomplished life of travel and leisure, leaving very little undone in my opinion and so it was with a sense of almost manifest destiny that I accepted our lot and was content to drift into an awaiting oblivion without so much as a curse or tear.

I was raised in the little waterfront New England town of Weston and had quit school at the age of sixteen to run away to join the great ships that sailed out to sea for long periods of time on awesome fishing expeditions that could take one anywhere. It was perfect for me. I had always been a loner of sorts and the sea offered the solace and solitude I so greatly relished in life as well as the chance to get out and explore the globe. I would spend my days fishing with a variety of sailors and when at port I could be found in the local taverns or soliciting company on the many docks I walked in various ports around the world. There are some who would consider my life incomplete, but it was the life that suited me and I couldn't have asked for a fuller or richer one than that which I had made for myself.

At some point I became cognizant of the sun. I have never in all my days looked upon the sun with such an air of menace and malice as I did now; cursing that wretched and accursed ball of impending destruction that hung over our heads like an angry and spiteful fire ready to consume everything in its insatiable appetite. It's little wonder why the ancients once prayed to such an awesome object and offered up sacrifices of blood and firstborns. But, on this vast expanse of open sea, the luxuries of the sane and civilized modern world were all but forgotten; swallowed by the reptilian instinct of survival ingrained deep within each one of us.

Suddenly and without expectation I reached the realization: I do not want to die. Not out here. Not like this.

Having been the first mate on the ship when it pulled out from port no less than a week earlier, I decided to assert my authority and attempt to bring a semblance of order to our small craft and offer what little hope I could. This proved to be easier than I had anticipated as the other three men seemed to me to be overly optimistic and had scarcely contemplated the peril of our plight. Apart from myself, there was Jim, who was new to our ship and had never sailed with any of us prior to this voyage. He was bulky and unkempt but appeared rugged enough to handle himself which would surely be a good attribute considering our present situation. I had thus far not had any dealings with Jim but on first assessment he seemed a capable man and not opposed to my assuming a leadership role.

Jerry on the other hand was another story altogether. He appeared unfit for work on even the smallest of fishing vessels and it caused me no shortage of wonder as to how he had come to find himself on our ship. He told us he had never sailed before and that this had been his first trip to sea and looking at him with his tiny frame and well-kept appearance I judged him far from his element and all but wrote him off as doomed. He was a small man and looked like he had spent his life in an office building or perhaps had even come fresh from college.

Finally, there was Thomas. Thomas was a well-seasoned fisherman and had sailed with me on many a ship and many adventures. No stranger to turmoil or even peril, it was Thomas who promised the best chance of survival aside from me. He stood six feet tall and was well equipped to handle himself in dangerous situations as he had been on another ship that had gone down somewhere off the coast of Haiti many years earlier before joining our ranks. He survived that twelve day ordeal at sea and was finally rescued by a British Navy vessel.

There was one glaring benefit to his twelve days at sea that we did not have, and that was adequate supplies for a sustained drift. The terrifying reality was that the human body cannot last in excess of six days without water and perhaps nine days without food... and we had neither. Taking into account the extreme and constant assault of the sun above, I figured we would be lucky to survive the next three days, if you could call that luck.

We drifted along under that unbearable and increasingly hostile sun for a length of time that was soon lost in the ensuing bouts of delirium that we began to suffer. Just how long we suffered under the punishment of that glowing yellow God is impossible to estimate. Consciousness came and went as did wild ravings and accusations made by all men on that tiny raft as we drifted ever deeper into the ocean and ever deeper into madness. Something would have to be done. I sat against the rubber backing of the small craft and surveyed the condition of the crew. They were in bad shape and we would have to do something. Soon!

I remember little of those next few days at sea. I remember water. The endless sight of water stretching out as far as the eye could see in every direction. Bouts of vertigo would come if you stared too long and the horizon and the surface of the sea would appear to merge into a single menacing entity in league with the sun bent on our destruction. Not a drop of rain did we see and nary a cloud formed to shade us from the relentless onslaught of the sun. Hope was long since abandoned and I had again come to terms with the inevitable, though far less calmly than I had previously accepted it. Of other signs of life on the water, we saw none. Not a ship, nor a schooner and not so much as a single plane did we see. We were completely alone and at the mercy of the wilds of the open sea.

It was the sound of Thomas' voice I next remember from that haze of suffering by which I had been overwhelmed and consumed. He was looking in my direction and I could see his mouth moving and could vaguely interpret the sound of his voice but I was quite unable to make out the individual syllables that his mouth formed and it took me several minutes to digest what he had said, and even then it was not until he repeated himself that it finally crawled into my mind and made itself understood, the horrifying realization of just how mad we had all become.

"We are going to have to draw straws to decide who it will be," he repeated, still keeping his eyes locked on mine. I never quite made out what he had said prior to this statement but it was unmistakable as to what it had been. He meant to kill a member of our survivors and resort to cannibalism. Had I the strength at that moment, I would have seized him by the throat and choked the very life out of him. What madness had he been reduced to? What insane madness did he expect us to take part in? I would have nothing to do with it. I resolved then and there to die in the sea when my time came and spare myself being eaten by this savage I had thought I knew and once called my friend.

***

48

GOD HELP US ALL! We ate Jim today. We continued to drift aimlessly toward destinations unknown when Jim first took up the argument Thomas had first broached, no pun intended. Ah, what I would not have given to have had a broach available to me when we took it upon ourselves to engage in that monstrous deed of savagery. I will spare you the disgusting details of what it was like to indulge ourselves on our fellow man without the aid of either fire for roast or drugs to numb the act. Suffice it to say it was dreadful to say the very least. But as I was saying, irony of all ironies, it would be Jim that was first to take up the cause Thomas first put forth so many sun-baked hours previous. With the sun finally setting behind us he spoke for the first time since our cherished ship had gone down in a barrage of unprovoked and hostile fire by nameless assailants for reasons unexplained and little fathomable. He said simply, in a squeaky and childlike voice, that we should draw straws. Nothing more. We should draw straws. And with that one briefest of statements this poor little man had sealed his own fate and not even known it.

I found myself too tired to give voice to my strong opposition to such a barbaric and vile exploit as the one these two civilized men had now openly advocated and merely sat perplexed and dumbfounded as the others openly discussed the terms of selecting who would be chosen. At one point I looked up and all parties were staring at me and had all fallen silent. I had not followed their conversation and must admit I was more than a little alarmed to glance up and see these weather worn men all directing their scared and hungry eyes in my direction.

It was Thomas who spoke then and reminded me that as the captain I would have to be the one who held the dread utensils of fate. I recognized in their faces that refusal was not an option and to do so would very likely result in a unanimous decision on their part and very likely have been the end of my narrative right then and there. I reluctantly agreed. It would be cigarettes that were to serve as the dire apparatus and we tore the end off of one and each selected in turn. Jim drew the short and before anyone could scarce utter a single word, Thomas drew a blade from its sheath and plunged it into the gut of the poor man. I had been witness in my years at sea to many an untimely death, but never had I watched an act of brazen and wanton murder happen before my very eyes. It all happened so very quickly. The blade was withdrawn and he went to scooping the mess that had spilled into our raft and hurling it over the side and into the sea where the sharks would surely make quick disappearance of it.

I turned away from the brutal scene playing out before me so as not to have to observe the carving and divvying up of the human being that had just been savagely butchered before my eyes. The sound alone was too much to bear and at some point blessed unconsciousness overtook me.

When I came to the two men were partaking of the horrendous meal and I took notice of rations that had been placed before me. I turned away in disgust and promised myself I would not, nay I could not be a party to what was going on here. This was carnage. And yet what choice was I afforded? There would come a point when I would be forced to eat or I would die here and no doubt be ingested by these carnivorous degenerates. Engulfed in shame and horror but with a desire not to fall victim myself, I ate my share. God have mercy on my soul.

***

I WRESTLED TO COME to terms and justify what I had done for many long and quiet hours at sea after the heinous act was behind us. The meat would not hold for long and we ate what we could and drank what we salvaged before pitching the remains overboard to feed the surrounding sea creatures. In the end, I know and understand there was no choice left to us. It was eat or all perish on this dismal and cursed floating jail cell on which I was desperately clinging to the hopes of rescue. The idea of having to face my fellow man again after having partaken in such acts of human cruelty and desperation were not at all appealing to me however and no matter the justification I harbored a secret desire to see us all die here and spare us the resulting humiliation and condemnation of the civilized world. One could argue that anyone in my situation would have committed the same unspeakable crimes, but I'm not so sure and am prone to believe that a hero, a stronger man, a leader would have chosen to perish with his honor and integrity still intact. I believe I acted in a moment of weakness, and having been overcome with fear and hunger, I sacrificed my humanity to prolong my life for only a little longer. I often wondered during those long hours at sea what it was that separates man from his fellow animal and just how much more evolved we truly are when forced into situations like the one I found myself in. We inherently resort to our animal instincts and baser instincts of survival, but what makes my sole survival of any more importance than any man amongst this wind-blown and current-carried craft? Perhaps we should all have starved to death rather than resort to such primitive and bestial means. For what would take place next only further confirms these initial suspicions.

Time was of little meaning out here on the vast wasteland of open and merciless sea and I had no recollection of the day or just how long we had been afloat at the mercy of the elements. But I know it was dawn when Thomas next spoke to me, though of what day on our journey I haven't the faintest clue. We had spoken not a word, any of us since we had engaged in our act of brutal treachery against our fellow cast mate until that fateful dawn when

Thomas broke the still silence to address me whilst Jerry slept unbeknownst of the plan soon to be hatched against him. His next whispered words will be forever burned into my memory and I believe them to be the very words that transformed us into what I believe we became. Rather than survivors we would now forever be considered cannibals. Killers. And God help me, I took part in his scheme.

He suggested we kill Jerry while he slept in order to ensure food for the two of us to carry us through the next several days' leg of our trip. No fairness. No straws. Just the cold blooded survival of the two of us at the expense of this sleeping man and his life to prolong our own for just a little while longer. I wish I could say that I took no part in this hastily laid and devious plot, but alas my silence and lack of opposition helped events to unfold as they would and serve to condemn our eternal and immortal souls in the process. And in all honesty after taking that first inhuman and ghastly step to survival, I no longer wished to perish since having crossed the line already. What matter did it make now that we kill this sleeping innocent rather than take the risk of drawing that abysmal short straw and being gutted like the proverbial fish and possibly eaten by him rather than consuming him first. Besides that, who would know upon our rescue, assuming we were saved from our disturbing predicament, that more than the two of us had escaped the fate of that ship anyways? Is it such a leap in character to lie about the survivors after having consumed several of them afterwards? I had all but made up my mind that nobody need know the measures we took to ensure our survival and with a little creative change in time, which was confusing anyways, nobody would ever have to know how long we sat adrift or what we had been forced to engage in to stay alive.   And so I sat and watched as Thomas grabbed the sleeping man and forced his head beneath the salty waters surrounding us on all sides. He drowned him and we consumed him as we had done to Jim before him, only he had not been afforded the luxury of a chance at survival that the drawing of straws would have given him. We had crossed a new line and I had become an accomplice to murder. But I would not die that day. Not of starvation or dehydration at any rate. I had simply done what I needed to do in order to ensure my own survival and that of my first mate. That night I slept well for the first time since having to abandon my ship.

**

AND SO THE DAYS would pass without rescue. We spotted nary a sea going vessel nor even a single plane on the horizon and our hopes were again dashed that any saving grace was forthcoming. Our death at sea was inevitable and yet I could not come to terms with this fact as I had been able to when first faced with our dilemma. I did not like the way Thomas had begun to look at me either. I would see him stealing sideways glances at me out of the corner of his eye and I could detect an air of malice and instinctual menace in his peering. He could not or simply would not, look at me directly but rather chose to steal looks when he thought my attention was directed elsewhere. I knew then that I mustn't sleep. Survival had kicked in fully and I knew that to doze off would be at my own peril for Thomas had made up his mind to kill me when I slept. I knew this as surely as I knew the reverse to be true. This had regressed into a graphic game of survival and I planned to win and escape with my life or be the last to die and do so on my own terms. I would sooner pitch myself into the briny deep than be eaten by this grotesque savage I no longer recognized. I would wait him out. He would have to sleep sooner or later and when he did...

**

WEAKNESS HAS OVERCOME ME and I feel he will attempt to take me any time now. Time ha! Time has lost all semblance of meaning to me now and I could not even begin to estimate just how long we have been adrift. Left out here to the tide and the elements it is only a matter of time now until we both succumb to the ravages of Mother Nature. Just a matter of time. There's that word again. Funny how often the word is tossed around in modern life without the slightest comprehension of its nature. But I am rambling now. It grows hard to stay alert and focused with this incessant growling and churning in my guts. I am so hungry. I hope he sleeps soon. God please, let him sleep soon or I shall be forced to attempt to take him while he waits and watches. He is a big man and I am unsure whether I can get the better of him when he is expecting it and waiting to do the same to me should I fall asleep or let my guard down for even an instant. But he must be growing desperate as well and it's only a matter of time until hunger will dictate his actions. Time.

***

HOPE OF ALL HOPE, we spotted land today! Far off in the approaching distance an island was spotted and grew considerably more visible as we drifted ever closer with each passing hour. Perhaps there is hope yet and we will not die on this raft after all. There are no words to express the jubilation we each felt and no longer did we eye each other with hostility or distrust. We used what little strength we had left to turn our hands into make-shift paddles and we steered with everything we had towards that blessed chunk of land that lay before us.

***

WE DID IT! WE made our landfall just as the sun was setting giving us scarcely an hour or two of light with which to set up a camp of sorts. We had several cigarettes left, a lighter and two knives which we put all to blessed use as we designed our little lean-to for some protection against the elements which we composed of sticks and the rubber of our raft which we cut up for maximum allowance. We were able then to build a fire and enjoy a cigarette for the first time in a long time as we revelled in the abundance of animal and plant life around us. Thomas had been able already to score two sea birds which we had already roasted and consumed while going about building our shelter. The island had yet to be explored by us and we had little idea just how large an area it was but judging from the mass as we had drifted closer earlier it looked to be of considerable size and it offered plenty in the way of survival.

As night descended upon us we were treated to the unmistakable sound of drums at some distance far in a direction behind us and through a thicket of trees and foliage we had yet to explore. We had plenty of time ahead for that now though. Time. Not such an ugly word tonight as it was in the days past. But it is no small comfort to know that this island sustains life. Human life at that, and judging from the amount of drumming that filled the cool night air, there were many of them. We must have stumbled upon some long forgotten South Pacific island tribe of some sorts perhaps.

Thomas turned to the sound, giddy with the prospect of what the tribe could offer us by way of survival, human contact and potential eventual rescue from this oceanic rock. It was then that I picked up a piece of drift wood we had dragged close to camp for future burning and bashed in the back of his skull with it, killing him instantly. As I sat warming myself, I cut him into small roastable pieces to add to the fire as I relaxed to the sounds of the continuous beatings of the savage drums. Thomas may have heard in those far distant percussions the hope of human contact and rescue by a potential trade vessel, but what I was listening to as I sat snug by the warm fire was the promise of a continuous source of food on this island for as long as I might be stranded here.

Thadd Presley Presents

Birds of a Feather
Charlotte Emma Gledson

"A beast dwells within us all..."

*SW3, Kensington, London 1998*Jonathan Moon

THE EMPTY HOUSE CREAKED despairingly as the wind wailed through the empty corridors and cracked windowpanes. The jagged glass from the third story bedroom window glimmered within the moonlight, exposing threatening teeth salivating from the harsh pelting rain. Trevor gulped another swig from his whisky bottle and cowered under the peeling windowsill. Tears welled within his bloodshot eyes. He shook, forcing his back hard against the cold brick wall in the delusional hope that he would fall through or dissolve into the shedding wallpaper. To his left, an antique teak door led out into a large corridor offering his only escape, but Trevor had neither energy nor courage to flee. *He knew he was about to die.* Fired with fear and fueled with alcohol, he shuffled his body against the dusty floorboards to avoid the threatening presence that was approaching. With two fingers he crossed himself as he stared into the gloom, whimpering his Hail Mary's under his stale sour breath.

A shrieking cry came from the bottom of the stairs causing him to gasp, his prayers held in terrified suspension.

A crescendo of footfalls ascended, Trevor's heartbeat became frantic. A guttural and inane squawk from some unknown, yet expected being hovered now outside the door. Perspiration trickled down the vagrant's furrowed brow along with the river of sweat from his malodorous armpits. The moisture traveled down his back like a leaking tap, mingling within the urine that had absorbed into his dirty jeans.

The door flew open. The vagrant recoiled in horror, digging his grubby fingernails deep within the palms of his hand. A tall bird like creature with a face resembling a Heron screeched out a terrifying scream. Its tiny feathered head angled as its enormous yellow speared beak yawned with anger. Trevor Giles, the lonely drunk that escaped life's reality with a bottle of malt released more urine, his lips dripping with bile and stale whisky. With no time to swallow the fluid back into his mouth, a long black sinewy wing wrapped and weaved itself around his cursed body, crushing his innards instantly. Blood splattered against the faded Victorian tiled fireplace, marbling the hearth in fresh vivid blood. Trevor's eyes bulged from within their sockets like crimson golf balls; his retinas bursting gelatinous fluid, coating the lapels of his shabby frayed jacket. He died quickly and with one swoop the beast and the vagrant soared up the chimney breast, leaving only soot and blood in their wake.

Within the channel of the chimney the menacing monstrosity, with its prey, sat on a wooden ledge. Wedged within the narrow brick walls of the chimney breast, the creature cradled his victim. After whistling a bizarre lullaby, the hunched bird spectre delved into the fleshy tissue of the alcoholic's chest with its razor-sharp beak and began to feed…

***

"SOME KIND OF DRUNK I'm guessing. But Jesus Christ, look at his face, he looks petrified!" The young officer retched, turning his head away from the mangled, blood drenched body.

"Well, Jones, his face is about all that's left of him. What a way to go..." The scruffy Detective Inspector placed his pen back into his upper pocket and studied the twisted and torn remains of the beggar as he lay discarded within the hearth of the black cast iron fireplace.

"Looks like somebody threw him down the chimney sir," Officer Jones observed.

"Possibly Jones, yes indeed. Head first by the looks." The DI pulled out a handkerchief from his trouser pocket and wiped his mouth. "So who found the body? A..." he referred to his small black police notebook, "Mrs. Dorothy Turner did you say?"

"Yes sir," The young officer confirmed. "She came to check the place over. She does most days as she plans to move in soon. She bought this property a couple of months ago and is waiting for some extra cash so she can do it up."

The middle-aged balding detective looked around and inhaled deeply. His rounding gut wobbled as he let out a large surge of air. "Yes it sure needs a facelift, but the house is so darn beautiful, even in this state. But my God, it stinks... Come on son; let's get out of here before I cough my lungs out. It's going to be a long day." He turned his face briefly to the vestiges of the middle aged vagrant and shuddered. "Poor bastard..."

The two men swiftly descended the stairs and into the large lobby, exiting through the heavy stained glass front doors.

From one of the exposed eaves at the top of the third floor, a pair of watchful eyes, dark and brooding with intelligence, studied the men as they left.

"Oh no. Not again! I wish she would just shut up!"

Daniel Carter clenched his fists angrily as his daughter's croaky cries filled the house once more.

"Daniel, stop saying that! Freya has a cold, you know that. You can't force a baby to stop crying at will!" Meg's brow furrowed with irritation. "I'm doing all I can Daniel. I have given her medicine and as soon as that kicks in, you can get your precious sleep." Meg was irked with her husband's selfish attitude. He insisted they all should be asleep by 8.30pm every night, impossible when you have two children under the tender age of three. "And if you are only worried about your precious lack of sleep," she continued, "then aren't *you* the *lucky* one. You heard about that body they found next door? Some kind of tramp was killed in one of the top rooms."

"Yes, I did hear," Daniel groused, punching his pillow fastidiously for more support. "I bet it was a bunch of druggies that did him over. An empty house is a perfect den for junkies; the loser probably deserved it anyway." Daniel closed his eyes as his wife turned to him in the bed, her expression incredulous.   "Daniel, how can you be so callous? Aren't you worried? It could have been one of us. There could be a murderer out there stalking our streets or watching us right now!" Meg's voice became shrill, but she soon bit her tongue when Daniel turned slowly to face her, his features shadowing with irritability.

"Look," Daniel hissed, "the house was empty; it was probably just a bunch of thugs getting a kick out of beating up an old drunk. Just check on Freya will you and shut her up then stop your incessant worrying, you make me sick woman." Wriggling deeper down into the bed, Daniel turned his back dismissively and closed his eyes once more. Meg cursed under her breath and slid off the bed to attend to their crying daughter, leaving her husband snoring like a pig.

***

MEG NOW SATISFIED FREYA was asleep and settled, padded down the plush carpeted stairs and entered the large kitchen. After pouring herself a glass of water, she sat herself down at the pine breakfast table and gazed out through the window. She felt vulnerable and she felt scared. But she also felt angry.

The street lights radiated a warm amber hue; a taxi blasted its horn interrupting her tangled thoughts. *What if the killer is watching me now? What if he is still lurking next door?* But another more urgent concern invaded her weary mind. *Why can't I find the strength to leave my bastard of a husband?* A melancholic wave enveloped her lackluster body. How could he be so childish and cruel? It was like living with a cantankerous old man, she put up with his dogmatic attitude to simply keep the peace. The fun had gone from their marriage years ago.

How can I possibly stay with someone who demeans me daily? But she knew why she didn't leave. Daniel was extremely wealthy. *And I would be too in the event of his death.* With these fanciful thoughts, she heaved herself up from the chair and checked that all her chores were complete. The dishwasher loaded, kitchen tidy, the cat fed. Good. *Daniel will now have no cause to moan at me,* she mused miserably.

As she reached to turn off the kitchen light, she heard a sound that startled her. From within the walls, she heard a labored heavy breath. A sudden unexpected scratching and scraping started to resonate around her.

"Hel… Hello?" Meg stuttered. She hovered between the kitchen and the hall, her arm still poised over the light switch. She heard another sound. A swooping gush moaned upwards, a distraught howl filled her ears. The strange noise then dwindled to another part of the house. Fleeing the kitchen, Meg ran upstairs.

"Daniel, Daniel! Did you hear that?" Her panicky voice travelled through the house as she bolted up the staircase. She reached the bedroom, panting. The door was open, the king size bed empty, their expensive duck-down duvet lay crumpled at the foot of the bed.

Daniel was nowhere in sight.

Amidst the bedding, a dark green feather fluttered around Daniel's dented pillow. Meg scoured the room. *Nothing.* Only a pile of soot and dust lay at the hearth of the brightly coloured tiled fireplace.

Meg's legs weakened as she strode towards her daughters' room, her stomach trembling with anxiety. The door was closed, just as she had left it. Meg fiddled nervously with her silver necklace and reached for the door handle with her slender shaking fingers. Cautiously she opened the door. Her short blonde hair began to stick to the back of her neck, as chilling perspiration prickled across her hairline. Chloe, her eldest daughter, who was almost three years of age, was sound asleep. In the murky shadows, she could see her delicate form. Her young chest rose up and down in the throes of innocent sleep. Meg turned her eyes to her ten month old daughter, Freya. She too was breathing soundly; her lyrical breath accompanied the soft snores that had been brought on by her cough and cold.

A sudden draft alerted Meg that something was amiss. *Maybe Daniel had already checked on the girls and gone to the bathroom? But why the mess in our room and how did that feather get there?*

With an overwhelming sense of dread, she suddenly felt that they were not alone in the bedroom. A light breath of wind touched her face again; she looked towards the bedroom curtains. They flapped briefly. Behind the floral fabric she noticed a tall slender silhouetted shape standing behind the wavering material.

"Daniel? Is that you?" Meg inquired guardedly, though she knew that it couldn't possibly have been. The curtain slowly stirred once more. In the gloomy room, with no significant moonlight to enhance her vision, she could barely make out the upright form that stood statically behind the cotton drapes. Meg's knees almost buckled, with terror churning inside her gut. The shadow stepped out from beneath the folds of material.

Silently, a tall bird with a long straight bill and a tiny pin like head, surmounted with a dark feathered crest, stared at Meg with its inky beady eyes. The creature stood on pale skeletal legs, its feet fanned with ugly black talons. It twitched then blinked, ruffles of sound came from its body as it quivered. A fleeting passage of emotion passed through them both as they scrutinized each other. Meg was horrified. She gazed at the extraordinary pointed yellow beak in disbelief as it started to snap open and shut, its slithery tongue flicking with earnest anticipation, darting in and out rapidly. Suddenly, it reached out a gangling wing and stretched out towards the sleeping child. Freya was swept from her cot and with a sudden leap, the creature rocketed up the chimney breast, embracing the baby within its feathery bony wing.

It was only then that Meg screamed, her cries awakening Chloe, who screamed in unanimity.

Soot and dust covered the rubbery pink torso of the bird-like creature; its skin cold and bumpy as a plucked chicken. However, a plumage of black and dark green feathers decorated its scrawny neck and head, with a scattering of random feathers nestled under its belly. The creature twitched inelegantly as it made its way through the narrow crevices of the building. Clutching the child to its chest, it glided swiftly along the network of chimney flues which ran through the internal structure of the terraced Georgian houses. As it dragged its body through several slender flues, it squawked and shrieked in annoyance. Freya blubbered as she was jolted and jerked within the wing's bristly grasp. Finally reaching the destination the creature scurried to its lair, which was a confined, though lengthy, chamber underneath the attic floor. It placed the coughing baby girl onto a sooty pile of rags. Freya's cries and spluttering gradually ceased as the bird fanned its wings to sweep the debris away, giving room for her to crawl and move around. The child raised her head to view her new surroundings, dragging her small fingers against the moist grimy walls with innocent inquisitiveness. Quietly burbling, Freya grabbed a single feather that lay abandoned on the filthy floor. It tickled her nose causing her to sneeze and a small giggle escaped from her lips. Amongst the detritus of dust, droppings and soot, the area was also littered with bones and tattered clothes. Fresh blood decorated one side of the crumbling wall, adding a fresh raspberry tinge to the depressing filthy pit. Glasses, jewelry, watches, credit cards and wallets were all placed in a neatly dug out hole near the nest. Freya crawled around the muck, then she picked up a small ankle bone, ramming it into her mouth. She sucked the rounded end gleefully. The bird looked on protectively, using its beak to remove a clump of abandoned bones that were scattered beside her.

Within the shadows at the far side of the hovel, a recent 'fresh' victim lay slumped against the soiled brick wall. Daniel Carter's dead eyes stared absently as the beast continued to study and tend to his daughter. Turning its head in a quick jerking manner, the bird faced its pending feast. Noticing the cold dead stare, it hopped onto Daniel's corpse and pecked at his bulbous eyes. Fresh glutinous liquid exploded against the grubby walls and dripped down the brickwork like glistening diamond and ruby stones from an elaborate necklace. Only hollow sockets remained once the bird creature had emptied the eye cavities.

Freya watched on, then crawled toward the corner where her father lay and gazed into the two naked holes, undeterred. Turning her head nonchalantly, she reached out fondly for her abductor and cooed softly. She crawled back to where the bird lurked, brooding within the shadows watching her. Freya rolled onto her back submissively. The lance like beak, now coated in a layer of sodden blood and soft tissue, stroked the soft stomach of the cheerful child. Smearing her white cotton sleep suit with dark red swirls, her nimble rounded belly resembled a pavlova dessert. It continued to fondle the youngster, but never once hurting her. In a playful tackle, it used its beak to roll her around on the filthy floor, examining her yielding form.

Suddenly it leant back distracted, craning its tiny head unexpectedly listening to a familiar voice echo through the empty chambers of the vacant house. Standing on its skeletal stringy legs, it arched its back, snapped its messy beak and squawked. Before it departed, the creature gathered a piece of shredded cloth from its nest and placed it upon the Freya's body, leaving her alone in the blood encrusted den.

The child turned her head from side to side, viewing her new play pen. Eying her father again, she crawled towards his lifeless, eyeless corpse. Soot, dust and dried blood rose up behind her in puffs as she shuffled across the floor on her hands and knees. He continued to gawk at his daughter like a battered, empty-eyed ventriloquist dummy. With the piece of pinstriped fabric still dangling from her back, Freya reached her father's carcass and gave him a dismissive poke. Unimpressed by the lack of response, she turned her head and reached out for her new friend, gurgling with amusement as she listened to it move within the inner cavities of the house.

"What have I told you?" A stern voice rang rampantly through the hallway. "I need more money, more jewelery.

Items I can sell goddammit! Come on you bloody fucking hideous fool, bring me what I want or I will send you back to where you bloody well came from: THE GUTTER OF HELL!"

Coughing after her outburst, the twisted lined face of a scraggy woman shouted louder up the stairs. "I can take you back to where you came from in an instant, and don't you forget it!"

Dot Turner slumped her coat and handbag onto the bottom step of the wide staircase, disturbing the dust as she did so. "Come out and show yourself! I had the bleedin' pigs here the other day. You made so much noise; some fucking neighbor rang the bastards." There was a silent pause. "You coming down or what?" The fifty year old woman had a thin mouth, crudely accentuated with a vibrant terracotta lipstick. She wore a tight purple T-shirt, emphasizing her flat chest and flaccid nipples. Vulgar gold earrings hung from her drooping earlobes, faded jeans clung desperately to her willowy legs. "COOEE! I *NEEEEED* YOU!"

Marching up the first three steps, she noticed that the creature was standing motionless at the top of the landing. She stopped in her tracks. With its lanky stork like legs astride, it analyzed Dot from the top of the staircase. Shadows circulated the bird beast giving it a foreboding presence. Raising its head in the air, it opened its obtruding beak and let out a hideous shriek.

"Stop your wailing! Now, what you got me this time? Better be worth sumin'. This ring you got was worth a few bob mind you, just had it valued…" She turned the platinum gold ring within her lined palm and smiled acquisitively. Before Dot could utter another word, the creature suddenly absconded, running along the upstairs corridors crowing in a painful screech. She waited impatiently, tapping her fingers against the mahogany banister. "Oh, come back here will you, I haven't got time for your petty games."

Only a shuffling bustle could be heard within the eaves of the house. Dot continued to climb the staircase huffing and wheezing, her asthma reawakened with the exertion. After a few minutes, the creature reappeared. Having eventually reached the top of the landing, Dot stopped short, irritation brewing within her like a pan of boiling milk. "What the... what the hell have you got there? A bloody baby?" She bellowed at the creature.

Adopting an insidious expression, the bird moved towards Dot slowly. It held out the baby to its mistress, whistling a trilling refrain.

"I don't want a fucking baby! Give it here." Striding towards the creature, she grabbed Freya and threw her to the ground. She was about to stomp upon her tiny frame when the creature squealed with an agonized wail, then launched itself towards Dot. It rammed its sharp beak into her flushed cheek. Thin threads of skin hung from the murderous bill. Dot fought back feebly, scratching at the sides of the bird's head, lumps of skin and feather became embedded deep underneath her false finger nails, causing them to snap and fall to the ground. Freya screamed, her breathing becoming erratic and out of sync, her cries filling the landing with echoing squeals. Blood gushing from Dot's wounds, splashed onto her legs, saturating her jeans like seeping spilled ink.

Slipping on her own sticky blood, she fell to the ground and the beast quickly straddled her and began to stab its elongated beak deep into the screaming woman's belly manically, like a woodpecker battering the bark of a birch tree. Her cries were pained and tortuous, Freya howled, trying desperately to crawl away and escape the carnage. The cacophony of screams filled the empty house causing the walls to reverberate with the sound, dust and plaster flaking like crumbling pastry.

The large front doors suddenly burst open. Bitter

night air breezed into the spacious hallway, a frosty mist clouded around the three individuals. Standing at the mouth of the doorway, Meg and two police officers stood rooted to the spot. Reaching for his weapon the younger officer yelled, "ARMED POLICE!"

Standing focused and motionless, Jones aimed the gun. The frenzied beast stopped its demented attack and gazed directly down at the officer. Meg instinctively launched up the stairs for her daughter, the need to protect her child prevailed over the fear of the terrifying animal. The giant bird turned briskly from side to side, then stooped low and placed its blood stained wing around the tiny child's body holding it close to its featherless, blood-stained breast. Freya was sobbing, but her cries diminished as soon as the embrace enfolded her. She gurgled softly, a smile filling her grubby face. Meg watched in horror.

Officer Jones fired.

Meg froze.

The bird creature's head exploded in a red cloud of bone and tissue, causing it to crumple to the ground like a collapsing chimney. Rolling out from under the creature's wing, Freya fell to the floor with a soft bump.

In a blind panic, Meg scooped up her daughter. "No! That creature was protecting my daughter!" shrieked Meg.

Officer Jones, now standing at the top of the stairwell with his colleague Officer Wilkins at his side, fired three more shots in quick succession blasting the trunk of the abomination into a soup of gore and entrails. A flurry of gun smoke, blood, and feathers filled the width of the hallway in a canvas of bloody matter. Meg screamed hysterically. Wilkins darted towards Meg and wrapped a protective arm around her and the baby, feeling her body spasm in shock. Wriggling out from the officer's embrace, she stepped back; wrapping her distressed daughter within the warmth of her cashmere cardigan, she used the woollen material to wipe away the blood and soot that cased her face.

"You alright? The baby?" Jones asked as he rushed to Meg's side, fixing his eyes on the tear stained child, then turning to the traumatized mother enquiringly.

"Yes, we're… both are fine. There's… there's not a mark on her…" Meg answered in a small trembling voice. She inspected her daughter again, though bloodstained and dirty, she was totally unscathed. "What the hell has been happening here." She pointed. "I mean look!" Meg swiveled around, eyes wide, viewing the aftermath and the bloodbath around her. Meg let out a desperate sob, feigning off the panic attack that was stirring within her.

Jones walked towards the creature and kicked its side to make sure it was dead, but by looking at the bloody disarray, he knew the beast was well and truly annihilated.

Wilkins joined him and stood by his side, stunned. "Where on earth did this *thing* come from Jones? Any idea who the victim could be," he inquired. His voice wavered, the shock of the last few minutes only just sinking in.

"Some kind of mutation that went haywire?" Jones answered. "I haven't got the bloody faintest! The deceased I am sure is Dot Turner, we interviewed her the other day. I recognize the earrings and handbag. We can check the contents to confirm." Jones responded and a trickle of sweat dripped off his upper lip. He wiped it away whilst screwing his face into a look of disgust. He studied Dot's body closer, suppressing the inner shakes that threatened to emerge. He recalled the abhorrent remains of the vagrant he witnessed the other day and let out a deep sigh, then shuddered. On closer inspection he noticed a large black tattoo of a five pointed star visible on the inside of Dot's bloodied wrist, he lowered his head closer to view the markings. The word *Diabolus* was neatly scripted underneath the icon. "Maybe she *does have* something to do with this. Looks like she may have dabbled in Black Magic," Jones queried, as he raised the woman's limp wrist with the tip of his gun.

"Who knows, maybe? But at least *that* thing is dead," Wilkins answered. "I think there are going to be many unanswered questions in this case Jones. Do you know what this Diabolus means?"

"It means Devil in Latin." Jones flopped her arm back to the ground and let out a silent gag, the smell of death finally absorbed within his nostrils.

Still holding Freya protectively, Meg joined the two officers making sure Freya's head was buried deep within her shoulder. Her daughter had witnessed enough already. Scrutinizing the creature and the shredded body of Dot Turner, she suppressed the buildup of bile that swam inside her belly. It was then she noticed a glint of silver, lying close to a bloodied fingernail. Tears began to settle within her stinging eyes, her stomach flipped.

"Look!" Meg pointed. "Next to her fingernail, near the earring. There," she bent closer, "by her foot. This thing must have had Daniel, my husband… It's his wedding ring. But where is *he*?" Still pointing out the ring to Jones, Meg's expression sported a mere smile, but guilt soon devoured her capricious thoughts.

The officers examined the evidence closely. "I'm so sorry Mrs. Carter…" Jones said, placing his hand onto Meg's shaking arm reassuringly and then radioed for backup. A cloak of heavy silence hung in the air as if they were standing in a mausoleum. They waited for the ambulance and support in silence. As they waited, rain battered against the stained glass doors. The three of them stared down at the mysterious creature and the mutilated leftovers of Dot Turner. Freya let out a feeble mew. Meg turned from the massacre and descended the stairs and sat on the bottom step, near to Dot's handbag and neglected Mac. Only then, did she cry into her daughter's downy hair, trying hard to make sense of the last harrowing 48 hours along with the new notion of living a life without her officious and conceited husband…

From within a dingy nest, roosted at the highest point of the empty house, a signal mottled egg cracked open and a sharp yellow beak peeked through the chitinous shell, tasting its first breath of natural air…

Thadd Presley Presents

Heart of an Angel
Jonathan Moon

I HAVE THE HEART of an angel.

I keep it in an old rusty bird cage on my table. There's a perch in the cage where the demon parakeet used to sit but the angel heart doesn't take advantage of it. It just floats there glowing like the un-light from a dead star keeping my old cabin an uncomfortable, eerie warm.

The demon parakeet never did anything but howl and curse, froth and spit, and occasionally make all the meat in the cabin go rotten all at once. Sometimes I miss the hateful bastard.

The angel heart convinced all the dogs to up and kill themselves all on the same damn day. Dead dog days take a lot out of a person. The day the dogs died the angel heart kept me up all night with a barking, weeping fit. Tendrils, strands of pure light, reached from its pulsing surface through the cage at me. I burned their tips with my Zippo lighter. Heavenly heart fingers are no match for butane and flame.

During a fierce high mountain windstorm the angel heart tried to make me do myself in. It hummed and glowed all loving and creepy while it sprouted a white hot beard of tendrils. The tiny tentacles danced before my tired eyes and convinced me I needed the sensation of brisk wind upon my face. My legs walked me through the old wooden door. I could vaguely hear it slam as I walked away as if it didn't want to be left alone with the angel heart. My legs walked me to the edge of the ridge and the angel heart spoke to me with a voice like long suffering coral and told me it was a nice day for a glide.

My toes dislodged rocks and pebbles and they danced down the steep ridge face. I was very close to jumping, with mind numbing faith, and falling to a terrible doom. But, luckily for me, my eyes saw through the trance and took sight of the carving I'd once made across the wide trunk of an old pine tree of a man and his dogs chasing down a legless dragon. It was the carving I was working on when I saw the angel crash to earth in a clutter of light, love, and feathers. I remember the day with uncharacteristic clarity. The demon parakeet smelt the unconscious angel and talked one of the dogs into opening the cage, most likely by threat of rotten meat. The parakeet then took on it's much less flattering natural form as it dove onto the angel broken on the rocks below. I tell you now you haven't seen degradation until you've seen how a demon really fucks an angel.

I clutched the tree I was carving upon. Splinters dug into the soft flesh of my cheeks and forehead but I couldn't watch the terribly violent copulation at the bottom of the ridge. Finally, I heard the demon flap away hellishly content. Perhaps he flew off to become a parakeet again to howl and curse, froth and spit, and spoil someone else's meat. I looked around the tree, blood and sap smeared all over my face, and beheld the mutilated corpse below. The angel's chest was torn wide open; it's devastated rib cage releasing that eerie glow through shards of splintered bone. I scurried down the ridge to see why the corpse was glowing and saw the angel heart blackening as the body died. I stabbed it with a stick and carried it home holding it out a distance in front of me. I was planning on eating it since all the meat had maggots swimming through it but the angel heart purred when I sat it in the demon parakeet's vacated cage. I watched it pulse and twitch until it began floating.

The dogs howled their disapproval but I didn't want to touch the angel heart once it resurrected. It stayed in the cage and eventually talked the disapproving dogs to death. It won't get me I warned it the day I buried my dogs. Its tendrils flicked love and understanding at me but my own heart has grown cold even in its cursed warm glow.

The angel heart will never understand that some of us don't want salvation; we just want our rotten meat back.

Thadd Presley Presents

Closed Captioned
Nate D. Burleigh

Closed Caption: [*The gruesome murder of yet another hearing impaired individual has the city's deaf community gripped with terror.*]

TERRANCE LOOKED AT HIS wife Misty and signed, "Another one, I can't believe it. This is really getting out of hand." His eyes darted back to the television screen.

A newswoman stood in front of a two-story house with a gray BMW parked in the driveway. Bright-yellow police tape lining the perimeter of the house flapped in the evening breeze. People bustled in and out of the house. She continued her interview with one of the neighbors.

Closed Caption: [*It was an absolute nightmare. He came home from work yesterday. I waved to him, like I always do, and he went into the house. I didn't hear or see anything. This morning his brother came to pick him up for work and... I guess that's when he found the body. It's been really hard around here ever since. Police have blocked off the entire street and they've been questioning everyone in the neighborhood.*]

Terrance felt Misty's soft hand on his shoulder. He turned.

"I agree," she signed and spoke out loud at the same time so he could read her lips. "How many is that now?"

"Four that we know of," he signed.

"Were all of them hearing impaired?"

75

"I believe so." He put his hand on her knee.

Even though they'd been married only four years, he felt as if he'd known her his entire life. He couldn't believe his luck. To have found a woman of her age who had never been married before — who could fluently sign — made him feel like he'd won the lotto.

"Does it make you nervous?" she asked.

"Kind of, but I won't let it get to me. You forget; I'm a black belt in *Jiu-Jitsu*, reigning tri-cities champ in the senior III category." He kissed her gently on the cheek.

"I know. I guess I'm just worried, that's all. I'll be able to sleep better when they find this psycho and throw his ass behind bars. Are you sure it doesn't stir up too many memories?"

A cavalcade of surreptitious thoughts flooded his mind. He had barely learned to sign when the man in the orange jump suit burst through the locked sliding glass door in his family's kitchen. Shards of glass had skipped across the floor in front of young Terrance. He stood rigid with fear as the intruder stalked behind his unsuspecting mother and grabbed her by the waist with his massive, grease-ridden hands. The rest of the incident came in jumbled blurs and shattered images as he watched the escaped convict brutally rape, torture and murder his mother. He tucked the images back into the recesses of his subconscious.

"I'm sorry, honey. I didn't mean to dredge up old memories."

He watched her dainty, slightly wrinkled hands, flow with the sign. But still a little dazed, he missed most of what she said.

"What?"

"I said I'm really sorry about bringing *that* up."

"It's okay. The sonofabitch never got caught. Anyway, he's probably dead by now. That was over fifty years ago," he signed with an exclamation point.

"Oh, shit!" Misty said, signing frantically. "Look at the time. I've got to get to work. I'll see you when I get home. Please keep the doors locked." She kissed him quickly on the lips, grabbed her stethoscope from the kitchen counter and hurried off to work.

Terrance had retired from being a sign language professor at the university a couple of months earlier. He'd started several projects since then, some woodworking, fixing an old car, and painting. What he'd ended up doing (and loving) was writing. He started with a love story which blossomed into a beautiful Harlequin Romance. He had to admit, he'd always been a sucker for those kinds of novels. He sat down at the computer to delve into the next chapter of his book, but curiosity kicked at him with a steel-toed boot and he decided he'd watch the news to see if the police had come up with anything yet.

He clicked on the television in the bedroom and then thumbed through several channels before landing on one that had the hunt for the newest serial killer scrolling across the bottom.

The police chief stood at a podium. It looked like a re-broadcast of a press conference.

Closed Captioned: [*This morning around eight o'clock Pacific Standard Time, Jeremy Litchfield was found dead in his home.*]

A reporter jumped into the conversation [*Chief, Pete Lozano here with Action News Twelve. Does the evidence show this crime is related to the other slayings?*]

The camera panned back to the Chief. [*We have reason to believe that the incidents are related, yes.*]

The reporter continued, [*Do the victims have anything else in common, other than being deaf? Because Action News Twelve has learned that the victims were alumni of the University's School for the Hearing Impaired. Is that true?*]

[*No, comment,*] the Police Chief said.

Panic tore at his gut. As an alumnus of the University's program, he realized that he could be next on the killer's list. He went through the house, making sure the windows were shut and the doors locked. In the hall closet he rummaged through box after box, searching for the only thing that would make him feel safe: his .38 pistol. After thoroughly searching the house he remembered that he'd stored it in the shed.

Armed with a nine-iron, he opened the kitchen's sliding glass door. The Sun blinded him for a moment. After gaining his bearings he followed the small cobblestone walkway, his eyes scanning, confirming the area devoid of psycho killers. It had been a long time since he'd opened the door to the shed. It took him a minute to remember where he'd hidden the key. Next to the door there stood a large empty vase. He crouched. Cobwebs entangled his fingers when he reached behind the vase and started palming the area for the key. He yanked his hand out and examined it, making sure no spiders had hitched a ride.

He scratched his head. *Where the hell did I put that?* It hadn't occurred to him that the door might be unlocked. He twisted the knob and the door swung open. He rooted through some piled up boxes under the window and moved to another stack when something in the back corner of the shed caught his eye. He walked over and moved an old tire out of the way. A door latch in the floor gleamed in the sunlight peeping through the shed window. He couldn't understand why he'd never noticed it before, and they had lived in that house for four years.

The latch slid over and he opened the door, revealing a ladder. He glanced around the shed and found a flashlight. With several sweeps of the light he saw that the ladder led to a room under the shed. He saw a light switch halfway down the ladder on the wall.

Terrance couldn't figure out where the room had come from and why he hadn't seen it before. Curiosity willed him to climb down the stairs. At the halfway point he flicked the light switch. A small bulb dangling from a precarious wire flickered to life. The ceiling of the rectangular room was an arm's length above his head. Handmade workbenches lined the three sides of the walls opposite the ladder. On one side of the room a small television sat on the workbench. On the other side, a red tool box and what looked like a safe decorated the bench. He figured he'd check the safe first…. *just to be safe,* he thought in an attempt to alleviate his nervous anxiety. He chuckled.

Much to his surprise the safe wasn't locked. He opened it, revealing a pile of papers. There were old newspaper clippings, torn out magazine pages, some other nondescript documents. He read the first headline and nearly went into shock when he read it.

Young boy committed to psychiatric care following his mother's brutal slaying.

"Young Terrance Maxwell was committed to Worthington Psychiatric Hospital after seeing his mother's brutal attack, rape, and murder…"

He nearly dropped the stack of papers in his hand. Somehow he didn't have any recollection of being committed to a psychiatric institute. But he also couldn't remember most of his childhood. He tossed the clipping to the side and went on to the next: an incident at the psychiatric hospital where another child had been brutally stabbed to death. The next three clippings had him sitting on the ground, shocked. They were clippings of the three deaf people who had been recently found slaughtered in their homes.

A lump welled in his throat. His stomach felt like someone had cranked a vice on it. Taking a few long breaths, he got hold of his emotions. This stuff wasn't his. So whose was it? The only logical explanation was… *Misty.* He'd only known her for a few months before he proposed to her. Maybe he didn't know her well enough. Why would she keep all these things hidden? Why would she collect old articles about his past? None of it made much sense.

He pulled himself to his feet and noticed a small drawer in the side of the workbench. Cautiously, he opened it. A swarm of flies flew out. He turned to avoid getting one up his nose. Something wrapped in a red cloth lay across the bottom of the drawer. He pulled the object out and knew immediately what it was from the weight and feel of it. He placed it on the work bench and unwrapped it.

The waving light glinted off the parts of the cold steel that weren't covered in a drying, brown substance. Terrance knew the knife. He'd been given it as a gift from Misty on their first anniversary. "The perfect carving knife," she once said. The blade curved outward and ended with two separate points, usually used for gouging the meat on the barbecue to flip or aerate it. He couldn't remember when he'd last used it.

Wires led from the TV to a small cabinet next to it. He opened it and saw that the TV was plugged into a surge protector. Next to the outlet sat a VCR with a tape half pushed in. He turned the TV on and a cloud of white snow bounced shadows off the walls. He pushed the tape in.

The TV screen flickered to life.

Someone carrying a video camera filmed as a man signed *good-bye* to a woman and children who were piling into a minivan. After they pulled out of the driveway, the man picked the newspaper off the sidewalk and went into the house. The camera went blank for a moment. When it came back on, it focused in on the man. He frantically rocked back and forth, lunging against the duct tape that bound his arms to a wooden chair. His ankles taped tightly against the front legs. The assailant waved the blade back and forth in front of the man. Tears streamed down his face. He had a long surface laceration across his bare chest. Light trickles of blood dripped from several small puncture wounds above his left nipple. Then, the screen went gray.

The video started. The unexplainable look of terror in the man's eyes sent waves of gooseflesh up and down Terrance's spine. A steady stream of blood flowed down the right side of the man's head and neck as he stared intently at something in his lap. The camera tilted down, zooming in on the object. The man's ear bounced around as he squirmed in his seat. The assailant waved the knife several more times. Blood oozed off the blade. Terrance couldn't see the hands of the perpetrator but somehow he knew who it was.

The TV screen blacked out and came back on. He dared not look, but he couldn't help himself. The hilt of the knife protruded from the man's chest and he'd gone completely limp. Blood pooled over the linoleum floor. Terrance knew the man had been murdered.

He rummaged through the papers in his lap until he found the picture of the man and the article detailing his brutal attack. He glanced at the TV. Another unfortunate soul with something more than panic in his eyes sat helpless as the intruder slowly tortured and killed him.

Terrance turned the TV off. How could she have done this? How could anyone be so cruel and why would she choose hearing impaired men? She'd married one for crying out loud. Would he be the last one on her list? He had no clue, but really didn't want to wait and find out.

In his rush to get to the trap door, the papers slipped out of his hands and fluttered to the floor. He knelt, gathered them into a neat pile and then noticed another videotape tucked under the workbench. Lying flat on his stomach he retrieved the tape. With trembling hands, he pushed it into the VCR.

It looked like old black and white footage; possibly an old reel video that had been transferred to VHS. A young boy played with toy trucks in the sand while someone videotaped him. He kept looking up and laughing and his lips were moving. Slowly, at the bottom of the screen, a closed caption appeared, [*Look at me, Mommy.*]

A man sauntered into the scene. At first, all Terrance saw were the man's khaki jeans. Then he crouched, wrapping his arms around the boy.

Terrance's heart felt as if it would burst through his ribs. He recognized the man; the man from his nightmares who'd made him watch as he gutted his mother. He kissed the boy on the cheek. The boy, he'd seen pictures of in his family album.

The man appeared to be talking to young Terrance. And while he knew that he couldn't hear, young Terrance seemed to be responding. A closed caption appeared,

[*Don't you have the nicest trucks, Terry?*] And then the man signed and spoke into the camera, "*Isn't Terry the best driver ever, Mommy?*"

Young Terry stood with his trucks and drove them around in the air. His lips looked like they were moving — talking.

Terrance felt beads of sweat building on his brow. His heart thumped against his chest and he felt faint. *This is it; you're having a heart attack. It'll all be over soon*, he thought. The room darkened as the scene changed. The dangling bulb above him sparked and went out. On screen, little Terry drove his toy trucks in circles around his father: the murderer.

Terrance felt a cold chill creep up his spine. He tried the switch several times, but the light had burned out. He could still see fairly well by the glow of the television and decided to look at the article a little closer, the one about the child who'd been institutionalized.

Dr. Livingston, the boy's psychiatrist, said: "It's an amazing transformation. He went from a perfectly healthy, happy, hearing child, to completely deaf overnight. We call it an Acute Traumatic Somatic Reaction. The interesting thing is that the boy seems to come in and out of it. Although, when he speaks, he refers to himself as Terry and when he uses sign language, he calls himself Terrance. It was almost as if he had dual personalities, although, Terry is very distraught and speaks about revenge and killing anyone who can't hear. He knows about the "other one" and thinks if he kills enough deaf people, he will somehow break free of his deaf-self, Terrance."

Terrance dropped the papers. He backed toward the entrance and started up the ladder. The door slammed shut above him. He pushed against it, but it wouldn't open. He felt trapped. No food, no water, no way out. Incessant pounding had no effect and he dropped back to the floor, defeated.

Then he remembered the knife. The seven-inch steel blade wedged under the door, made just enough of a crack where he could see the floor of the shed. He exerted more pressure to widen the gap and lost his grip. His right hand slid forward over the blade, severing the insides of his fingers. He fell to the ground, clenching his hand as blood gushed between the mangled digits.

He felt light-headed and the room swam around him. After securing the wound with the towel the knife had been wrapped in, he thought the TV would make a good battering-ram. He turned to unplug the television and felt something hit the back of his head. With a flash of light, everything went black.

Terrance awoke to find himself sitting on his living room sofa. His eyes darted left and right until they rested on the item in his lap. The knife soaked streaks of crimson into his khaki trousers. Tears streamed down his face, horror creasing every line as he read the blood-written words on the wall above Misty's twisted and mutilated body.

You did this!!

Love, Terry!

Thadd Presley Presents

It's up to You, New York
JD Stone

TWO A.M. ON THE number 7 train, flickering fluorescence, ghouls of the city all tucked in for bed, and Rez didn't want to stop his terrible singing. Smoker's voice still puffing away as a curdled lump of cancer nibbles the voice box, teeth grating across guitar strings, spitting lyrics like stones at Delilah's head.

"Here we go again!"

If her band Electric Orchid was meant to be brutalized in this fashion, Delilah would have never signed up for the glitter and darkness of the stage, the slipping of time through the golden crescendo of keyboard and guitar, double bass peddle marching into the void of hands and faces enchanted by their tunes.

"I'm getting better," Rez said as he ran the brass pick across the strings again like a maniac, head banging his tuft black hair.

The train hummed on, soulless, the colorless ground slipping past without any sense of direction: one quiet Pennsylvania girl on the verge of insanity and a city boy inspired by the night. Bonded by blood, separated at birth, but now back together, the two shared a love for mischief, and that's what they were up to right now. Delilah prayed that none of her dream-demons could break through the aluminum walls to stop her mid-morning mission; the smell of the murky river would surely make them turn their dead, cold hands away. They'd done such a good job of chasing Rez his entire life that they were nearly unavoidable, but tonight was a night to call back the past, to venture into the dreamlands again.

The silver handrails gleamed like fingers wet with blood and sweat; decadent advertisements for Jameson whiskey lay juxtaposed stupidly next to food stamps. She couldn't make sense of it; Delilah thought it all looked childish, but she'd been riding these trains for a long time now so she was quite used to all of the secret madness of the city. It lay in things one didn't easily understand.

"We've got the first stop," Rez yelled.

The candy colored lights of Citi Field blasted through the windows, illuminating the unstirred swamp of Flushing Bay below. That was where she needed to be. Nobody but her and Rez and the chill of autumn air. Then the back door opened and a coal-faced hobo came skidding into the train, begging for chump change, crying about his doomed life of bedsores eating away the skin on his ass from being wheelchair bound.

"Just one dollah' would set me straight," he said moving across the train in a jagged fashion. "You got any money, little *strange* girl?" He mouthed at her with cracked lips and a filthy begging hand.

"No."

Delilah knew that he'd put himself in that chair with the bottle and needle. She could see the mosquito bite track marks running up his trembling arm, so her empathy ended right there. Just as he was wheeling himself away, Rez flicked a nickel and a PBR to the bum. Delilah began to pace back and forth awaiting the stop, listening to the haunting roars of the metal wheels against the taut metal tracks. Her lipstick was black in the window's reflection, eyes puffy and bruised giving way to her soft young face, blue-black dreads streaked with pink lightning and whipping like angry snakes.

"And I'll say it again, as I said before; this is my *personal hell...*" Rez stopped singing and sipped his PBR. "Ah, carbonated piss."

"Enough already... butchering my music," Delilah said.

"Want another tune?"

"Please... no."

Rez pulled out the guitar pick out anyway and began to pick the strings of the Warlock again, his black nail polish stripping off at every strum of what he thought was a chord, every slide he made with his thumb across the neck sounded like he was using butter knives. Rez was torturing her, but lovingly of course because they were siblings. He was playing one of those prideful kinds of tunes that Delilah just didn't get. Pride was one of those sins that religion talked about, a major sin that all religions practiced like bowing at the altar. Rez pulled off the rhythm delightfully well, each note rising and falling as if he was writing a musical scale in midair. His perpetual bad luck had all of a sudden changed into inspiration, but for Delilah these times had turned back into inescapable nightmares laced with liquor and sticky summer nights spent in dreary clubs.

"I want to wake up, in the city that doesn't sleep. And find I'm king of the hill, top of the heap. A number 1!"

"You got the lyrics wrong," Delilah said as she sipped from a small flask, enjoying the whiskey burn and electric aftertaste.

"I'm just having a good time. Want one of these?" Rez pulled out a tightly rolled joint.

"No, and you can't light that on the train. You should know that, Mr. New Yorker."

"It's only me, you and the night, who cares. It's good old Haze. You know you want it."

Rez looked around him and sparked the joint to life with his green Zippo lighter. The spicy cloud shrouded his face, his tiny sapphire eyes darkened by makeup, features twisting into his signature mask of wonder and amusement. Then Rez folded the guitar back into its case as Delilah watched his thin spider fingers, careful not to damage the steel tuning knobs and body, or Jimmy Knox and his psychotic yellow afro would certainly beat his ass for scratching his baby up. Rez was better with his pen and notebook by far, churning out short stories week after week, but he was open to trying new things unlike Delilah who was comfortable in knowing she was a master at her art, her singing, and in no need of any other creative outlet.

Now the guitar was on his back and the train doors were opening like silver lips. The two rushed out into the night, swallowed by the dimly lit station, down narrow steel stairs, rubbing fingers across paint chips and gum drops, settling into the jungle of green metal pillars and open road that held the train up in the air. Delilah wished she hadn't been led here, but it was the only way to the answer.

*****

DELILAH DREAMED OF SWIMMING, leaving the world behind and letting cold ugly water drown her, washing the sins of her life away. Left only would be music, she was sure of it. But she couldn't do that here. North Queens was a squalid, smelly place she had never been too, and the water was horribly rancid. She came into the land via her dreams, a gift she had since she was a little girl, riding waves of shadow into the night, walking its uneven terrain looking for nothing special.

Plagued by garbage and graffiti, the water swelled and relaxed as if a bayou haunted by Katrina, glowing black in the night and snake twisting through the puzzle of overgrown grass and highways around her. It was a sulfurous mass; it was definitely hungry.

She was told this was Flushing Bay, *dead water* to the locals, a place where Korean packing industries and Chinese newspaper factories dumped their trash, where coal ash was buried a century before, bone dust and chemicals mixing dangerously, forming a mucky excuse for soil. She trekked closer to the shore, wondering what would happen if she stuck her hand in. Would it come back out the same? Would she get an extra finger, or would the water poison her blood? The mud smelled rancid, something between chunky milk and spoiled meat, clumpy with engine oil and boat fuel.

This place was the death of dreams.

Her mind sailed over the smelly waves, into the deepest part of the bay. She could walk right into the cold stretch if she felt like it. She loved to swim. Delilah wanted to know what mutant faces of fish lie beneath the water now, what thing could easily come up and swallow her because this place bred potent poison. Delilah wanted to seek out aberrant inspirations for music writing. The lights of the city were lost this far out, and the smell hit her with a ton of memories: Flushing Bay was the reason for that god awful stink inside the 7 train heading in or out of Main Street, a body of water seemingly slumped off the side of the earth, a wide spot forgotten by the city around it, the city that never sleeps.

She planted her body atop the metal side rails holding the land above it, tattooed with cryptic graffiti, swirling shapes that began as things she knew, but ended as things she was better off not knowing. It was the perfect place to work out music and lyrics, to stretch her vocals to no end, where no grumpy asshole would ask her to quiet down, where no bustle of the boroughs could stop her. She was in need of new songs, and the grit and grime that inspired her, the loneliness made her happy.

From this black vista a huge metal globe glittered argent, the skeleton of the earth for everything and everyone to see. Two flying saucers of the despaired New York Pavilion lay rusting to a dying orange, not the place to see the sights of Queens anymore, just another run down gem waiting to be crushed by gentrification. The moon was a big white gold ball filtering generous light to her.

And then there's the splash at the foot of the tarry shore.

A waft of foul smelling tide hit Delilah in the face, forcing her eyes to the pale spot lucid in the dark. It wasn't a light, not a reflection of a star or moon, nor a shadow of something angelic. She put her notebook of putrid poetry and lustful lyrics back into her messenger bag and forced her Docs south to the area. She came up to the thing on the left, no longer pale, but the skin bruised as if a dark lily blooming inside its blood. If looked at hard enough, its blood could be taken for purple. A beaked shape mouth opened to a row of flat square teeth and one fang, eyes as black and stern as an owl's. Its four paws stretched flat like flippers; a limp rat's tail hung limp at the end of the crooked spine. It looked like a big cat or small raccoon, the smell as red and brown as rotten cinnamon.

A mutation of some sort, for sure.

And then she saw the symbols.

Ornate symbols twisting in the water, all around the creature engraved into the murky sand, star-shaped ideograms, intricate as dream catchers and pentacles spotlighted by the wavy grey moon and the wretched stars. But the dark comes back for vengeance, stealing the light away, not letting her see if the thing was alive, if the water had chewed it up and spit it out like a bad snack. Delilah didn't care, it was an animal and it needed her help. Her heart remained in a catatonic state for everything except animals. As she went to grab the creature, two blue-black dreadlocks brushed the water and curled upward as if cringing at the smell. She brought it to her chest, walking away thinking what a mess she has gotten herself into, but how happy she was that she found new inspiration. Music would be written, and soon.

***

"WHERE'RE WE WALKING TO?" Rez asked, skate shoes scraping against the concrete from the tacks he stuck into the soles.

"To where I found it," Delilah said, loving the silence and chill of the mid-morning mission.

"It was here? That thing, that animal?"

"Well… more towards the bay. But I just want to see something over here by the park."

"Ew. Dead water."

"Who cares!"

"Is that thing really going to help you write a new song?"

"Yes, it is. You don't get it. I need new inspiration."

In her dream Delilah's body wasn't her own. She had left it back in the 7 train, held safe only by a thin opaque line attached to her head that she was sure was her soul. She'd always been able to astral project, but over the past year she was perfecting the practice, and she could bring anyone along now as long as she focused her mind hard enough, as long as she didn't lose control. Rez came to show her to the park because he knew the way. Her sense of direction in New York was still sharpening. And plus, everything in the astral world was skewed. Simple things looked like pictures in a book, items such as a smashed street light or a stop sign took on a new light, a new darkened perspective. She needed a native of the city to see her through. Rez was that person.

The park was the only place Delilah could imagine answers lay, something to explain the creature-corpse she'd been keeping. There had to be some portal or some spotty silver void that could transport them back through time to when and how such an unknown thing could have been washed upon the slow murky shore of Flushing Bay. Maybe she'd even find more symbols. There was a nightmare the other night of a lonely boy who provided a lot of light, an angel of sorts, but not from heaven, not even from hell, but from elsewhere; a simple boy with tri-colored hair and a peaked face who wrote down symbols just like the ones at the bay. Delilah had tried to grab him, but he was gone, left behind was his hollow chrysalis.

The overgrown weeds crunched beneath her Docs, cluttering the ground was more garbage, a needle's dusty shine and faint loathsome vampire grin; it tested her patience from the distance. It was laughing at her. They jumped over construction gates and Rez sliced his arm on the way down across a razor-ring, his blood dripping like a descending butterfly to the cement. Delilah hated when Rez got hurt, she was his older sister by milliseconds and it made her very protective.

"If we keep going this way, we're going to run out of light."

"That's why we have you," she said.

"Me?"

"In this place, you're like a flashlight," she assured him.

"What are you, psychic?" Rez moved in front of Delilah and stopped her, pulling his thick dark hair in many directions. "This isn't the safest neighborhood, especially for kids like us. These people here think we're the freaks that need to disappear."

"I'm feeling very psychic these days. And let them come, Rez, if they want to fight..."

Delilah lifted an X-acto blade out of her messenger bag. It had a sleek grey handle and a bit of rust on the thin edge, but Rez could tell that the thing could do damage when touching human skin. She'd used the same blade to tear into her skin as a teenager, leaving spidery scary scars behind across her forearm.

"Ouch!" Rez held his one ear of piercings and his crotch as a pet peeve reflex.

"This blade can open human skin like a can with a pull top."

Blade to unwilling skin, to rich scarlet flow...

The passageway turned thin, shaded by dust. The seldom tree grabbed for them with its black arms and rotted leaves hanging like tooth decay; glittering glass was strewn like gems looped on an endless garland across the pavement. Delilah had Rez's hand entwined in hers now; she didn't want him to fall behind because his poor little legs just couldn't keep up with hers. For a city boy he was very slow. The train roared behind them as if a giant steel worm out for food; the sound was like an explosion, and Delilah loved it, though in this dream it was a bit evil.

"I used to live in this borough with my foster family."

"I know."

"Yea, but," Rez pulled the joint from his pocket and lit it with his green flame zippo lighter, "they'd probably kill me if they knew I was back here."

"You've been gone for over five years, they wouldn't even remember you."

"I cut their paycheck down by leaving. I know they want me back, for the moneyyyy!"

The New York Pavilion was coming upon the

onyx sky on the left, two copper space ships certain to have dropped that creature off at the shore; maybe the atmosphere of the earth had killed it. But Rez had talked about genetic mutations, and how that was much scarier than some stupid thing from a remote deep dark universe. To have real people—scientists—grow new limbs and mouths in places where they weren't given by nature was something Delilah didn't know how to make sense of. It was worse than Rez's bad luck; worse than her screaming nightmares. All she knew was that her National Geographic collection couldn't explain it, and the internet called it a *Montauk Monster*, but she knew her creature was none of that.

Every single picture she took with her digital camera brought back a distorted image, a shape-shifted thing that her eyes couldn't adjust too. Its sandpaper skin left rashes across her body. She'd spent nights petting it, feeling every crease and wrinkle of its body. This led to her dreams becoming monsters themselves, her mind jumbling thoughts crazily. Was this price to pay for inspiration? The creature was metamorphosing even in its death as if trying to vanish from this planet. The thing influenced her like a bad hallucinogenic. It was making her crazy.

"I'm going to sit. You go ahead. I want to practice my strumming," Rez said, speech slurring a bit.

Rez sat down on the smooth edge of the fountain, fucking around with the Warlock again. His strumming was getting better, but he might as well have been playing the guitar with claws. His wretched throaty voice was echoing awesome, but the colliding sounds were like music being raped.

And then Delilah saw the boy playing in the pile of dried autumn leaves.

Pale spot.

Blind spot like a roundabout.

Rez's music made the strange boy with the tri-colored hair lift his peaked face in the air, stop his drawing on the ground and smile the blackest smile Delilah had ever seen. His eyes were huge and limitless; his hands were flippers. Delilah moved to talk to him, but he began to quickly wash the symbols away, ones that looked like the glyphs etched into the monster's skin. Before she knew it, the boy was swimming in the air, leaving a trace smell of bad cinnamon.

"Stop," she said as she got closer. "You're messing things up."

Rez stopped. "There's a nightclub I want you to see. The last of its kind."

"Did you see him?"

"See who?"

"The boy."

"I saw nobody."

Delilah gave up, pulling herself out of dream world and was back on the train in a flash, ready to rest her brain.

***

THIS SIDE OF THE borough is tricky. The streets yawn wide and the people move passed like black wisps of wind, heads bowed and covered by wiry hair, nervous fingers clutching cigarettes and sticky bottles of rotgut liquor. You can meet your best friend here, or encounter a solid rock star without noticing; the atmosphere itself takes your mind out of reality and pulls it into its own dimension.

Rez and Delilah found themselves traversing its half cobblestone, half blacktop streets looking for the club. The weeks had been languorous on Delilah. She'd broken her back at the laptop trying to find clues about what the creature was; she learned to sleep with one eye open while projecting her body into dreamland to find the boy again, but failing miserably. She watched the creature's descent into its new body carefully: tortured limbs frozen in broken angles, beak and tongue bitter blue with age, eyes gauged open, hurt.

Even her pet bat Zazo didn't like it. He'd made it his business to stay away from wherever the creature was. Delilah even noticed now that the warts on her hand were getting worse, wondered if this meant she was turning into a new being as if some mutating cells growing her a new skin. That would be wicked!

The club was a smudge of stretched neon and tendrils of pot smoke when looked at from far away, like bad streaks in a window you just can't clean. It lay between crumbling tenements that seemed to be built from charcoal. The corner bars sold dollar PBR's through the smashed window panes for half that rate, hoping for any idiot patron to come inside. In the distance, a metal slinking sound of a train stopped at a station.

As they slipped through the door Rez noticed a dark pink veve and dream catcher logo glowing under the black light above. He tried to alert Delilah because she kept talking about the fucked up symbols and how they were going to influence her new music, and about some boy who was an alien invader with limitless potential. But her mind focused only on the riotous sounds of the music. Immediately the smell of whiskey and wine crept up the cement stairs as they descended. Not even the faintest trace of oxygen could surely flow here. There was dead light everywhere, glass chinking and chains covered in lace slung across the walls. The floor opened up into stroboscopic maze of bleached hair, fangs, fishnet and nameless obscurities scrawled along the stone walls. This was a culture that people believed was a dead trend, but alive in the basement of the city right.

Delilah's spidery hair reflected the light; her face appeared rotted from the inside, skin so translucent Rez could see the row of teeth beneath her lips as if some kind of x-ray. Some people passed around blotter acid from in neat little sheets. Rez took one, not accepting the one from a lion-faced girl who offered it with her tongue. As the crowd thickened so did their tempers and it separated Rez and Delilah. Rez went around touching everything he could: the obscene grime built upon dust, insignias of magic and delirium, and band patches stapled to the lone billboard.

If he stood still long enough, the feedback from the guitars could surely swallow him like a mouth full of static, or make his brain explode within his head. This place would surely be haunted when the sun rose, when the kids filtered out to hibernate from daylight. The battered stage was streaked with paint like tinsel; a band was blowing fire from their mouths while drinking chartreuse out of scarlet goblets. They announced a new tune and their name, *Sodom's Sanctuary*, the lead singer's face bleached pale with sharp teeth as he grinned, pointed finger nails forming a cut into his wrist.

The kids jeered for more. The boundless joy of Psilocybin mushrooms with a chaser of absinthe guided their night-world of smoky mayhem. Then the music jangled, filling the room with a fear and loathing. Rez watched the band run through two sketchy songs before being confronted by a short boy with tri-colored hair, torso covered in fishnet, and a funny looking peaked face. He reached for Rez and pulled him close, and Rez noticed the strangest kind of hand he'd ever seen: slimy like fish skin, almost like a penguin flipper. The boy's one eye was a pool of blood, the other brown. *Delilah would like him*, he thought. *Alex would too.* The boy gave Rez an eighth of a mushroom and he nearly choked on the squalid taste, but the burn of vodka with a splash of red bull took the bitterness away. The drug hit Rez in almost an instant; it had been a while since he'd taken a hallucinogenic.

The room moved around him like a wave pool, colors

mixing before his eyes and bursting like a supernova as the crescendo of music came alive. Things felt very mixed up. The boys and girls went stiff around him, as if walking in line to the apocalypse. That's when the boy pulled Rez to the bar, slicked in beer and the purple glitter strobe of the black lights. It all left him unable to see straight, didn't let him hear the mindless conversations sifting through the loud music about voodoo and the occult. He felt brainwashed. But the boy held Rez's hand tight, nasty-slimed flipper fingers copping an all too sneaky feel. And then Rez heard it, a voice introducing a new rock and roll riot: Delilah.

"Straight from Pennsylvania, here to *caress us* with her vocals, DELILAH!"

The people didn't make any noise for her at first, not like she looked like she cared anyway. Rez knew that Delilah didn't need anyone to like her music in order to get her to sing. He knew she'd blow all of them away. The music cued and Delilah began to hum behind the keyboard's spiking rhythm that boarded on the insane, the drums that beat slow and mischievous in time with her. The guitarist crept up to the chorus pressing various distortion pedals. When Delilah opened her mouth the crowd seemed to sober up and stood attentive, their graceless hands moved into the air and began to clap. Her voice was the magic of a great goddess.

"I know she's been wanting to see me," the boy said to Rez leaning on the bar.

"What?"

The boy turned to the bar and ordered two goblets that came with green liquor inside, passed one to Rez and as their fingers kissed Rez felt his cold touch again, reminding him of instant death, an unearthly feeling, not like he imagined his warm tongue.

"What do you mean?"

The boy's eyebrows arched into straight V's. "She's

been marking me like a dog at a fire hydrant in her little dreamland."

He began to scrawl with a small pencil on a bar napkin, and Rez turned away to watch Delilah cast her magic. She was doing an original *Electric Orchid* tune. How *Sodom's Sanctuary* knew her music was a guess all of its own, but *Electric Orchid* had gotten popular enough in the New York underground scene for other bands to know their music. Rez pulled his slouched shoulders straight, like a rope tightened into a knot, and lifted his head above the crowd to hear Delilah end her song. She walked off the stage and everyone scampered out of her way quickly, afraid of her feminine brutality. She found Rez and he ordered her a gin and lime gimlet, served in a beer mug.

"That one's free for the lady singer," the bartender said. "Radical song."

She thanked him and nearly choked on it the minute she turned her head and saw the boy. Her eyes flushed into the color of inquisition, solemn as night. Rez knew it was her instant, curious look of approval.

"You," she said.

"Nilea, Delilah, the name's Nilea." The boy looked right through Delilah, still scribbling on his napkin.

"That's a chick's name," said Delilah.

"Actually where I come from, male names end in A."

"Where's that, exactly?"

"Never mind that. You've been looking for me in your dreams, haven't you?"

"Yes."

The boy's thin nostrils went wide. "Ah, the smell, I can smell it. It's feels like home."

Delilah's eyes sharpened, and even in the devilish light it made her seem innocent.

"Like home?"

The boy mumbled ancient words as he read from

his napkin. Delilah looked at Rez and almost broke out in a careful laughter. She had found weird symbols on the internet that were related to those words. It came from a deceased language recorded as the mother of all diachronic tongues. It was rumored that aliens had taught the human race this language.

"I *know* those words…"

"Of course you do, Delilah." The boy licked his lips. "I can see your dreams, see them well. The faces in the dark, the hands waving, and the symbols from the bay. My symbols and my language. I was once a lost puppy, but now I'm going home."

"Where is that?"

"And this rash on your hand," the boy moved his cold-slicked finger over hers, "this means you've touched something that doesn't belong to you."

"What? I just wanted some new inspiration."

"But you shouldn't steal. Isn't that what the law says?"

Delilah froze as if she wanted to scream, fists clenched; the bumps on her hand began to pulse. Rez knew she was on the verge of attack for being made a fool. She always had a hidden rage that was waiting to boil over; such is why she carried her X-acto in hand. Rez threw more drinks down his throat, unable to speak. If Delilah was lost for words, the situation was more than strange, it was preternatural.

"What language?" Rez asked.

"Sumerian," he said in a monotone, turning to leave.

"Hey! Where're you going?" Delilah yelled.

"You can thank me later. Consider this our first and last engagement."

The boy vanished through the people and spiraling yellow smoke. Delilah asked for another gimlet and put a cigarette to her lips, lighting it and staring into the orange burning sphere as if it could suck her soul away. Her anger calmed as the boy's eerie essence grew weaker and weaker. Random death-heads and metal kids asked Delilah to play again, their hair covering their baby pale eyes. But Delilah decided to leave after she read what the boy had drawn on the napkin, crumbling it and throwing it to the floor. When Rez looked at it, he saw the symbols she had found online, drawn in plain black and white as if the boy could read her mind. And perhaps he did.

***

BACK AT REZ'S APARTMENT Delilah was doing her typical antsy pacing back and forth, barefoot, her toenails painted red with swirls of black in it. She had Rosetta Stoned stuck in her head, and Maynard James Keenan's growling voice were piercing the delicate tissues of her inner ear.

ET revealed to me his singular purpose... he said you are the chosen one. The one who'll deliver the message to those who choose to hear it, and a warning to those who do not.

"Stop moving around, it's gotta be here," Rez yelled as he rummaged through cabinets, throwing plastic tupperware and beer cans all over the place.

"It was under the bed... I swear I put it under the bed."

They both stormed to the bedroom again, the first time nothing was touched or out of place, the lamp was lit, the air thick as summer soup, the posters were still thumb tacked in place, and the curtains were pulled shut. But this time, with the lights off and the only shine from outside, there were the symbols. They were streaked like paint, sagging from the ceiling as if a crop circle dying its last day, or a dried sponge with fingerprints still sunk into it.

"It was that fucking asshole kid! He took my animal!"

"No, Delilah. You're wrong."

"Where's the guitar, I'm gunna' smash it over your head!"

"He *was* the animal."

"All that work down the drain. All that research. Gone! How can I focus?"

"Are you paying attention?"

"I was going to write a fucking song about it. Just like how I wrote my lyrics for *28 Days*. Remember that movie?"

"Of course."

"Inspiration… gone now."

Delilah could have forced herself to sleep, taking her body back to the bay in the other world to lay patient for the boy to come again from his space-hell land, but Delilah didn't want to do that, she'd given up. Inspiration would have to come in other forms. Instead she bashed the cardboard box where she kept the creature against the wall until a beam of light bolted from it, and at the same time Zazo came swooping down and cradled itself in her breast. A symbol shot like a star out of the box, drawing slow moving shapes onto the ceiling, and they were exactly like the ones from the sand Flushing Bay: Sumerian hieroglyphics that she could not decipher.

The language of the aliens!

Nilea… Nilea… Alien!

In a simple flash the box was gone, left only was the cellophane wrapping still fresh with the creature's rotted essence. Delilah would not sleep tonight, perhaps not ever. And that was okay because Rez loved nights. Somewhere in her head Delilah heard new lyrics.

I'm about to make a brand new start of it, right there in old New York.

Thadd Presley Presents

The Conscience of Janice Clovell
S. Wayne Roberts

THE CLOCK STRUCK 7:14PM as the strongest portion of the autumn evening fell upon this small town. Sitting in his car, he couldn't help but look up at the sky, wishing for an answer to why he was there. Though it was not out of the ordinary to be parked outside of that house, this particular evening there was an extra party involved whom made everything all the more complicated.

"How long has this been going on?"

Shaun happened to catch his reflection in the mirror. He could barely stand the sight of what he saw. The salt and pepper hair that laid at shoulder length and the thick brown glasses that Shaun had always assumed where the ugliest pair to have ever been made. His 5 o'clock shadow was getting the best of him, as the clock ticked on and on passed 7pm.

Fourteen Twenty-Seven Lancaster Drive was the home of Kenneth Brady, who had been Shaun's best friend for years. Normally this house was where he would go to avoid his wife, but today it was the one he followed her to. All he could do was speculate on what was taking place inside, even though Shaun was able to see them occasionally walk past a window.

What if I am wrong? Shaun questioned. *What if this is*

completely innocent and I am just overreacting?

Aware of how embarrassing this would be if he burst in with his false accusations, screaming and fighting without the slightest bit of proof, he slowly slid out of his car. He crept up to the nearest window, carefully and quietly to avoid the nearby neighbors. From within Ken's azaleas he could see them, stripped naked and on top of each other on Ken's couch.

Shaun felt as if he would be sick, yet he couldn't take his eyes off of his jezebel wife and traitor friend. On and on he watched their sensual movements, until he finally lost his lunch in the flower bed.

***

WHIPPING DOWN THE SIDE streets, Shaun's mind was racing and his eyes were fixed on his left hand. The occasional horn blowing from a passerby was about all that broke him from his obsession. He never took off his wedding band, not even when he showered. Today it seemed to be burning his finger, as well as his soul. He quickly ripped it from his finger and threw it into the ashtray.

Well, that solved that then.

Shaun turned on the radio in hopes of a good song, only to be let down by commercials. Beaming from his car speakers was an ad about marriage statistics and how only through God could marriage last. The last thing Shaun needed was an overdose of televangelism, but the ad seemed to capture the fragile man.

"Listen to me, my Brothers and Sisters. Hear my voice and know that I speak the truth. A moral and lawful marriage can work, though all of this premarital fornication flooding this already sin filled world is saddening to the eyes of God, for He loves you," Brother Billy J. Colewell said with a southern accent.

That'll be enough of that. Shaun turned off the radio and its nonsense.

By the time Shaun was done with the radio broadcast, he noticed that he had covered a great distance and was nearly home. This was lucky for Shaun to have noticed, beyond other obvious reasons, he had almost missed his turn. Turning onto Woodland Boulevard was nothing short of daily routine, though Shaun had never felt such sadness while pulling toward his home. Passing house after identical house, Shaun pulled up to his own. With a deep breath and a hanging head, Shaun pulled his car toward the center of the street, took another deep breath and proceeded to back into the driveway.

Sitting there in his car, he couldn't help but think about Wendy. Think about what she might have been doing at Ken's house. The usual excuse of working late or a girl's night out was enough for Shaun, though a funny feeling and stealthy driving brought him to them. To 1427 Lancaster Drive, where he would often pick up Ken for a hard night of drinking and harmless flirting with waitresses.

"Working late? Is that what they call it now?" Shaun mumbled as he turned off the engine. He opened the car door with a shove, with keys in hand; he swung his legs out angrily. "Girls night out? But I always assumed that Ken was the pitcher in his relationships."

Jingling the keys in his hand as he approached the door, he noticed a mailbox with the number 37 printed on the front of it, which was no doubt stuffed with bills. With no interest in reading his mail or even picking it up, he just left it in the box as he slipped his key in the door. A quick turn of the wrist and the door swung open to his home. The one he bought for her after their wedding, also being the one that he could just barely afford.

"Honey, I'm home!" Shaun yelled as he entered the doorway, closing the door behind him.

Though there was nobody to hear him, he still liked to do it. It made him feel like the happy husband from the old movies, though he never had the housewife meeting him at the door. Never walked into his home and smelled the sweet scent of dinner on the stove. Shaun was not the sexist type who wanted the desperate housewife, he just wanted a wife. One who didn't physically live in a cubical and emotionally strive for his best friend.

With his keys on the hook and his jacket on the rack, Shaun made his way through the foyer and on to the kitchen for his post-work beer. Shaun popped the top, his mouth had become very dry and he couldn't wait for that ice cold liquid to hit his lips. Though it quenched his thirst, it wasn't as sensational as his mind had made it out to be. Shaun took a couple more big drinks, belched, grabbed another can and tossed his empty in the trash.

Upon making his way back through the foyer and into the living room, Shaun flopped down in his dark blue recliner. It was probably the only piece of furniture in the house that he liked. The rest of it Wendy picked out, which was fancy and nice, though hard enough to make your butt go numb. The color of the rest of the living room furniture confused Shaun, both because it was completely white and it somehow never got ruined. Thinking back to it, Shaun had to fight hard to even get this chair into the room, which is why it's off to the corner where it was only a minor eyesore.

As Shaun put the chair back and his legs up, he opened his beer and reached for the TV remote. Though his mind was racing and he could hardly care about television, he flipped on the news and then just closed his eyes.

"Police still have no suspects in the murder of Janice Clovell, whom was found dead in her home early this morning," announced the news anchor for the evening news.

Janice Clovell? Where do I know that name?

The report caused Shaun to sit up in his chair, eyes wide and listening intently. He clicked rewind on the remote and searched back to the beginning with his DVR. Twice more he listened to the sterile voice calmly stating Janice's untimely demise, and then finally it hit him.

Shaun sprang from his chair, spilling his drink in the process as he ran from the living room. He went through the foyer, up the stairs and into the master bedroom, which brought him to the closet.

"C'mon now, I know that it's here," Shaun mumbled to himself as he searched the closet.

A small white box with a red ribbon normally sat on the top shelf, though it was nowhere to be found. The box contained many pictures and videos of the family. Mostly full of Wendy's family, Shaun knew that he had a few of his own photos jammed in there.

It isn't here?! What the hell?! His anger was finally beginning to catch up to him.

He stuffed the junk back in the closet, slammed the door shut and then turned to give the room a once over. For a moment he just stood there, stewing in his emotions and cursing that damn white box with the red ribbon

"Where is my box? For that matter, who the hell is Janice Clovell?" Shaun questioned, expecting no answer.

The box was nowhere to be found upstairs, which infuriated Shaun. Not knowing if his wife misplaced it or even threw it away, plus the burning question of Janice Clovell was haunting him. Shaun needed answers for far too many questions today and he knew that he wouldn't get any by standing in the bedroom alone, so he made his way back down stairs.

As Shaun reached the bottom of the steps, he heard the front door slam. Instead of announcing his presence, he just peered around the corner of the wall at his wife. Her shoulder length blond hair was a bit messy and her white button up shirt was wrinkled, which was the total opposite of how it looked in the morning. Wendy looked very tired, which could be from a long day's work or a sinful evening with Kenneth. He ducked back behind the wall, freezing in place as he listened to his wife hang up her coat.

The tapping of her high heels on the floor told Shaun that she was drawing near. Still unable to move and unaware of what to say when he did, he just stood there and she walked right in front of him. She nearly walked right past him, but caught a glimpse out of the corner of her eye and gasped. She dropped all of the stuff in her hands, including the little white box with a red ribbon.

"What the hell, Shaun?" Wendy shouted.

"I'm sorry. I didn't notice you were here," Shaun explained, disgusted that he had said sorry out of habit.

"Even so, why were you hiding on the stairs?"

"I wasn't hiding, I was walking down them."

"Whatever Shaun, I don't want to play your games. Please, just help me clean this up."

Without another word, Shaun stepped down off the steps and began to gather the stuff off of the floor. First her purse and date book, which Wendy snatched from him. Then he began to clean up the box of photos and videos. Once completely gathered and closed up, Shaun stood up with the box, though not extending it to Wendy.

"Did you need this for work?" Shaun asked with a smirk on his face.

"Why would that matter? They are mine anyway," Wendy answered with a dismissive shrug.

"It's ours actually. You didn't marry yourself, did you?"

"If only that were possible."

"Wendy, I didn't ask to be possessive. I simply need to know how I know Janice Clovell."

"Why?"

"Because she was found dead this morning."

Without another word, Wendy covered her mouth and rushed up the stairs. Instead of chasing her, Shaun continued into the kitchen with the box. Shaun grabbed a beer from the refrigerator, opening it as he sat down in front of the box.

"The answer must be here," Shaun said to himself as he skimmed through the photos.

To find her would be easy, assuming that she is in the photos. Wendy always marked the back of her photos with names, dates and times, which seemed to be a bit much until now. It took a few minutes. Shaun even had time to finish his beer before he saw it. There it was right in front of him, on April 12, 2002 at 2:43, there was a picture of Wendy and another of her cousin Janice. The picture looked familiar, though he could have passed her on the street without notice. There was no reason, as far as this picture could explain, for Shaun to remember Janice. He *did*, though. She wasn't very attractive, being middle-aged and a bit overweight with glasses, her curly shoulder length brown hair didn't do much for Shaun either.

Think you idiot, think, Shaun thought. He thumped himself on the forehead with his palm.

Leaning back in his chair with his palm against his forehead, Shaun noticed the red light on the phone charger was blinking. The red light was only on if the cordless was charging and blinking if the phone was in use. The cordless was not on the charger that hung on the kitchen wall. Slowly, Shaun turned in his chair as he sat up right, thinking of who his wife could have called.

Shaun got up and began to tiptoe up the stairs, which is where the only other phone in the house was kept. The cordless, being the universal phone of the house could be found sitting in any room. There was an old phone with a cord in the hallway, in case of emergency. Step by step, Shaun somehow made it without making a single noise. Slowly, he removed the phone from off the hook and places it to his ear.

"What did I tell you, Wendy? Didn't I tell you not to worry," Ken asked.

"Yes, I know, but this is serious. Not only was she found, but Shaun is also asking questions," Wendy explained, the anxiety was clear in her voice.

"Shaun? Don't worry about Shaun, he's an idiot." Ken chuckled as he tried to assure Wendy.

"Stop telling me not to worry! I think Shaun may really be on to us."

"Wendy, please just trust me."

"O.K. I'm trying. Can we meet now? I need to see you."

"Yeah, sure, the motel like we discussed."

"OK, I love you."

"I love you, too."

Shaun could barely believe what he is hearing. How could it be that his wife and best friend got together, not only to fool around but to commit a murder? He waited for them both to hang up before he did, then quietly stood there, staring at the bedroom that his wife was calling from. Suddenly Shaun heard a lot of commotion coming from the bedroom, so he quickly rushed down the stairs, just barely making it to the kitchen before the bedroom door swung open.

"Shaun?" Wendy called out as she walked down the stairs.

"Yes?" Shaun answered as he walked from the kitchen.

"I just received a called and I need to get back to the office." Wendy explained, while rushing toward the door.

Standing there for a moment, not sure of what to say, Shaun watched Wendy put on her coat and swing her purse over her shoulder. Shaun cleared his throat just as Wendy turned the doorknob, which caused her to stop for a moment.

"The phone didn't ring," he said with a smile.

"What?"

"The phone."

"Oh, well maybe you just didn't..." Wendy tried to explain.

"I heard your phone call. I heard all of the call with Ken."

"You're mistaken. That wasn't Ken, you're..."

For the first time in their marriage, Shaun had been the one to leave Wendy completely speechless, which felt really good. He couldn't help but smile.

Wendy's jaw hung half open as she stood frozen. Refusing to keep eye contact with him, it looked as if Wendy was searching for the right thing to say. Before she could say anything, Shaun turned back toward the stairs.

"I am sorry Wendy; I am just tired and likely mistaken. Do have a safe drive and decent time at work, my dear," Shaun said, just before running upstairs.

How could she lie to me, even when she has been caught red handed? Well, I haven't caught her red handed, at least not yet.

That thought made him run faster up the steps. All of the stress of the day seemed to be filling Shaun. He could feel his face going numb and a burning pain in his stomach. The discomfort made him want to follow her even more.

Once at the top of the steps, Shaun began to pace back and forth in the hallway. He knew what he had to do, but had no clue how to do it. He had to follow them to this motel that Ken spoke of, but if they were capable of murder then this could be dangerous.

Shaun walked into the bedroom. His anger grew with every step. Then the nightstand caught his eye and he remembered his 9mm pistol that he kept for protection.

Am I really ready to take this step? Shaun asked himself.

Then he shook off the feeling of doubt, knowing that he had to do this and quick. Shaun rushed over to the nightstand, removed the pistol and checked the clip. A full clip was a relief to Shaun, though he hoped to only use it as a scare tactic. Gun in hand, Shaun ran from the room and down the stairs.

"Calm down, I just forgot my keys!" Wendy screamed, as she noticed the gun.

"Oh, I'm sorry. I guess I had fallen asleep and got scared." Shaun explained.

"Well, be careful, guns and alcohol don't mix, you know." Wendy added with a smile.

Without a verbal response, Shaun turned to the kitchen and grabbed her keys. After handing them to her, he watched her walk out the door. Once the door closed, he ran over to it and looked out. As Wendy started her engine, Shaun snuck from the home and crept toward his car. Once she started to take off down the street, Shaun jumped in his car and quickly whipped it out of the driveway.

With his gun in the passenger seat Shaun quickly sped down the street, trying to make sure that he didn't lose her. Finally catching her at the stop sign just at the end of their street, Shaun did a rolling stop, and then made a right turn behind his wife.

A right? This place must be in the middle of nowhere. Shaun thought to himself.

He followed closely, though not close enough to be spotted. All along the way his mind was racing. Anger and betrayal caused alien thoughts he never imagined before. With every second he spent staring into the red glow of her taillights his fury grew and his thoughts grow darker. Shaun grew so angry that he didn't notice until long after that they had went passed Ken's street.

Marley lodge was Shaun's guess, but only time would tell. Marley Lodge was some run down motel at the edge of town, standing in the middle of nothing but trees.

"I always knew that Ken was a man of substance." Shaun mumbled snidely. "This is sure to be a classy place that he picked out."

The Marley Lodge motel was a single level resort with about 12 rooms; Wendy pulled into a parking space halfway down the row. Shaun followed, not parking too close. He sat within view as she got out of her car and quickly approached room number 6, looked around and then entered.

Wow, this was well planned. Except they thought I'm too stupid to follow. Shaun smirked.

Shaun knew that he was the better man this time. He refused to allow himself to run off with his tail between his legs. He killed the engine, and then began to step out of the car. Keys in hand, he locked it with his remote. He tucked his gun in the waistband of his pants. Ducking down, he ran toward room number 6 and his mischievous wife.

Upon reaching the door, Shaun was overcome with the greatest stomach cramp he had ever felt. On one hand he would love to burst in and hurt them, yet he also had a strong love for both of them. It seemed so easy to imagine the conflict while behind the wheel, yet it became complicated once the decisions were now lying before him. Shaun felt a couple tears roll down his cheeks as he gripped the handle of his gun, which felt now more than ever like his only hope.

The faint sound of Wendy's moaning voice could be heard from the room, which caused Shaun's whole body to begin to shake. One hand still on the grip, he grabbed the doorknob with the other and twisted it hard, only to find the door locked.

"Locked out?" asked the night manager.

The voice startled Shaun, which nearly made him jerk his gun from his pants. Pulling his shirt down over the gun he turned around to greet the chunky old man.

"I am sorry, did I scare you," questioned the night manager with a smile.

"Yes, no, umm... I *am* locked out," Shaun stammered.

"Oh, well I have keys. Boy oh boy, it sounds like a wild party in there."

"Yes, it is. I am here to surprise them."

"Oh, well maybe I had better knock first. You know, just to make sure."

"No! Listen to me, that is my wife and my best friend in there, they're expecting me."

"Oh? Oh… I see. To each his own I guess. A bit too kinky for my taste, but I ain't one to judge."

Shaun forced himself to laugh as the old man searched for the key. His palms began to sweat as he anticipated the moment that now was just heart beats away.

"Actually, here's the key. I don't want to ruin the mood by opening the door in front of you."

"Thank you, sir."

"Hey, the name is Larry."

"Shaun."

"Well, have fun in there, Shaun."

Shaun watched as Larry made his way toward the office. He then stuck the key in the door. One twist of the wrist and the door began to open. Shaun eased the door open and stuck his head in. The first thing that Shaun was able to see was his wife on top of his best friend, completely naked and screaming.

Unable to contain himself, Shaun burst into the room reaching for the light switch. As soon as the lights can on, Wendy leaped from the bed, wrestling for the blankets as she hit the floor. Ken, with his short brown buzz cut, sat up and placed a pillow in front to cover him.

"Oh God, Shaun," Wendy said with her head in her hands.

"Shaun, buddy, this isn't what you think." Ken explained.

"Oh really? Then please, tell me what it this. Tell me, because all I see is my wife fucking my best friend!" Shaun screamed.

"Shaun, man, I don't know what to say. I just…" Ken tried to explain.

"You just what, you thought she needed it? Am I all wrong, did she trip and fall on your dick?" Shaun demanded.

"Shaun, I'm sorry."

"What for, Ken? For fucking my wife or for getting caught?"

Before Ken or Wendy could answer, Shaun pulled his gun from his waistband. He thrust his pistol at Ken, as if daring him to make his move. He then turned his gun to his darling wife. Wendy started to scream, and then placed her hand over her mouth as Shaun cocked the gun and rushed a couple steps toward her.

"Shaun, this is crazy. What are you doing?" Ken asked.

"Crazy? I'm crazy, am I?" Shaun screamed as he pointed the gun at Ken.

"Shaun, please stop this," Wendy pleaded through her tears.

"Shut up!"

As Shaun screamed at Wendy, he pointed the gun at her and began to approach her. Ken got up and tried to jump toward Shaun. As he stood up Shaun fired once. Ken fell against the wall, twisting in pain as blood poured from his gut. He grabbed the spot where the bullet put the wound. His pale fingers were painted red as he dug at the exposed tissue.

Wendy let out a loud scream. Shaun rushed over and hit her in the face with the butt of his gun. Wendy fell limp to the floor as he turned his attention back to Ken.

"Look at me."

"Please, Shaun, call for help. Please, man, please!"

"I said fucking *look at me!*"

Ken did as he was told.

"I'm sorry." Shaun said as he placed the gun against Ken's head. "You sealed your fate when you screwed my wife. You fired the bullet the first time you put your dick in her, it just took this long for it to kill your worthless ass."

Shaun closed his eyes and squeezed the trigger. He felt the moist splatter of his Heterosexual life partner's brains on the front of his shirt. He opened his eyes and wiped a splatter of blood from one of his haggard cheeks.

Ken's neck was leaned back at an odd angle. The entry wound just above Ken's right eye didn't seem big enough to have killed him, but upon further inspection Shaun found a softball sized exit wound at the top of his crown.

Shaun looked at Ken for only a moment before it occurred to him that Larry would have heard the shots.

Quickly, he leapt over the bed and grabbed Wendy by the hair, forcing her up onto her feet. Half out of it from the blow, she tried to fight him off by pulling his hair. Shaun grabbed her by her throat and began to choke her. He squeezed with all his might, feeling the life leave her body, just as new life rush flowed through his own. Then he delivered two more blows to her face, which caused her to fall to her knees. Her cheek burst open as the second blow landed. The flap of skin and tissue fell away from the cracked bone. Her head lolled despite his firm hold on her hair.

He stuffed his gun back in his pants as he picked her up and lifted her over his shoulder.

Very paranoid as to what might have been outside waiting, Shaun peaked around the corner. The parking lot was deserted. Without another moments thought, Shaun began to race toward his car. Keys in hand, he unlocked the doors with his remote and threw Wendy in the passenger side. He got in and put on their seat belts.

Shaun looked around for any sign of Larry, as to make sure he still went unnoticed. Now without a moment to lose, Shaun whipped the car backwards, and then turned around toward the highway.

Speeding down Marley highway, going the opposite direction from their home, Shaun swerved past a few 18 wheelers. He only took his eyes off the road to see if Wendy regained consciousness. He continually sped toward an unknown destination.

"Wendy, wake up," Shaun yelled as he shook her.

"Shaun, where are we going?" Wendy asked as she came conscience.

"I haven't thought of that yet. Now tell me, what happened to Janice Clovell?" Shaun questioned.

"Why do you care?"

"Damn it, Wendy. Tell me now! She was your damn cousin, why did you kill her?"

An awkward silence fell over the car as Wendy stared a hole into Shaun, while he passed around another truck. The only thing to break her gaze was the gun resting in the front of Shaun's pants. He noticed that she was staring toward his lap so he quickly grabbed his pistol. He brandished his gun in her face, mocking her like a child.

"What's wrong Wendy, did Ken not measure up to what I'm packing?" Shaun asked with a laugh. "Start fucking talking, darling. I'm tired of looking at your ugly face."

"It was Ken." Wendy said.

"Ken killed Janice, but why?" Shaun asked

"Janice was a life insurance salesperson and Ken tried to get her to go along with killing you."

"Wait a minute, back up a second. Killing me?"

"Yes. Ken thought that Janice could help hide your murder and then we could collect on a policy that she would set up."

"Janice had a conscience?"

"Yes."

"At least somebody did."

"Hey, speak for yourself. I am the only person in this car who isn't a murderer."

Shaun couldn't find the words to even begin to respond to that. Even if Ken wanted to kill Shaun, it was still an act of murder. This whole situation had turned Shaun into a monster and he was finally aware of it.

Shaun tossed the gun into the backseat and then placed both hands tightly on the steering wheel. He was forced to slow down based on a car in front of them and an 18 wheeler gaining speed in the oncoming lane.

"Shaun, listen to me. It is not too late for us, we can just run. The two of us could be so happy."

Shaun didn't respond with words. He reached over and ripped the torn flesh from her bleeding face. As she screamed he pressed down on the gas and merged into the oncoming lane. Gaining speed and closing in on the 18 wheeler, Shaun closed his eyes and Wendy screamed louder than ever.

"Shaun, what are you doing? Stop it, Shaun!"

The collision of his small car and the big rig was comparable to a train's collision with a go-kart. Glass flying, airbags bursting and lives fading. The world was likely to blame Shaun for all the deaths. He didn't care anymore. He had to put an end to the monstrosity known as his life. He opened his eyes at the last moment.

Unbeknownst to the world or even to Shaun was the logical explanation for all the mayhem. Logic went out the window with his marriage.

The last sound to be heard by Shaun was that of his

wife's screams.

His last sight was of bright headlights of his oncoming doom.

His last feeling was that of death's icy grip.

Thadd Presley Presents

The Old Fishin' Hole
Todd Martin

"SLOW DOWN, ASSHOLE!" DENNIS gasped as he struggled up the hill behind Justin.

Justin turned and faced him, fighting the urge to tell him that he probably wouldn't be having such a difficult time keeping up if he wasn't so fat and out of shape.

Dennis was a rather plump eleven-year-old, and if he didn't change his eating habits soon he was certain to tip the scales at two hundred pounds or more by his twelfth birthday.

"Jesus Christ, where the hell is this pond again?" Dennis asked as he tried to catch his breath.

"We're almost there; it's just down at the foot of this hill a little bit." Justin replied, watching in a combination of disbelief and disgust as Dennis took out a cigarette and lit it.

Dennis took a long drag off of the cigarette and immediately went into a violent coughing fit. He gagged and choked for a few moments and then to Justin's surprise he proceeded to take another hit off of it, making him cough even harder.

"You want one?" Dennis asked, wiping at his eyes that were watering like there was no tomorrow.

"No thanks, I don't smoke and neither should you."

Justin replied proudly (he knew mostly from watching GI Joe cartoons that smoking was bad).

"Why not, you scared?"

"No, I just don't want to do it. It isn't for me. I don't want to put that kind of crap in my body."

"Whatever, more for me then."

"Where'd you get them anyway?"

"I swiped a couple from your dad."

"What? Why would you do something like that?" Justin asked, feeling himself become scared as well as angry, "He's going to know that some are missing and he'll know that you took them!"

"Just relax, he was passed out dog drunk on the couch, he'll never know they're gone," Dennis said, throwing what was left of the cigarette he was smoking on the ground and stepping on it, "quit being such a fucking baby."

Justin didn't respond and instead just stood there wondering to himself why he ever hang out with Dennis in the first place. He was three years younger and a hell of a lot more mature, and he just didn't really care for him in general. He thought that he was an obnoxious fat ass who thought that he knew everything and tried to act like he was some sort of tough guy even though in reality he was a big wimp who was afraid of his own shadow. He was a spoiled rotten brat and his parents always bought him whatever he wanted, a fact that he always threw in Justin's face. It was no secret that Dennis didn't really have any friends his own age (most of his classmates hated him and picked on him unmercifully), so he hung out with Justin because no one else wanted to have anything to do with him.

They had lived next door to each other for years and more than once Justin had prayed that Dennis' family would move away so that he wouldn't have to spend time with him anymore. Most of the members of Justin's family shared his hatred of Dennis (both of his older brothers had beaten him up a number of times) with the exception of his little sister who had a crush on him (but Justin was willing to forgive her since she was only six and didn't know any better).

They made their way down the hill with their fishing poles and tackle boxes (Dennis had a much easier time going down the hill) and Justin pointed toward the small pond in the distance.

"There it is, just like I said." Justin said, feeling the excitement building up in his chest.

"I didn't even know that there was a pond back here," Dennis said, taking Justin completely by surprise since he had never before admitted that he didn't know something. "How'd you find it?"

"Me and Jamie Cooper came across it a few months ago when we were camping out here."

"Jamie Cooper? That's that weird ass kid who is all obsessed with the military, isn't it?"

"He isn't weird!"

"Like hell he isn't. He walks around wearing camouflage and talks like he's a soldier or something. What the hell is wrong with him anyway?"

"There's nothing wrong with him, he's just really into the Army and stuff."

"What happened to him anyway? Didn't he like go missing or something?"

"Yeah," Justin replied quietly, not really wanting to talk about it.

"I heard that he ran away from home because his dickhead step dad was diddling him or something."

"I don't know."

"Some guys I go to school with even think that his step dad killed him so he wouldn't tell anybody he was

fucking him and buried him out in the woods. What do you
think? Is that true?"

"I really don't know, can we talk about something else?"

"What are you acting so funny about it for?" Dennis asked, eyeing him suspiciously, "You know where he is, don't you?"

"No I don't."

"Yeah you do, I can tell by the way you're acting. You better tell if you know something. I really don't give a shit if he's alive or dead myself but if you know where he is and don't tell anybody you can get in trouble."

"Look, I don't know where he is, OK? I wish I did but I don't. He's been missing for almost a month now and his mom is worrying herself to death about it. If I knew anything don't you think I would tell her?"

"OK, OK, don't piss your diapers or anything," Dennis snorted, "I don't care what you say, I think there's something you aren't telling me."

They walked the rest of the way to the pond in silence and once they reached it they sat down to bait their fishing poles. They'd dug up some worms earlier underneath Dennis' porch (actually Justin had done it as Dennis had been afraid to touch the worms because he'd just seen a movie about worms that ate people that scared him senseless) and had gathered quite a few to use as bait.

"You're sure there's some fish in here?" Dennis asked as he handed his pole to Justin so he could put a worm on the hook for him.

"Oh yeah, this pond is loaded with fish." he replied, impaling the worm through the midsection with the point of the hook.

"There better be, I'd hate to think I walked all the way out here in the middle of nowhere for nothing!"

"Don't worry! There's fish in there, I promise!"

They both cast their lines out into the water and sat waiting anxiously for their bobbers to disappear under the surface of the water, the signal that a fish had taken the bait. They had only been sitting there for a few minutes when Dennis got antsy and started complaining.

"This sucks! Where are all the fish you were talking about that were supposed to be in this pond?"

"You have to be patient. Sometimes it just takes them a little while before they start biting."

"Well I wish they'd hurry up, this is boring as hell. When we went to Florida last year we went deep sea fishing and it was a lot more exciting than this. I almost caught a shark that made Jaws look like a baby!"

"I think we're going to go to Florida this year. I bet Dad will take us out deep sea fishing too.

"Bullshit," Dennis snorted, "you're family's too poor to go to Florida. Even if you were able to scrape together enough money to go you'd never be able to afford to go deep see fishing. It's way too expensive for you guys."

Before Justin could respond Dennis' bobber was pulled under the water with tremendous force. He didn't even have time to set the hook before the line was tugged so hard that the fishing rod was ripped out of his hands and disappeared into the murky water of the pond.

"Holy shit!" Dennis exclaimed, jumping to his feet, "Did you just see that?"

"I sure did." Justin said, standing up and reaching over to pick up a large, thick branch that was on the ground behind Dennis.

"What the fuck is in there? I mean, what kind of fish could've done…" Dennis started but never got the chance to finish as Justin struck him in the back of the head with the branch, knocking him forward to the ground.

He surprised Justin by getting back up and turning to

face him, his eyes burning with anger. He took a menacing step toward him and he swung the branch again, connecting this time with a blow to the face that no doubt broke his nose and made him cry out in pain as he fell back into the pond. The sound of his obese body hitting the water made Justin think of a giant turd being dropped in a huge toilet and he couldn't help but laugh at the image in his head (which was appropriate he thought since he considered Dennis to be a piece of shit).

Dennis stood up in the waist-deep water holding his face. He was crying not just because his nose was broken and one of his front teeth had been knocked out but because he had gotten water in his ear as well (he was such a big baby when it came to getting water in his ears). Justin saw the water behind him ripple and smiled when he thought about how Dennis was about to really have something to cry about.

"You little shit!" Dennis managed to scream between sobs, "I'm going to rip your fucking head off and spit down your neck!"

He never got the chance to follow through on his threat as a tentacle with sharp prongs in its underside shot out of the water and wrapped around his head, shredding his face.

Justin had a weak stomach and closed his eyes, but not fast enough to not see several more tentacles wrap around various parts of Dennis and rip him in half at the waist. What was left of the upper half of him disappeared under the surface and the water soon turned red with his blood seconds later as they fed on him.

He saw one of Dennis' arms floating around on the top of the water and one of the things that lived in the pond jumped up out of the water to retrieve it in its mouth. Just the sight of one of them made his blood turn to ice and while he'd never seen one up close he prayed that he would never have to.

He didn't know what the things in the pond were or where they came from, but he knew that they were vicious and ravenous carnivores. They were about the size of his hand and had bodies that resembled catfish with the exception of the fact that they had tentacles and rows of razor sharp teeth similar to those of a shark's.

They had sharp, bony protrusions on their heads and eyes that were dark as night. There didn't seem to be a set color for them as he's seen a couple of red ones, green ones, and even a black one. He didn't even know how many of them lived in the pond and as far as he knew there could possibly be hundreds of them.

He wondered if they were some sort of prehistoric fish that somehow managed to survive all this time or if they were normal at one time and somehow became mutated due to exposure to some nuclear waste or something. The thought that they could be alien beings from another planet also crossed his mind but he thought that it was a little far-fetched. He wanted to catch one and take it to his science teacher to study but he was afraid if he did they would find pieces of Jamie (and now Dennis as well) inside of it.

Justin stood there looking at the pond for several minutes until the thrashing of the water stopped, meaning that the fish were done feasting and were satisfied for the moment. Since Dennis was a lot fatter than Jamie had been he hoped that they were so full that he wouldn't have to feed them for a while.

He picked up his fishing pole and started walking back home, trying to think of what he was going to tell Dennis' parents when he showed up at their house all alone. He knew that he was going to have to make himself cry if they were going to believe him so he thought about sad movies and the time his dog Herbie ran away so he would be able to produce some tears.

As he made his way back he thought about the next time he would have to feed the fish and wondered how he was going to get his dad (who was nothing but an abusive drunk) to come to the pond. If nothing else he could always get his annoying little sister to come out with him as he didn't think it would be that hard since she had the bad habit of wanting to follow him wherever he went. He hated to do it to his dad or sister but he really didn't have any other choice. The fish had to be fed and since he was the only person in the world that knew about them it meant that he was the only one who could do it.

Thadd Presley Presents

Allie, Advantageous
S. Wayne Roberts

1

IT'S ENTIRELY UNKNOWN, EVEN to myself, as to how long I've felt this way, though to my recollection it's always been this way. I don't completely hate the way I've felt, it's normal to me, but I must confess that I often wonder just how it might be if I were different.

If I were normal.

Maybe I would've had a mother and a father, the old white picket fence where my siblings and I spent our days playing with the family dog as supper simmered on the stove. Maybe I could've graduated from high school as the football star, move on to college for nothing but success. Maybe marriage and children with my high school sweetheart, maybe not. None of this happened, in fact, I have no living siblings, I was no good at sports or girls, the family dog quickly met a tragic end and the only attention I got from dear old mommy and daddy was the occasional cigarette to the neck or stiletto to the back.

But none-the-less, I live my life the way that the typical styling's of the everyday, normal world demands of me. I go to work and am quite efficient at that. I show up on time and work in my little cubical covered in quirky little Sunday paper comic clippings that I, myself lack the ability to understand, though it gets a chuckle or two from the occasional co-workers. I answer my phone with much enthusiasm and not only sell my companies product, but I sell myself to not only be normal, but quite charming to boot.

The exact product that my fairly paying job sells is trivial at this moment, though I should say that it's basically all that I have to keep myself hidden. Hidden from my co-workers, hidden from passer-by's on the street and their occasional judgmental stares and hidden even from myself from time to time. I, myself even have moments where I suppress my inner truths, but the ticking face on the wall is a constant reminder of how I long for nothing more than to clock out.

I live alone in a quaint, one bedroom apartment with a fairly sized television, computer with a slow, but sufficient internet access and boat-loads of books. There is barely a gap between the occasional piece of furniture that doesn't possess make shift book shelves on the walls. I need these things to feel connected to the world, to feel knowledgeable. Knowledge and education is power, I crave the power. I need it.

I think it's fair to say that every man has his hobby, a special activity to pass the time in between the trivial necessities of life. Sometimes a secret selective leisure pursuit for one to hone his abilities and to gain a sense of superiority. A sense of power.

Some people find what they seek in simple games, others collecting whatever may catch their eye, but my game kind of incorporates a lot of the fundamentals of different hobbies, but is slightly different in the sense that I can never share my rules with anybody, well, anybody who intends to live very long. I'm something like a hunter, collector or even a bit of an explorer, but not in the conceivable sense of the average man. My hobby is therapeutic, a way to truly be myself and get all the things weighing on me off of my chest. I have never expected a single living soul to understand that which I do, but before the end I do make them respect it.

I kill people and I like it.

It's that simple.

***

NOW, BEFORE YOU GO and decide what kind of man I am based on your preconceived notions, please, do listen to all that I've got to say before you snip, snarl or snatch me up with a lynch mob. You may well know what kind of a person I am, but I do know this, you've never seen her. With all that you think that you know in your pathetic little existence, you've not experienced the unmitigated bliss that is her eyes. The flow of her hair, the bitter sweet taste of her kiss, nor the sensual, silky smooth feel of her skin against your skin.

Oh, and I know what you're thinking, but it's she who stalked me like a hopeless gazelle aimlessly sprinting for its life with lion toeing on heel.

I never meant to hurt her, I never wanted it to end — I was in love — but just as the ever-so-haunting smug face of twelve sits on the wall, a constant reminder of life's imperfection and the infinite marching pattern of time, things between us; they too, had to end.

But I had her; if nothing else stands evident in this world I know this much to be true.

The night was cold, wind chill nipping at my bear skin like tiny bee stings. I was lonely; self-conscious of my imperfections, but willing to give this night and this world a shot. I needed somebody else to fulfill my needs, though nobody was ever around for me. Therefore I had to seek out conversation, simple touch and maybe even a cheap thrill or two.

I knew of the perfect place for this, for I had been successful in the past. A dinky, little, hole in the wall kind of place just around the corner of my apartment, one filled with lost souls and occasional persons like me. The lonely ones.

Now I confess that I was looking to lose myself as I entered the bar, but that in itself is no crime.

I scanned the bar for peers of my liking; somebody to sit next to and associate with, somebody to partake in a moment's monotonous deliberation based upon common likes and dislikes and of course come to a certitude on the demanding query of her bed or mine.

That, of course, is when I first set eyes on her. As others sat and drank, wallowing in their own decadence, she stood alone on a small stage, dancing in a way that would seemingly demanded the attention of all around her as she swished and swayed her youthful curves. She couldn't have been more than 22-years-old, nor could she have stood taller than 5'3", but her body's movements told a different story. It begged for the attention of one longing for love, of one like me.

Now keep in mind that this rat shack commissioned no dancers, but this foxy young lady just felt like dancing and chose the stage on which they held Tuesday night karaoke. Her shoulder length blonde hair flipped from side to side with every movement, much like the rest of her supple body.

I must have wondered over to the bar whilst entranced by her, for the next thing I knew I was being asked by the same old pudgy bartender to order my drink. I got two shots of whiskey and a pitcher of fuzzy navels, and then slowly made my way to the closest table by the stage.

I took my first shot and continued to watch her unnoticed, though only for a second.

Her fine, soft cheeks a flush, rosy red as she hopped down from the stage and approached me fearlessly.

"Enjoying the show?" She asked in the softest, most innocent angelic voice I'd ever heard.

"I'm sorry, I didn't mean to-"I paused. "My name is John." I lied.

"Allie." She replied, taking the seat across from me. "Is this pitcher for me?" she asked.

"Yes, I thought you might be-" I paused again, smiling as she promptly downed my whiskey shot. "Thirsty."

"A post-work out drink is always good, but now I feel cheated." Allie said.

"Oh?" I asked. "Now I'm truly interested." I was.

"Well, it seems that you got a free show, but here I sit without the same satisfaction." She smiled.

"You don't want me to dance do you, because that just might be an ugly sight." We both laughed.

I truly enjoyed her company and knew that I had her where I wanted her, but self-consciousness stood in the way of the one question I had to ask. As I smiled at her, looking deep within her eyes I knew that she had no idea of what lingered within my head. Such self-doubt.

I screamed the words within my head.

Say it damn you, say it! Would you like to get out of here? say it!

"So, umm, Allie-"

"Yes?"

"Would you like to get out of this place?" I asked, leaning in close for my answer.

Before I knew what hit me she thrust her body over the table, kissing me long and deep and causing a whirlwind of physical reaction and emotion. I knew nothing more in this world than the fact that I had to have her, Allie had to be mine. She would be.

"Your place, ok?" She asked, smiling her cute little smile.

"God yes." I replied, taking her hand and leading her from the bar.

***

THE FIRST INCLINATION OF mine was to take it slowly for this ingenuous and somewhat seemingly gullible little lady, though I clearly underestimated her petite form and faint giggle as she leapt into my arms forcing me backward onto my bed. Our constricting clothes were a faint memory as she peeled them from our bodies with ease, all the while maintaining the pure glow of the sweet girl I met in the bar, even as it became clear as to how it were little devil horns that held up that iconic halo.

My mind was racing as our perpetrating bodies danced entwine, exploring unknown odysseys and sampling the vigorous fruits of existence. I recall feeling inexplicably confused, though delighted at the insatiable sexual appetite of this young woman. One so brand new to life; aged at approximately half my time here on Earth, though also one who taught me things I never imagined.

Her luscious skin against mine created a warmth the likes I was far from accustomed to, her unspoiled, absolute dignitary figure in my hands fit perfect form, we spent hours covering and coveting every inch of each other as if we were connected as one. She and I, the perfect act with the perfect girl.

Allie emitted the most innocent love sounds atop of me, thrusting, grinding and squirming uncontrollably amidst genuine rapture and in ultimate satisfaction our vivacious physical forms flourished as one, shifting and shaking frenziedly in utmost ecstasy.

We both panted heavily as she fell to my side. She giggled slightly as I pulled her head to my chest, kissing her forehead and stroking her hair in admiration.

"Jesus Christ John, that was amazing." Allie shared, exhausted.

"Ditto."

Allie went on to say other random facts about random subjects that I couldn't possibly care less about, in fact, all I could focus on is how I'd broken so many rules in the name of lust. Granted she looked great in the bar, but it's a little known fact that they always lose their shine, their angelic glow post-ejaculation.

How could I have been so careless? To bring her home would make this process so much harder to handle, though not impossible. It was never impossible.

As she snored ever-so-softly into my chest I laid there, just lying and thinking. Planning on what it was that I would do with her. Something had to be done, obviously, but what? I knew nothing more in my life than the fact that this woman, here and now, would have to meet her untimely demise.

***

I TOLD YOU, DIDN'T I?

She found me without much effort at all, laying the bait that no man could resist. Hooked on her in the exact way that she intended, though she had no idea what it was that she happened to reel in. Sure, I bet she figured that she had me weighed and measured, mentally preparing to mount me on her wall.

No, not me.

I couldn't ever afford to let anybody get as close as this dame no doubt had planned, it wasn't conducive to my plans in life. Believe it or not, I had big plans for my time

134

here alive and it had nothing to do with the futile existence that lay before me. No, I couldn't ever settle in one place, I'd miss out on so much more while doing so.

Sights to see.

People to meet.

Time to kill.

Oh no, the thought of such a life was frightening to me. In fact, I'd rather not live at all for to give up on my hobbies, nay my life's work, would be the same as not breathing. Poor little Allie, if that was her real name, was not the first to tempt me with common life damnation, nor would she be the last. I'm young, fit and ready to move on to my next love in life, perhaps this time a red head. I've always been partial to their inner fiery nature. Perhaps I'd bring that fire out of her, scorching her body with lust, passion and gasoline.

Trash bag after trash bag I loaded my angel into the car, just barely beating the sun to rise was quite belated to my plans, but it'll do. She seemed a lot heavier when I was still under her spell, but in reality I didn't even have to double bag her after the cutting and proper division was applied. They'll never find her anyway, so I've got nothing to worry about.

I made a mental note that I'd just have to mop later.

I chuckled slightly to myself as I turned the key in the ignition, setting out for a morning drive, one that Allie wouldn't return from. Much like that defenseless dog in the old movie I watched as a kid, it was just about time for me to take ferocious little Allie out behind the barn and put her out of her misery. And that, in many ways, is what I did. Though it was by my hand that her misery came to pass, but then again she caused me great misery too. Rats like Allie live semi-successful lives every day, as too would she if only she'd kept out of the snake's pit.

Farther and farther out of town I drove my sweet

date until I found a sufficient place to bid her farewell. Out in the middle of the sticks, a small town a couple hours from mine that I'd never been to before and likely would never return to again. Something backwoods, dark and quiet. Probably ideal for hunters, hunters like Allie and I alike. We played our game well and no offense to Allie, I loved her dearly, but it truly was self-defense. Her or I, one of us would've had to die in that apartment and I took the high road by saving her all the work.

I pulled down an old dirt road which led into the woods, though worried that it might also lead to a residence I stopped at an ample amount of distance so that I could just barely see the road in my rear view, though I was still unable to identify one tree from the next that stand before me. I respect the trees for they stand their ground, never kneeling to the wind, nor do they ever avert from life's mission. It's never beneficial for one to forget their roots.

Bag after bag of the moist, misshaped mistress went into the brush. A ditch that lay open, though deep, seemed perfect for me, for I'd simply drop off her remains and kick some leaves on top of her before driving away. Which is exactly what I did with much haste, though I couldn't seem to just drive away. Something touched me in a way that I couldn't identify no matter how I racked my brain.

Was this feeling for Allie?

Perhaps I was overrun with guilt, though I doubt it. It wasn't lust, for frankly I'd had better. It couldn't be any unnecessary feelings of love, for I loved all my women the same. But none-the-less I couldn't shake this feeling in my gut, a faint rumbling that caused no discomfort or pain, but just steadily went on.

Was I losing my touch?

No, I mean I'd mutilated and dismembered women before, but I guess something was different about her. Something abnormally innocent that drove me wild about

Allie, though I do wish I knew more about her, something fact based to keep in mind when I think of her. The thought of not knowing was burning within my brain, overthrowing the stomach grumble and forcing all other thoughts from within my head.

Of course, how could I forget?

How foolish of me, indeed. I'd forgotten that one of the bags, in fact, the last bag I dropped into the ditch was her clothing. Surely she'd have an identification card or something, perhaps a driver's license to keep like I did with the others. How forgetful of me to even attempt to leave without something so precious. Maybe I am just getting old, or maybe Allie got to me. Regardless, I leapt from my car and downward to the ditch until I pulled a blood soaked pair of jeans from the bag.

"Ah ha." I announced profoundly as I removed her wallet.

I rummaged through it as I approached my driver's side door, though what I did find stopped me in my tracks. Among the remains of $12 and a library card sat both her learner's permit and school identification cards. No wonder she was hanging out in the corner instead of by the bar, this girl was only 16-years-old. No wonder Allie, which was her real name, seemed to stick to my mind so feverishly. She was my first minor, the only underage kill I'd ever bagged. A rush of excitement ran over me like a cool bath as I savored the elation of it all, which is until my fantasies were interrupted by that damned stomach grumble.

I knew right away what it was that I wanted more than anything else in the world after such a revelation.

I wanted pancakes.

***

SO THIS IS IT, huh?

My final destination was something I'd admittedly often dreamed about, but I guess I never imagined it would be lying on a cold, metal table surrounded by prison guards, a priest and a doctor. They caught me; somehow they caught me as I was returning home that day from my date with Allie. Somebody must have tipped them off for they had time to get a warrant and ransack my home before the pancakes settled. I had blueberry.

I'm told that I deserve death for what I did to that little girl, but I wonder if any of them could even begin to fathom just how devilish their precious little Allie truly was. An utter breast in the sack and a mastermind behind the rifle as she lay in wait for her prey, figuratively speaking.

Hell, maybe they're right, but one thing is for sure, they have no idea of exactly how much carnage I've caused in my lifetime.

I wrote a diary.

A little book that I started the day they put me in my cell. I've mailed it off to multiple publishing houses, as well as newspapers, so by the time that the guards search my cell it will be too late for them. Every schmo in the world will be at least one step ahead of them in this investigation, which is fine by me and I know they would thank me if they could. For let's face it, serial killers are as important and beloved in American society as any award winning actor, musician or athlete.

Books and movies, Hell, I'm a celebrity now and can't stop smiling.

"Any last words, son?" The doctor asked as he prepped my arm.

"How kind of you to ask." I replied, smiling wider than ever.

"Is this a joke to you, I mean c'mon, you're about to die here and-" The doctor paused, coming to a sudden realization. "My God, you're proud of what you did to that poor little girl aren't you?"

"Proud?" I asked, though expecting no answer.

"I don't take pride in what I did to precious little Allie-" I paused, inhaling deeply as the needle slipped into my arm. "But I am proud of all the other things I've done that led up to her. Tell the guards to gently search my cell, for the F.B.I. is going to have a field day when they count the bodies."

I don't recall much else after the needle entered my arm, which is except the shocked look on the doctor's face as I began to convulse. I believe they tried to resuscitate me after my revelations, but I got lucky.

I knew that I wouldn't die in vain, nor would they ever forget my life's work.

With death's glacial gasp upon me, I know one thing that they'll remember that above all is I died with a smile on my face.

The prison priest once told me that I'd go to Hell for what I did.

We'll see.

Thadd Presley Presents

Rain of Terror
Todd Martin

"LOOK, DADDY!" ERIN EXCLAIMED in her squeaky voice that Dane always found so endearing, "See how high up Kevin's kite is?"

"I see it, Princess," Dane replied with a smile. "He better be careful, if it goes any higher it's going to end up in outer space!"

Erin laughed at the comment and continued to watch Kevin fly his kite. Dane watched both of them for a moment and felt an incredible sadness well up inside him when he thought about how things were about to change for everyone.

"Are you sure we can't work through this," he asked in a soft tone, not wanting the kids to hear.

"I'm positive. Neither one of us is happy and I really don't see things ever getting any better," Sheryl answered, looking like she was about to start crying. "I just think it's better for everyone if we went our separate ways."

He wanted to tell her that she was wrong and that they could get through everything together. He wanted to tell her that he still loved her and that he didn't want their marriage of almost thirteen years to come to an end. He wanted to tell her that he didn't want to put the kids through the torment of having to see their parents get a divorce. He wanted to tell her that he didn't think that he could go on without having her in his life. He wanted to tell her a lot of things but instead he kept his mouth shut and just sat there trying to accept everything without breaking down and crying.

He glanced over at Kevin and Erin as they continued to fly the kite and wondered how they would react to the news that their parents were calling it quits. He thought that since Erin was only six she wouldn't quite understand why they were splitting up and hoped that Kevin could help her cope with everything. He was a wonderful big brother and was very mature to be only eleven, so Dane was pretty sure he would help take care of his little sister and do his best to make her understand.

"When should we break the news to them," Sheryl asked, almost as if she had read his mind.

"I don't know." He sighed, looking up at the sky. "I just don't know."

"Well, we better decide. We're going to have to tell them sooner or later and I just want to get it over with."

"Right. I think it's only fair that you are the one to tell them since this whole thing is your idea."

She started to say something but was interrupted by a loud crash of thunder. It was so loud that Dane jumped and a couple of cries of horror came from some of the people playing volleyball. Since Erin was terrified of storms Dane looked over at her to make sure that she was okay and saw a worried look on her face. He started to get up to comfort her but didn't have to as Kevin put his arm around her and attempted to calm her with some soothing words of comfort. Yes, Kevin really was a great big brother.

A huge streak of lightning lit up the sky and caused a skinny teenage boy with greasy hair and bad skin, who had been skateboarding down the sidewalk, to curse loudly. The sky started to grow dark and Dane got up from the picnic table as he figured that it was about to start pouring rain. He wanted to get everyone to the car before it started so they wouldn't get drenched.

Part of Dane was happy that it was about to storm since it meant the conversation he was having with Sheryl would have to be postponed until a later time. Still, he couldn't help but wonder why the weather had changed so suddenly in just a matter of moments. It just didn't seem natural to him. When they'd gotten to the park it was nice and sunny, making it a perfect day for a picnic. It was supposed to be nice and warm all weekend but he guessed the weather guy had just gotten it wrong, as usual.

The wind started to pick up, blowing paper plates and plastic cups off several picnic tables. As the thunder and lightning became more frequent the people playing volleyball decided to call off their game and began to make their way off of the court. The foul-mouthed kid on the skateboard and his pals started to head home as well, as the sky began to turn a weird yellowish-green color the hair on Dane's arms stood on end. He just had a feeling that something wasn't right, and all he wanted to do was to get his family together and get home where they would be safe.

Before he could tell Erin and Kevin that it was time to go, the rain — and the screaming — started.

Dane knew it wasn't normal rain when he saw it shred Kevin's kite. Instead of beads of water, it was shards of glass that started pouring from the sky. Sharp, pointed, jagged shards of glass that cut and stabbed anything (and anyone) it touched.

"What's happening?" Sheryl screamed as they both stood there helplessly watching, refusing to believe what they were seeing.

"I don't know," he replied, closing his eyes as the glass rained down on the skater kid and his buddies, ripping them all to shreds.

"We have to-" Sheryl began, but she never got the chance to finish as a large shard of glass fell from the sky and lodged itself in the top of her head with such impact the jagged point came out through the bottom of her chin.

Dane didn't have time to grieve for her death as he was too busy trying to dodge all the glass that was falling from the heavens, but he absently thought to himself that at least he wouldn't have to break the news to the kids that their parents were getting a divorce.

There were dead bodies everywhere and the grass was stained red with blood. There were severed body parts strewn everywhere and he nearly tripped over a still twitching leg wearing a blue Chuck Taylor All Star. As he tried to make his way toward where Kevin and Erin were many people were rushing to a nearby pavilion where they'd be shielded from the rain and the ones that managed to make it safely started screaming for Dane to join them but he ignored them. At the moment his own personal well-being was the last thing on his mind. All he wanted to do was to get to his kids and make sure that they got to a safe place. He was being cut to ribbons as the glass hit his flesh and blood from a nasty wound on his head was running into his eyes but he was still able to see Kevin lying on top of Erin to protect her. Always a good big brother.

He knew that Kevin was dead before he even touched him. There were several shards of glass sticking out of his back, the back of his head, and even the back of his arms and legs, making him look like a porcupine with glass quills. There was a pool of blood under him and Dane was terrified to roll him over for fear of what condition Erin might be in underneath him. He took a deep breath and moved his son's dead body, trying to ignore the fact that Kevin had soiled himself at some point.

Erin was completely covered in blood and Dane felt

his heart sink until he noticed that she was still breathing. She was lying face-down and sobbing uncontrollably, so he scooped her up quickly and made a run for the safety of the covered pavilion. Erin was hysterical and started screaming in his ear, but he did his best to ignore it as he darted across the park in a dead run.

Unfortunately they didn't make it too far as a shard of glass struck him in the calf, making him tumble to the ground. He fell on top of Erin but she was able to squirm out from under him and despite the searing pain in his leg he felt a wave of relief wash over him once he knew that she hadn't been hurt in the fall.

"Daddy get up!" she cried, grabbing his hand and trying to help him to his feet.

Before he could stand up a large shard impaled him through the back, pretty much fastening him to the ground. He tried to yell for his daughter to run but all that came out was a stream of bloody vomit, letting him know that he was indeed gravely injured. Several other pieces of glass rained down on top of him, slicing and slashing him all over his body.

As the darkness started to engulf him he saw one of the people who had been playing volleyball, an attractive blonde woman in her early twenties, run out from under the pavilion. Doing her best to protect herself, the woman picked up Erin (who was still screaming hysterically) and made her way back toward cover as her friends cheered her on, telling her to hurry and get back.

Right before Dane took his last breath he saw that they made it back to the pavilion where they were embraced by a group of survivors who were huddled together. He never knew it of course, but the woman who had bravely risked her life to save Erin only suffered minor lacerations due to her actions.

The rain stopped just as quickly as it had begun. By

the time it was over the death toll was in the thousands as it had taken place not only in the park, but over the entire town as well.

Rescue workers made it to the scene to tend to the injured (and remove the dead) and one EMT made the comment that it was the worst thing he'd ever seen in his entire life, which was saying something considering that he'd also responded to the Oklahoma City bombing years earlier. There was another worker who'd witnessed some of the worst accidents imaginable (one that really stood out and haunted her dreams being the time she was called to the scene where a farmer had been killed by a combine) who broke down into tears when she saw the countless bodies everywhere.

The local media arrived on the scene as well and it was only a matter of hours before the whole world was aware of the tragedy. Candlelight vigils were held across the globe and churches everywhere were crammed with people praying for the victims and survivors of the horrible incident. Flags were hung at half mass nationwide and the President addressed the nation, calling the day a national day of mourning. In general the entire country (and most of the world) was shocked and saddened by the occurrence.

There was however, at least one person happy about what had happened, and he was sure that he was going to make even more people equally pleased once he called in his report.

He sat in a van on the side of the street watching everything going on and smoking a cigarette. No one paid him any attention so he was certain that he hadn't aroused any suspicion. He dialed his phone and wasn't surprised when his military contact picked up on the first ring.

"Yes sir, Project 'Rain of Terror' was without a doubt a complete and total success," he said, "the people of Iraq will never know what hit them. Yes sir, I'm happy to hear that the President is satisfied with the results."

He listened to the instructions that the contact on the other line gave him without saying another word and then ended the call and drove away, eager for his next mission to begin. He felt a twinge of guilt when he thought about how he'd had a hand in all the death and destruction around him, but felt better once he told himself that it was all for the greater good. After all, every experiment needed to be tested if it was going to be successful.

Thadd Presley Presents

The Rock Garden
Stacy Bolli

I BECAME AWARE OF my power when I entered puberty, before that I was miserable. I had a patch of fiery red hair on my head that I texturally compared to cotton candy; then I discovered how sweet and irresistible cotton candy could be. In high school I learned to sway my hips just so when I walked and it would make the anxious, little boys drool with desire. My flowing sexuality graced me with a perfect GPA and supreme popularity; even the girls respected my presence. I was idolized. I graduated from a top university and my charm and charisma earned me a position with a lucrative advertising agency. I was on my way, but I was not sure which way.

I began to become dissatisfied with my sex life in my mid-twenties. I had tried everything to make it more gratifying. I painted my room black and adorned all my furniture with pieces red silk and roses, feeling it would give the room an air of erotic mystery. I desperately longed to reach that fabled, feminine peak and to cry those tears of victory as orgasm wracked my body, but no man has ever been able to lead me up that victorious peak. After sex I was often left broken, sitting upon my pretty silk bed, the thatch of fiery red hair between my legs still wet and limp with hunger. At times they seemed to squirm and cry out with a life of their own and I began to refer to them affectionately as "My Girls."

Some lonely nights I would feel them tickle the sides of my thighs and top of my belly as if searching for something. When their agitation seemed to reach a crescendo I would reach into my panties to pacify them with soft strokes and sweet lullabies. This would soothe us all into a relieving and empty slumber.

One brisk October day I arrived to work early. I was carrying my coffee across the hall when I noticed a new addition to our staff being given a tour of our office by the senior supervisor, Dave. Our new addition was electrifying. I had to know this man! The girls down below felt that tingle of electricity and began to wriggle out of control. I sauntered up to the two men and gave both my boss and the new recruit a sweet smile. I introduced myself and held out my hand in an offer of welcome. The man graciously took my hand into his and I felt a deep warm jolt slither up my arm into my chest, sending my heart into a flutter.

"Hello Roni, pleasure to meet you, my name is Benjamin." His chiseled features received my welcome with a genuine smile.

"Stay away from Roni," Dave warned with a joking tone to his voice, "She has a voracious appetite, but she is also my most esteemed employee. Heed the warning and interpret it for what you will."

Dave raised his eyebrows to me and gave me a twisted smirk. Dave's sexual preference was not a secret and this was his way of telling me to withdraw my claws.

"Don't let Dave here frighten you from speaking to me again in the future. I would be happy to show you the ropes and some hot spots around town if you are a newcomer." I smiled and added, "don't be a stranger, Benjamin."

"I won't be and please call me Ben."

I nodded to Ben with a coy smile, walked to my office and closed my door.   Behind closed doors the girls began to excitedly chatter among themselves.

"Shh, I will get him for us, I promise you that." I gave them a little pat to calm them down.

Later that afternoon, Ben approached me and we decided to have lunch together at a new Bistro down the block. Our conversation was smooth and never once was there one of those awkward moments of silence. I filled him in on the office gossip and all the rumors connected with each of our co-workers. He especially seemed shocked when he learned that Dave was gay.

"Well don't worry, I don't play on that side of the fence," Ben assured me with a flirtatious smile. "I moved here from Chicago and would love to see some of the nightlife here in Miami. You did offer to show me around, right?"

"I did and that offer still stands. In fact, I would be delighted."

"Well then how about Saturday?"

"It's a date." The girls did a rhythmic dance inside my pink silk panties and I swatted them under the table.

Work finished up very slowly that week and word got to Dave of our plans.

"Bitch," Dave whispered teasingly when we passed each other in the hall and gave me a tight smirk. "I will win the next one."

"We will see," I said and laughed, almost skipping in victory back to my office.

Saturday came and plans were made to meet at his apartment since my house was well over 30 miles past the outskirts of town. I loved to live my life in isolation and work on my private rock garden in the nude without the fear of being noticed. I collect geodes and odd colored river rocks, always on the prowl for new candidates. The entire right side of my house was devoted to this rectangular garden of unpolished, uncut gems and pieces of winding, convoluted driftwood. All the gems I gathered myself when vacationing in various places around the country. Geology was my passion, along with my girls. I credited them with my success in life.

Before the date I spent time carefully prepping and adding careful details to my bedroom and primping myself for the evening ahead. If all went well, I planned to be back here with Ben after dinner.

I slipped into my favorite little black dress that hugged my curves closely and showed the perfect amount of skin. I made sure my red hair was pulled back tightly from my face, wanting to accentuate my high cheek bones and wide set brown eyes.   Satisfied with my appearance I filled a spritzer with baby oil and placed it beside my bed. Baby oil can be quite an entertaining accessory if used correctly.

The date commenced smoothly and the food was delicious. There was a definite connection and often our gazes locked for minutes at a time. We started to play footsie under the table and when my toes inched between his legs I found him becoming aroused. Ben's breaths became deeper and he bent forward to take my hands within his.

"Let's leave," Ben whispered. He pulled my hands up to his thick lips and kissed them lightly.

I just nodded back to him, a little breathless myself. We climbed into my silver car and drove quickly in the direction of my house

"How far out in the sticks do you live," Ben asked in amazement.

I laughed and told him it was only fifteen more minutes away. I reached over to him and rubbed between his legs. To my delight I found him still aroused. I laughed and teased him with my tongue, flicking it back and forth between my teeth with the speed and precision of a viper.

"OK girl, you better stop or we will never make it to your house! I'm almost tempted to make you pull over here so we can hump like bears in the woods."

"No, we have to get back to my house. You will enjoy it. I worked very hard in perfecting the details for tonight."

"Oh, what makes you so confident I would have fallen for you? Are you that sure of yourself," Ben mocked affectionately.

"Who can say no to me? I'm the most unique woman you will ever meet and I can promise you the most intense and sensual night of your life."

Ben did not answer me. Instead he clutched the hand rest a little tighter. I could see his knuckles turning white with the added tension and I depressed the gas peddle a little harder and we sped into the night.

When we finally pulled up my gravel driveway Ben stepped out of the car and gaped at my rock garden. "What fantastic and unusual rocks! Where did you find them all?"

I shrugged. "Here and there, vacationing around the country. Some of this drift wood washed up along the banks of the river that runs in back of my house. Enough small talk," I said and smiled to him coyly.

I grabbed both of his sweaty hands and guided him into my house like a Black Widow pulling her prey deep into her web. As we walked hand in hand I felt the girls begin to vibrate between my legs. They knew their time to come out and play was drawing near.

I led Ben through my cold, white living room and directly into my bedroom. I closed the door behind me, isolating us into my playful and erotic set of seduction. I went around the room and lit the small tea candles strewn about the tops of my furniture. After the small flames filled my bedroom with their warm glow I turned the overhead light, immersing us in nature's light.

"This room is amazing, just like the woman who sleeps and dreams here," he whispered in awe, after taking it all in.

I put my finger to my lips to silence Ben's chatter and began to pull forcefully at his clothes. I needed to expose that rock hard chest of his, my tongue wanted to cavort along his sculpted abdomen.

After I unsheathed his body, I let his clothes fall to the floor and I kicked them under the bed. I placed my hands on both his shoulders and roughly pushed him backwards into my waiting silk sheets. Ben laughed a little nervously and leaned forward in an awkward attempt to kiss me.

"Not yet," I whispered and put my fingers to his lips and pushed his head back into the pillow.

Ben let out a small groan in frustration but remained recumbent in my silky nest.

I leaned over and opened my nightstand beside my bed. I took out several red, silk scarves and scattered them around Ben's perfect, Adonis body. I dropped a scarf over his penis and let gravity arrange it around his obvious eager state. I used several of the remaining scarves to secure his arms and legs tightly to my wrought iron bed frames. Ben just laid in silent anticipation, looking at me like a hungry puppy. I heard my girls begin to whisper and giggle.

"What is that?" Ben inquired with a smile. "Is this some kind of weird music?"

"No, you will find out soon enough," I promised.

I stood up and sauntered to the foot of my bed and began to pull down the straps of my little black dress. Ben's eyes widened at my little strip tease. I let the little black dress slip easily down my slender form and fall to the floor around my feet. I sashayed and twirled in circles to the side of the bed so Ben could get the whole effect of my nude body. I put in a lot of effort to my physique and I prided myself on my firm bottom and perky little breasts.

I reached into my nightstand and pulled out my trusty baby oil spritzer. I looked down to Ben laying upon my bed, so helpless and at my mercy. I turned my back to him, faced the wall and spayed the oil between my legs. The girls seemed to jump and catch the oil droplets in mid-air, as they became gravid with the oil and glistened like spun gold. I smiled, pleased with myself, and turned around.

Ben's eyes grew even wider. "I see you are a natural red head! That bush is as breathtaking as your rock garden." He squirmed reverently even more with impatience. I again placed my finger to my lips imploring for silence.

I walked back to the foot of my bed and slowly crawled up on Ben's muscular legs, massaging the oil up his midsection with my torso. Ben let his head fall to the pillow and let out a small little whimper of defeat. I rested my body on top of his and let the oil glide me around as if I were a hungry eel. Ben slowly opened his heavy eyes and looked to my face. I watched his gaze fall to my breasts and I slid down his body and sat up, straddling his legs so he could get a full view. His eyes finally reached to my girls down below. They were dancing in unison, with eager and starving with anticipation.

Ben's heavy eyes suddenly bulged in shock and his mouth worked silently for words. The bound Ben could do nothing but work his pitiful, useless lips and search for a scream his frozen lungs couldn't muster at that crucial moment. I smiled patiently at the silent creature, waiting for a sign of intelligence.

"What the hell is this, some kind of crazy STD," Ben whispered hoarsely when he finally found his voice. He then began to frantically twist his body back and forth in a futile attempt for freedom.

"Ben, be still, it will make it all move forward much easier."

I bent over him and tied a red scarf around his eyes.

As I was tying Ben strained and twisted his head around to bite my hands in a weak attempt at self defense. Finding he could not quite reach my flesh he then began to scream for help, begging me for mercy.

I shook my head at him, as if scolding a small child for being disobedient.

"No one can hear you. We are miles from no where, Ben. You know that."

Then Ben began to cry. I could see the tears gather below the red silk scarf tied around his eyes. This human and submissive act empowered me. I felt a deep arousal I had never felt before and I quickly mounted Ben. I took his flaccid penis within me and ground him deeply forward, it was an incredible moment. Despite his terror I felt Ben grow within me. I worked my hips frantically and I finally climbed to the top of that mysterious peak. The climax was just as sweet and victorious as I anticipated. I quickly withdrew, my muscles spent and exhausted. Ben remained erect and silent. Drool had gathered on the corners of his lips and trickled around his ears. I reached down and began to massage him. Men were such funny creatures, so easily aroused even in the face of death. I empathized with the betrayal he must be experiencing, betrayed by his own body.

I then felt a tugging and a sudden cold draft between my legs. I quickly spread my thighs and to my shock and horror "My Girls" detatched from my body. I watched in fascination as they inched their way up Ben's legs, like slender black worms and weave around his penis. They began to dance and circle his penis; the sight reminded me of children dancing around a may pole. Then Ben came, it showered all around the girls. They screeched and jumped to catch the spray but this did not satisfy them. They wriggled about in a fevered pitch and again Ben began to cry. They inched up to the tip of his penis and began to slip down his urethra. Ben began to scream frantically and writhe back and forth.

"Please, Roni make them stop! Pull them back! It's beginning to burn," he begged me pathetically.

"I can't, they have chosen you. I cannot stop them now. I am sorry..." I from top of him and down to the floor, a little afraid of what was going to happen next.

Close your eyes, Roni. You do not want to see this. The words reverberated in my head.

Sitting on the floor, I scuttled backwards until my back hit the wall. I closed my eyes and put my hands over my ears trying to muffle Ben's heart breaking screams.

I must of fallen asleep because when I awoke the girls were back in place, a little fatter for the wear, but in their proper place. I stood up and looked at the bed. I gasped and covered my mouth. Ben's body was totally drained of any fluid. His body resembled a burnt potato chip you sometimes came across while snacking. I walked over and poked him with my toe. His body lifted and fluttered back to the bed with the ease of a feather.

I got dressed and gathered the silk scarves from around my bed. I was able to roll Ben up into a little cylindrical tube. I gathered my red scarves and wrapped his dehydrated carcass up into a little red cocoon. I dropped the morbid cocoon into a plastic grocery bag and stepped outside my house. I picked up a few rocks from my garden and dropped them into the bag with Ben's cocoon. I tied the handles and walked quickly to the river. When I reached the banks I flung the bag over my head. It sailed towards the middle of the murky river and splashed into the water. I watched it smack the smooth surface. The air billowed out of the top of the bag as the rocks pulled it deep below the surface, down into the dark, icy water. Ben was gone.

I turned my back to the river and started back to the house. I felt my footing slip and I caught myself before I fell to the ground. I stood up and looked down to the culprit. It was a large smooth rock and I bent down and to pick it up. When I inspected it I could see small red crystals embedded into the grain, what a find! I slipped it into my pocket and continued home.

When I got inside the house I wrote Benjamin 2009 on the rock and went outside to place the small memorial in my fabulous rock garden.

Thadd Presley Presents

Grind
JD Stone

VOICES! COMING FROM ALL angles, long ones, short ones, full of secrets from the bowels of the underworld. They flew out of chattering mouths soft and deathly, rising to the crescendo of a shrieking jukebox. But it was the promise of a lover that drew him from the bar.

"She'll be there," Jonathan said with a devilish smile.

There were rains that had started last week, still washing the city down like a rabid cat. The ground was softening to mere mud between the buildings, to gunk on the edges of the boroughs. The sun hadn't been seen in over a week; gray was the color of days, sepia poisoned the night. Jonathan tugged a friend with him to follow into the maze of night streets, on their way to the graveyard in the middle of the city.

He was a rock and roll rebel possessed by barking at the moon and the frailty of darkness, the great glitzy BOOM! of sinister music and its promise of disaster. His name was Draven and he knew the ways of Obeah magic, knew the short cuts to the crypts and the language of the dead; ultimately he'd bring forth the lover of a thousand generations in heat.

It was nearing midnight and the bright lights of the dollar stores were clicking off as the ominous neon of nightlife clicked on, innervating the gushing water over the cobblestone with a spiral of colors; the deep glow was a hectic vortex into nowhere. Women of the night came clicking their stilettos, flesh swathed in fishnet, waiting to make a wage. The sky remained a permanent twilight, painting the saw toothed city a riotous purple, and Jonathan traced it along his arm as if some growing tattoo as viral as weeds in a field.

When the rains came last week a shrill vibration was felt, the skyscrapers swayed, the offices shook with the premonition of destruction: an infinitesimal earthquake opening its eyes, clawing chitinous pincers toward the earth's fiery core and cradling it like the fine dome of an infant skull. The steady movement was gossiped between hushed voices as a train passing deep and dark in the subway, of metal veins pumping oily blood. But Jonathan saw the clouds crash from his bedroom window, felt the foundation of his tenement shiver, and he knew it was time to go the graveyard. Draven saw the first giblets of angry water coming down like smoldering razors.

It was night now and they pushed passed bodies squeaking in rubbery coats, vicious umbrellas dripping acid rain onto the next unsuspecting person. Their boots splashed a few inches deep in the cold water; makeup ran down their faces like sludge and hair gel tasted of melted plastic on their lips. Jonathan didn't care much for his appearance anymore: good-bye costume jewelry, black nail polish and rainbow contact lenses. A dead lover would not need to sulk in the indecencies of outer beauty. They would only need the energy from a youthful heart beating as fast as bee's wings.

Draven pushed them through backstreets where a veritable darkness slithered like serpents lapping at their feet looking for a master. A soulless part of the city where all hell could break loose in the manner of a second, where people with beady eyes and razors in their shoes battled egos, their mannerisms long since decayed of any class. It was a glossy wall of darkness, and what could be seen through the columns of buildings and quivering roadways was not formidable enough to describe: a shimmering shadow of ectoplasm and dripping dust. Cars seldom passed and the angry pedestrian caught in the blaze of weather kept their heads bowed and their hands buried deep in their raincoats protecting their money, their cheap jewels.

A rosary was snapped in two, black jewels succumbing to the sewer, Christ and his impossible faith drowning to the power of nature. A hand shot out of the alley begging for change, murky fingers gripping a Styrofoam cup about to burst with water, crimson-veined eyes fighting sleep, hidden beneath a million drugs habits. Draven passed him off, unmoved; Jonathan threw him his last quarter and he watched it splash into the cup, the bum's smile stretching like he'd found out the secret to a grand stash of priceless poisons.

An alleyway that bore nothing but evil splashed before them, a puddle of disastrous garbage and runny graffiti. Draven dragged Jonathan into it by the hand and their black pants soaked up to nearly the knee. Jonathan saw a billion drops of scintillating silver rain above, clotheslines zipping window to window as if ancient Europe holding torn undergarments, heads of half burnt dolls with blank looks in their eyes dangling like cocoons in a spider's web; a famed city rat that had been the size of a small cat hung by its gossamer tail clawing for escape or nearly enjoying its upside down water torture.

"We wait for the bus and take it to the last stop," Draven said pushing his black hair away from his knife-like features.

"What will we pass going across town?" Jonathan

asked. "I'm deathly curious."

"Strange dwellings. But it's the cemetery we're after. Everything is wet and vulnerable. Mud makes it easier to dig."

The bus arrived at the spot with its headlights calling for a caped crusader, yellow beams cut like a thousand shards of light through the rain. They stepped on, paid their fair in wet nickels, and sat alone in the back where a huge window gave them full view of the dark flooding city. There were no passengers other than a small woman mumbling about being alone, dirty as a baby tasting its first breath of air. She was curled so tight into her seat that Jonathan thought she might want to get back into the womb.

The treacherous blocks passed and most of them could not be seen other than the flash of a doorway opening to a phantom knocker, faint spots of pale rain illuminated by smashed street lamps. Draven closed his eyes and hummed a song of sorcery to himself, his face thrown into a shadowy place. It was of a band swathed in black and who had absinthe for blood. The drum of the bus weaseled into Jonathan's muscles; the smog kept him at bay to not fall asleep for fear he'd never wake up. A dozen towns passed quickly, languages written in characters streaked psychedelically across the bus windows. A wild train track loomed above, metal beams bending to the will of Mother Nature.

Chinese characters blasted gold and red, grease vapors claiming the inside of the bus, coating the boy's throats. Jonathan could taste steamed rice and the rich red barbeque sauce glazed over pork belly in his mouth; frog legs and live squid served deep inside a shimmering Dozo. He remembered a stray cat that had landed on the stoop of one of his Chinese neighbors waiting for a bowl of water, and two small white hands welcoming it inside the hallway. He never saw it again, and perhaps that was its viscera hanging there, insidiously camouflaged by oily red sauce.

The town faded fast, a couple blocks of dreary blackness, and then a great hellacious fist of curried goat washed over their senses. Ancient Indian text was scrolled from window to window in Henna paint as if from the withered hand of a King. A huge golden temple remained solid against the rain. Blurry and ambiguous, no one could decipher the scrolls, for what language was written in curlicues of dots and swooping slashes?

An Irish section passed by like a smeared tapestry of beer and bar room brawls, so said the flashing police lights. Tiny little green bodies with flames of orange hair huddled around their pots of gold (the beer taps), Nazi-blue eyes snarling at any stranger that would pass. Draven and Jonathan stared in hope for a fight to break out.

It became dark again, and the lights in the buss puttered as if about to die. Then they were passing a calm neighborhood of brownstone houses suffering from a blackout and a minor flood. The windows were lit by kerosene lamps and cheap votive candles. A great surging wave came upon them, and Jonathan thought the bus would stall, forcing them to swim to the graveyard, but the bus pummeled through the water like a monster truck over old cars.

Draven's eyes took in all the colors of the night, all the protesting neon and sparkling rain spatters against the window. He opened his small black cigarette case and handed Jonathan a small square tab of blotter acid which promised the most decadent sights as it was an inner city blend. Jonathan let it sizzle into nothing over his tongue, washing it down with the Dogfish Head craft beer he lifted from the little dark bar. They'd done enough drinking to satiate any old soul, but their night of fun was far from over.

They'd spent a few nights in the south camping by a bay that was said to be used by pirates in the colonial times, where it was rumored the alligators were huge as dinosaurs. They shared Wild Turkey by the moonlight with a few southern belles, waited patiently for the beady black eyes of the gators to show, the elegant roar, but nothing ever came. The belles didn't give it up either. It all left Jonathan sick to his stomach for weeks, an amber haze claiming his vision. He never wanted to go back to the south.

"The rain was like we saw in the marshes down south," Jonathan said.

"Ah yes, decadence and girls in lace tops who hated the sun. Good times. NO gators though."

"Girls, girls, girls! We'll never have to worry once we make it to the cemetery."

"My feelings for this are harsh," Draven said with the ghost of black lipstick fading on his mouth. "I've never succeeded in trying to make this kind of craft a reality."

"On a night where the rain doesn't stop, we're bound for success."

The bus came to a grueling halt and the blubbery driver called LAST STOP and the boys were off the bus, sucked out like a vacuum into the wild night. The ground was sopping with three inches of water. A giant iron green gate towered on both sides of the street, bolted into brick pillars, creating the doors. The road cutting through the middle was a water slide into the pits of hell. Draven had a safety pin and a small skeleton key with him and he moved like a bat to one of the gates and opened it up with two easy clicks.

Jonathan was taken aback by a few thoughts: there were no more lights, no more food wafting their weird odors. Who would know they were here? Who would come help them if they needed it? He then realized that he was feeling a little fuzzy; his eyes made images bleed before him; his brain was cushion of meat inside his head. Somewhere, he heard the agonizing ticker of an AM radio…

"Get in!" Draven called, closing the screeching gate behind them.

The cemetery ground was soft as hot butter as their feet met it. They had to drag their boots hard; their smoker's lungs puffed and wheezed like an old man's. The rains became so heavy at one point that Draven turned into a head full of hair and warbling white eyes as they discussed the plans: they were lonely, hadn't had a female lover in some time. They were sick of one another's body; the pointed curve of their hips were too sharp; the pulsing white serpents between their legs were deemed too boring. They wanted a sweet woman who had aged like fine wine, fermented as beer forgotten in the barrel.

They were known as freaks throughout junior high school and beyond. They sharpened their nails to points, wore fishing hook bracelets and rubber black bands on their wrists, each one bearing a perverse significance, though they all looked the same. Most kids thought they were born on planet X and had possessed the bodies of two human boys to live amongst the sheep here.

They kept themselves draped in funeral attire and high top converses scribbled with morbid pictures. They spoke about getting *closer to* god, of worshipping *the beautiful people*. The dead were much better friends, much better lovers. They had no mouths to ramble about nonsense imagery, no bullet opinions to permanently scar another person. Dead brains were cooked to goo as if put in a microwave for hours on end, and they could keep secrets for eternity: the living only wanted to smash that kind of trust.

Amongst the cemetery crowd here were angels with stone wings like razors; their hands were frozen spiders waiting to attack. Opal puddles of water turned the ground loose and vulnerable, so the angels and saints were hunched over as if listening in on ghostly conversations. Centurion caskets had been sent to the surface, wavering and floating to an unknown destination; marble tombs that had once imprisoned the deceased to an eternity of claustrophobia were opened by quick fingers. Sepulchers softened and the bodies rose with the smell of swamp gas to taste air again. *Their dead souls*, Jonathan thought.

"They're coming to life!" Jonathan said.

"This will be a night of celebration indeed, Jonathan."

Draven drew Jonathan close to him and let his cold thin lips press against Jonathan's. It would be their last kiss because they had to save the energy for their new lover. They marched along a path that seemed an arid land of wasted trees and odd stones with names carved in the jutting stones that could not be pronounced. There was a crooked oak tree, huge and limitless in the night sky, and it towered over the tombstone of choice. The letters were filled with dark moss and encroaching vines like venomous veins; the rest was eaten away by the sun and bad weather. Draven stuck his hand in the mud, and Jonathan closed his eyes, dreaming of her.

***

THE WEATHER MORPHED BACK into temperate patterns and the clocks began to tell time again after its long stand still. The air was just beginning to lose its fine coat of demise before they brought her into the mausoleum. She was wrapped in a sopping quilt, stiff body protected by a morgue shroud made of ancient plastic: a tight grey chrysalis stretched from head to toe, tucked so strong that even when Draven dropped her to the marble floor she was still wrapped like a gaudy present. She was almost demanding to be freed the way her knees were pulling up to her chest. It was frightened position. She smelled faintly cankered.

"What do we do with her," Jonathan asked.

"Johnny boy, we simply unwrap her like an X-mas gift most desired!" Draven drew a long piece of hair into mouth, biting it with a curious affection.

"No, we must tour the grounds, we must drink to the night. We must celebrate before we do what the movies war against."

"If that's what you wish, we could go poke around at the wild names marked on the stones. We could try to set up a tent and sleep here for all eternity. The rains will come back again so maybe we should build an ark!"

Draven had ways with his speech which were influenced from the books he read, from the television shows about horrid mysteries unsolved, of UFO intelligence and cult phenomena brain washing people throughout the country. He led them both out through the entrance of the mausoleum, filing back out the double glass doors, leaving the body in the center of the scarlet carpet so they could explore more.

The outside was still black with the scent of night-mud and fetor. The skeletons of hopeless dead were slouched across the great lawns, their head bobbling on long stems of spine, fingers clutching nothing but their own wasted palms. Draven bent over and collected a finger that came away with a crack and a fine spray of dust, putting it inside a small glass vile.

For a moment Jonathan caught the glimmer of two garish black orbs in the sockets, spinning like a marble rolling down a hill. He blinked and it was gone, just the face of a man dead since 1896 so said the stone he was brushed up against; a clear gunshot wound had splintered the forehead. Jonathan imagined brains like oatmeal leaking out through his ears.

Then the sound of the ticker happened again. Jonathan could hear it, knew he wasn't going crazy, but where the fuck was it coming from? Draven said he was hearing things and the thought of being in tune to poltergeist activity made blood rush to Jonathan's crotch. That would mean he was a mystic of some sort. The psychic at the café always said he had a queer talent for darkness, but he could never pin point it. But it was none of that at all, yet the conviction that the deceased could come and talk to him was a thought he did not let go of.

A muddy path Draven had taken them on was quiet as a morgue. No more voices. But the ticker still sent static through the hills and valleys of Jonathan's brain. It was a grinding sound like no other, and it made him think of cogs rusted metal turning in a swarming circus attraction, a theme park coaster gone mad.

Then the light at the end of the tunnel!

At the foot of the hill there were heavy duty curtains pulled up into a teepee where smoke and mirrors reflected bane light into the wet cemetery, up into the trees and over the green spire gates. A long line of bodies were shuffling inside making monsters with their shadows, a crescendo in the dying light. It was music that Draven knew, that Jonathan had once worshiped. The bodies were all gyrating sexually behind the teepee. Jonathan saw wild hair styles, guitar necks and a drum set. But the music wasn't a live show, it was coming out of the amps piled like a mountain, and the ticker noise was simply feedback.

It was a graveyard party!

"I told you there was a ticker sound!" Jonathan hissed.

"Want to crash it?"

"Are we dressed appropriately?"

It was always a game of outer beauty in their crowd,

of the dark nature, naturally.

"We look like wet rats, but there will be beer," Draven said. "They'll probably have the shells I need to see if that woman could be used."

"Shells?"

"With Obeah the shells speak. The tiny teeth line the edgings like a mouth full of razors. If you touch them the wrong way, you can be bitten."

Jonathan nodded his head, entranced by the smell of the smoke; the taste of liquor was rotten on his palate. Then he realized through a smoky blur that he was biting his nails, and that he had touched the shroud. He was *tasting* her! Jonathan immediately took his hands from his mouth and hoped for that cold beer.

The tent was open a sliver, and Draven parted it carefully with his long white fingers. A strobe light was making everything move slow, all limbs contracting, swaying to the beats blowing out the amps. The jargon was depressed; the eyes swam around like sentinels. They reminded Jonathan of Zombies. It even smelled faintly sweet, sweet at the freshly risen dead. Draven slipped inside and moved instantly to the table lined with a fine array of juices. Cartons of nameless drinks reflected the sweet faces of missing children, most likely turned to bones by now and lying unrested in this cemetery.

Draven shared conversations with kids in costume jewelry and faces powdered moth-white. They had peacock hair dos and barely smiled. They were an insidious bunch, but they didn't move Jonathan's mind from the woman a single bit. He imagined himself slicing the shroud open from head to toe, the fetor of the underground belching up at him green and slimy. He would wrench her legs open like that of a real girl and see the pleasures of a woman's sex open like a carrion plant, long since dried of its life, like flower petals falling from a wilted stem.

Her skin would be mottled; her eyes would be dried grey prunes of flesh in sockets that he could stare into all night and wonder what her last thoughts were. Her tongue would loll and roll out of her mouth wet, long and dark like an ornate carpet before an emperor. It would be cankered and festering. He imagined her hair, curled and fair with age, and her cold-slimed hand reaching, sliding between and up his thighs. Then Draven tapped him on the shoulder and his blistering fantasy was popped like a righteous pin hitting a balloon.

"This kid here wants to know about it," Draven said.

"Are you a one too?" The shadowy kid asked, perhaps Draven's long lost cousin.

"I'm looking for love in all the wrong places."

The boy cocked his head back and laughed. "You'll find it here. Take a *drink*. Take a hit."

"What it is it?"

"A nice surprise."

It was a long brown blunt and a plastic cup filled with a thick red juice. When he took the entire thing down Jonathan thought that the drink tasted rather meaty, rather like a handful of coins were thrown into the mix. *Blood.* And it tasted of her, Jonathan knew. Dead blood. The boy nodded to Jonathan now with an unsure Cheshire smile stretched ear to ear, and his stomach almost turned when he saw in the back of the tent that some kids were cutting their wrists and draining them into milk cartons.

"Now you've tasted the decadence," another long smile, and Jonathan saw the apex tip of canine teeth.

Draven moved them to another part of the tent where a young girl sat staring into a portrait where a figure was fixed between two carcasses of meat, its long white stripes of rib shown, its paunch bejeweled across a meat hook meant for a large extinct creature. It was a Francis Bacon original, and it seemed to be their monument of worship.

She passed Draven a small black velvet bag with a red tie at the top. When he shook it the sound of a million glass shards could be heard.

"These are the shells!" Draven said. "It's time to get back in the mausoleum."

***

WHEN THEY ENTERED THE mausoleum for the second time that night the doors had been pushed open by some sort of tool. A hammer had perhaps wedged between, or slammed against it, forcing the doors open, so said the bent metal. It was a metal frown with a jagged lip and a huge chunk bitten out of it. There was broken glass and fluted marble chips scattered across the carpet. The Italian language robot directory kept repeating itself over and over like a hypnotizing technique. Someone had smashed the screen, looking for precious metals, a good mother board to sell. Grave looters, drunken idiots wanting to deface a place of worship. Whether for the dead or not, the entire mausoleum reeked of Catholicism.

That's when Jonathan noticed that the girl was missing. They jetted up the stairs and into the center of worship, finding her laid out, but this time in a more maniacal position. The room was candle-dark as the electricity had been knocked out by gusts of wind. Through the small lights Jonathan saw her limbs spread in all the positions of the clock: ten, two, five and seven. The shroud was even tighter, suctioned to her form like Christ betrayed on the cross gloaming above. Jonathan thought he saw the faint bobble of her head, but a small wind was blowing up the stairs as the storm had come again.

This time Draven was ready to open it, ready with his shells to lead him to the future. He jumbled them in his grip and let them fly out, landing on the tiled plateau washed in all colors of the church, in frankincense and the pay as you go votives held in blood red holders. *The blood of Christ*, Jonathan thought, *shelling the prayers of a million lifetimes, a million missed souls.* The shells landed right side up, teeth showing, marking the sign of a hex.

"It's real." Draven said.

"We can make her ours?"

"The scent of a lover never dies. The stars will always burn in their eyes."

Jonathan clicked open a disposable razor and ran the silver tip carefully over the shroud. It was an easy job. He'd practiced this at home, flicking the blade back and forth over his own arm, precise enough to not draw blood as he sliced tight shirts from his own pale flesh. Down the center and rushing over the bump of breasts, Jonathan had made a clear vertical line from head to toe, though it seemed she had no feet to speak of.

The shroud sucked away with a gooey sound as they lifted it. They discovered a desiccated body, curvy, and with prepubescent breasts where two purple nipples were pinched beyond repair like raisins in the sun. The smell was not that of archaic mud or the collected essence of dead insects burrowed into her brain, for Jonathan knew that scent would be wicked. It was a milky smell, white as the skin that covered the body, white as the beads of sweat that ran from its pores. She had no breath to speak of; her torso was rock solid, though it was hollow as Jonathan laid his head on it to listen for a dead heartbeat.

"Show me the face!" Jonathan demanded.

Draven peeled the last part of the shroud off carefully as if a cleansing face wash made of acid so that if you pulled if off too quickly all that would remain would be a skeletal mask made of melting tissue. The cloth came way just as Jonathan searched the inside of her legs with his fingers, the skin passing for warm was more like cheese left out at room temperature. Her vagina was an arid zone of black and grey.

The knee twitched and Jonathan pulled back.

"Just a reflex," Draved said passively.

This was when he pulled the last of the cloth away from her face. She was mentally handicapped in her lifetime. She had the lip droop of a down syndrome baby, but the cleft of a third world rescue. Her hair swayed moistly behind her head, a brown that should have been grey and wasted by now. This was when Jonathan was finally able to loosen her rigor mortis limbs and funnel his fingers into her vagina. The dark lips crackled away at his grip, the brittle hair turned to dust. As his thumb made it in all the blood in his body had went to his penis, and his head felt faint.

Then something bit him, hard.

He pulled his hand out and there was a shell latched on his pointer finger. Draven shrieked about the hex, running for his life as the body began to move upward. Her face morphed into a painter's easel of dark smears, lips churning chop meat between her teeth. One oily eye rolled toward Draven, and a languid hand reached for him before he ran off. Jonathan hoped that hand was coming for him.

Draven vanished in a screaming arc of terror. For all the death Draven revered, all the nights he spent watching the stars and wishing to be part of some ancient cemetery family, he was gone without even a good-bye.

Jonathan's head filled with an image: the girl's sluggish tongue lapping at her lips for his blood; her contorted lip growing teeth all its own. It reminded Jonathan of the blood he drank back at the tent. Then she was standing with her hair covering her breasts, but Jonathan's vision kept scrambling. An explosion of colors and the threat of passing out was upon him. Suddenly her chest was sunken in, a breast was missing and her rib cage jutted at broken angles through her grey skin. He saw shriveled organs and spiders crawling out of an aperture. It was the mark of her death, by fire from some thrashing car accident.

When Jonathan opened his eyes she was already pulling him down by his tough dyed hair, her breath tinged with blood and rot, stretching his neck upward so he could see the glass roof and the last of the expensive marble.

Her mouth opened with a grind, full of sharp metal.

Open. Dark. Endless.

Thadd Presley Presents

You'd Better Learn
Thadd Presley

"THIS ISN'T HOW IT has to be," John told the man with the bolt cutters. "I'm tryin' my best t' hold everythin' together." He looked toward his wife. "And just look!" Slowly lifting his hand, pointing at his wife. "Look at what I come home to find."

Blood was dripping from his hand and running in streams down his forearm, when he focused on the blood, he felt a wave of confusion flow from his head to his mid-section. "She's here smokin' up the profits while I'm out working. That's where your money's goin', man."

The black man held the mouth of the cutters out, waiting for John's ring finger. His grey eyes focused on the woman huddled in the corner crying. "That true? You and this crack-head stealin' Big Daddy's dope? You smokin' up your man's money and making him late on his payments?"

She started to say something, but her voice failed.

"Tell me somethin' John," the black man asked, "do I take another finger or do I take one of hers?"

"Just give me more time. I'll have his money."

"Time's up. Daddy don't want money now. He wants you t'know that he's finished with you."

These words meant more to John than losing his pinky finger. He couldn't survive without Big Daddy's help. "Come on, man. Take the finger. Just..."

Then, in a snapping motion, the executioner cut the ring finger from John's hand. John screamed and his wife joined him. Lying on the blood covered ground was John's finger. It twitched, as if trying to crawl away. John's wedding ring was on the finger.

"My job's done here, John."

John looked up. "Do I still have to pay?"

The black man laughed. It was hardy, amused laugh. "Pay? Don't tell me you haven't learned anything from this, John. You owe Big Daddy money. Big money. Don't you think you should pay up?"

"But my fingers? God!!"

"God?" The black man slapped him. "Say it again."

John lowered his head.

"I'll not have you takin' my Lord's name in vain."

"So, I have to pay Big Daddy?"

***

"JOHN, SO HELP ME. You'd better have the money or next time I'll bring a gun and shoot your wife in the stomach." He looked over at her. "She's your problem anyway, right?"

John looked at her as well. She was high and slouching now, more that cowering in the corner. John's eyes focused on the floor in front of her, resisting the urge to look at his fingers. For some reason, the urge was too much and he couldn't take his eyes off of them. Is this really happening, he thought. Am I really...

The executioner slapped John hard in the back of the head. "Right?"

John couldn't remember what the man had asked, but he answered. "Yeah, right. You're right." A shutter went through his body. "You're right." He mumbled again.

"Now, get to a hospital."

"What do I say?"

"Tell them you got your fingers cut off because you owe for drugs."

"Really?" John was getting light headed. The world was growing dim. Things seemed to warble around him.

"Woman," the executioner said as he kicked her outstretched foot, "get your man to the hospital."

She looked up, her eyes were yellow and dull. "What do I tell them?"

"Tell them you brought him to the hospital because if you didn't a big black man said he was going to kill you."

Her eyes flickered, showing the smallest recognition of life. "Really?"

"Yeah, really."

Slowly she stood up and started toward her husband. He wasn't looking at the ground anymore. He was limp. His head flopped back, eyes glaring at the ceiling. "Do you think he is dead?"

"Yes."

Grief came over her face, but then the executioner saw relief. "I'm going to miss him so much," she said. "He was my high school love."

The moment was lost when the executioner spoke. "Big Daddy wants his money. Don't let this man's life go needlessly. I'll be back in a week."

"What!! I can't –"

"But I can. Just know, I'll be back in a week."

"I'll don't know how to come up with twelve thousand –"

"You better learn," said the man walking out of the door.

Thadd Presley Presents

Fallow Ground
Thadd Presley

"ALREADY DEAD," EZEKIEL SAID under his breath, "Fallow. Damn ground is ruined." And only after four years. The day had been spent looking through fields of stunted corn and flat hills of potatoes. He walked the fields with his two young boys, who were still young enough to enjoy digging through dirt to find potatoes and chop down corn in a race to the end of the row. It was a measly harvest, Ezekiel knew it; the year was about up and the land taxes would be due. If the pumpkins didn't come in good and strong, the year will have been wasted.

"Pa," Aaron spoke from a stooped position, using a hoe to uncover the small potatoes he'd found. "A man is coming down the farm road."

Aaron was Ezekiel's youngest son and usually left the talking to his older brother, Thomas, who usually knew what to say when it came to their father's temper and moods. "See, Pa, is that a banker?"

Ezekiel raised his head from his empty potato hill and squinted into the distance. He reset his hat, a habit, and waited, leaning on his walking stick until he could see who it might be. Sweat was pouring from his brow and he dabbed it with a red hanker chief.

The man in the distance was on horseback and

dressed like an undertaker, all in black. Even the horse he rode was black, not a spot on it. He pulled a large wagon behind him that swayed with every bump in the road. The wagon was ornately decorated in silver and some white type of metal. As he got closer, Ezekiel could see that the carvings depicted men and women writhing together, naked and tangled in knots of three and four. There was even more on in the designs that Ezekiel wished he couldn't make out; depraved sins that Ezekiel didn't want his boys being subjected to. They would learn this all too soon.

Across the horse's flank, was a brown burlap bag that the man lifted onto his lap as he pulled up close to the three in the field. Thomas watched the bag intently. He felt as if this could be a rich man come to help their family. It could be gold, he thought, and smiled. He couldn't wait to see what the man had brought. But, his hoped were dashed as the man started to get off his horse. There was a look on the man's face and Ezekiel spoke up.

"You boys go on home now. Go help your Ma with the chores until I get there."

"Who is it, Pa?" Thomas wanted to know "What's in the bag?"

"What did I just tell you? Now get!" Ezekiel raised his hand and started toward Thomas.

Thomas knew better than to run. He would take a lickin' if he was due one. But, Ezekiel put his hand down and tried to smile. "This has nothing to do with the likes of you boys." And, even though he tried to smile, the look in their father's eyes told both the boys they had best do as he said. Neither boy had a habit of back talking or disrespecting their father in any way. The man had a fierce anger and didn't put up with insolent children.

The boys said, "Yes sir," in unison and made their way through the field running as they went, sometimes touching each other and yelling "tag your it."

Then they entered the woods.

Once in the woods, Thomas stopped running and put his hand out to stop Aaron.

"You're it," Aaron yelled as he suddenly was able to reach the back of his brothers shirt.

"Hold on," Thomas said. "That don't count anyway. I want to see who that man is."

"Do you think Pa's sick and that's the doctor coming to tell him."

"Ain't no doctor. He didn't even have a doctorin' bag. Plus, doc Traverse mostly comes in the church wagon."

"But, that's not the church wagon."

"So, who is it, then?"

Both boys watched as the man got off his horse and walked closer to their Pa. The two men did not speak to each other. But, once close enough, the man in black gave the farmer the brown bag and in return the farmer took out his pocket knife and cut his thumb. Both the boys watched with wide eyes, even from that distance, they could see their father drop some blood on the paper.

"Damn," Thomas said.

"Don't cus, Tom. You'll go to hell." The words caused Tom's eyes to go wide.

"Who says? That old baptist down at the church who I see drunk all the time. You know, he even told Susan after she was caught kissing Brody that if she kissed him God would forgive her."

"Did she do it?"

"Yeah, of course. She kissed him and then she told her Ma that she did it so she wouldn't go to hell. That's why her Pa went down there and burned the church. Remember that?"

Aaron nodded his head. "Yeah, I didn't know why though. Thought it was an accident."

"Well, that's why 'ol preacher Carson ain't around

no more."

"Where did he go?"

"I heard he was in the church. Anyway, Ma said, Susan's Pa sent him to hell in a hand basket."

Thomas' watched his father in the field, but Aaron didn't seem to care anymore about the man or the bag. He was thinking about the church that had burned.

Thomas couldn't stop wondering what was in the bag his pa had bought. Coming from a man like that — all dressed up and with a tall hat — it could be anything. But, he knew there was something wrong because usually when men did business they shook hands. Thomas didn't see these men shake hands. Only that, when it was over, the man rolled up the piece of paper and got back on his horse. Then he rode away back the way he came.

Whatever the business was and whatever idea Thomas tried to form changed the moment Ezekiel untied the top of the bag and pulled it down. It was hard to believe what he saw pulled from the bag. Thomas did everything in his power to fight it, but he had to believe it.

The baby was crying so loud anyone would know.

Just some kind of animal, Thomas tried to tell himself. But then there was just no doubting it being a child.

"Is that..." Aaron started, but Thomas put his hand over his younger brother's mouth.

"Shh."

Then their Pa took the child, who couldn't have been more than two years old — it was hard to tell from where they watched behind the tree — and stabbed his knife into the child's neck. With this done, Ezekiel walked around the field shaking the blood here and there. Thomas wasn't sure if he could hear his Pa talking or singing, but he could hear something. He thought for a second that the child was still crying.

"Pa's singing," Aaron said. "Like in church."

"Shh..."

With the sprinkling done, Ezekiel dropped the now dead child on the ground and walked to his wheel barrow and took from it a hatchet and shovel. Then, proceeded to cut the child's arms and legs off. The sounds of the axe blows could be heard by the two boys. Tha-whop. Tha-whop. Tha-whop.

The last thing to be chopped off was the head.

Then, picking the pieces of the toddler up, he walked to all four corners of his field and buried a leg here, then an arm there, and on and on like that until he went to the very center of the field. Instead of digging a hole and burying the remains, he gathered chaff and put the remains of the child in it and lit it on fire.

When the fire started going, their pa started singing again. The boys found their chance and ran back to their home. When they got there they smelled their mother's cooking and carefully went inside.

"Not again," Aaron said. "I hate taters." Then, carefully, he asked his older brother. "What was pa doin'"

"Don't worry about that." He thought about to the child, the one he felt was a girl by the way of her cries. She only screamed once and he would never forget it. "Pa wasn't doing anything. You imagined it. Little boys do that."

"But, you..."

"Not me. Not nothin'. Pa didn't do anything."

Aaron knew not to cross his brother, so he didn't say anymore.

***

AN HOUR LATER, EZEKIEL returned to the cabin and washed up at the well pump. He finally came in and sat down at the head of the table. Without a word for anyone, he put his hands together. "Great God, who art in heaven, forgive us sinners for our transgressions against you and your immaculate image. We are a sinful lot. Please bless the lives, families and the fields of our neighbors. You know the importance of the harvest and you know the hearts of us all. Find it is your eternal love to bless and keep us. Bless the sick, the down and out, and help those who do not know you to find their way to your life giving salvation. Amen."

The others said Amen and dinner began.

The first words spoken were from Ma. "You boys worked late in the field today didn't you. I am glad to see our boys are such a help to you Zeke."

Pa looked up. "I sent the boys home three hours ago." He then looked to Thomas, did you not bring your brother home like I'd asked?"

Thomas knew it would be bad to lie, but even worse to not answer and give Aaron something to build on. "No, sir, we came by the house, but after we played at the cabin a minute or two, we went to the meadow to look at the creek."

"So you disobeyed me." Ezekiel rose from the table and started to undo his belt.

"Please, Zeke," their mother interrupted. "Not now. Let the boys eat, then punish them."

"I'd rather have a beating as to eat more of these taters." Aaron said.

At this Ma started to laugh and it brought an evil look from Pa. "If you don't like what the lord has provided, then go to your room."

Aaron hung his head. "No, sir. I'll eat it."

The rest of the meal was ate in silence.

When the dessert was brought out, smiles came on Thomas and Aaron's face. It had been a long time since they'd had a dessert. Blackberry cobbler was the favorite dish of the house and it never failed that Ma would make dessert.

Pa looked at the delicious cobbler and looked up at Ma. "Those weren't here this morning. If you had them you would have put some in the grits."

"I picked them today down by the field. I spent the better part of the afternoon there.

Pa started to open his mouth, but Ma started to cry. "I want you to eat them Zeke. I want to know that I did one good thing for you before I have to send you to judgement."

"Send me to what, woman." Ezekiel started to stand.

From her apron Ma produced pa's pistol. "I saw what you did in the field and I believe these boys saw it too." She sobbed. "How could you?"

"Did you boys see me..." But pa's voice was cut short by a blast that knocked him back out of his chair.

"I'm sorry boys. But, you Pa was consorting with the devil."

"Was that man in black the devil?" Aaron asked.

"Shh..." Ma said. "Now, you eat your cobbler while I take your Pa's body to the field and give him the same burial he gave that child.

Thadd Presley Presents

Born To Fight... Commanded To Kill
Jason Hughes

BLASTING BOMBS AND GRENADES littered the night air. Forest green and jet black choppers swarmed over the chaos and carnage that unfolded beneath them. Sherman tanks crawled like massive iron animals, taking out and crushing anything or anyone in their path. Sirens of medical vehicles and alert towers whistled in disoriented harmony from all directions.

Lieutenant Mac Ledford and his assigned men of platoon six were deep below the ground in their protective bunker. Although they felt secure many feet below the Earth's surface, they had a swirling feeling in their guts and a mandatory mindset that any one of them could be wasted at any given moment. An ominous demise watched over them all. Many men and women had suffered and been snuffed without remorse on this blood drenched soil. Most were sworn enemies that had died by the trained hands among them.

"Lieutenant! It's brutal Hell up there! Our men are dropping off like flies splattered on a fucking windshield!" General Irving said as he began to turn pale. "I... I have a family to go home to! I... I can't die down here like a rat trapped in a cage! I have to go home," he said as he looked around at the rest of the troops. Most of the men seemed to have their fearless heads on straight, but they had just as much fright within their bleeding hearts and battered minds as the general. They'd witnessed more than anyone could imagine, some, on single occasions and others, on multiple. Morbid images were burned into their minds and their memories were scarred and damaged. Several lingering souls roamed free within the vicinity of the ground in which enemy blood was shed on a daily basis.

"You signed on to this team, General. You knew and now it's your God given duty to protect the country and take it like a man. Do you hear me," Lieutenant Ledford replied with eyes of raging fire. The underground fortress they occupied began to vibrate, from the enemy planted land mines being set off a few feet above the giant sized manhole. Small pebbles and grains of sand sprinkled through the cracks in the makeshift ceiling.

"Lieutenant, they're all dying up there. Some of us have got to go and take the front lines. We *have* to." Ralph Peterson said in a demanding but timid tone.

"You're right, Peterson. You have just volunteered. Get up there and make us proud, soldier. Thomson will be right behind you," Lieutenant Ledford replied.

"Me? Shit, man... I didn't..."

"*Thomson*! Do as I say! That's an *order... from my lungs, to your ears*! Do you *hear* me? *Get* your ass up there, *now*!" Lieutenant Ledford roared in a shroud of reigning dominance.

"Colonel Hodges is wounded up there!" Major Walter Jacobs shouted as the other men bickered amongst one another. "I just got confirmation through the wire, Sir!"

"Shit... Oh, shit," Ralph said under his quivering breath, as he geared up and prepared to join the others dying above on the surface. His heart raced as his palms became drenched in perspiration. He felt as if a steaming locomotive was running through his quaking skeletal structure. He could feel his knees and legs dissolving into jelly as he strapped on his last belt of ammunition. A visual cephalic tug of war between returning to Wellington, Virginia to his wife and children at home and meeting his last breath in mere minutes was shifting in his mind. *All I have to do is get to the top of this ladder, stab myself in the fucking neck and come tumbling back down here and... I'll be sent home, maybe even with a Purple Heart;* he thought to himself as he approached the ascending stairway to a nightmarish Hell that was far from imaginary.

As Ralph reached the top and cracked open the hatch, he saw the ruins of who Colonel Hodges used to be. The man who had once been appointed as his mentor upon arrival to the force was now face down in a pool of crimson honor. His legs had been blown off at the knees and he was shot twice in the back of the head. His cracked and weathered helmet was beside him and the United States flag beside him was smeared in fresh blood. Adrenaline-fueled courage and heart-pounding dread began to surge through Ralph's body. He was well aware that at any given moment and within a few petite steps, just as the Colonel before his very eyes, he could be at his terminal stand. Ralph looked below him one last time and saw Gerald Thomson a few feet behind him, shaking in his boots. Gerald was looking up at him with a gaze of cowardly wonder. He could see the medics run by with stretchers transporting mangled, dangling bodies to either the first aid station, or the morgue. As a medic ran past him, he had a hallucinatory vision of his own face looking back at him on the transported body.

Bullets whizzed by Ralph's skull as he looked down at Colonel Hodges' spattered and lifeless shell. His men were scrambling around him in a frenzied panic, dodging, and returning fire. F-18 Fighter jets soared through the night air, cutting through the clouds like fierce razor blades.

The entire surrounding surface was a growing cemetery, both beneath and above the expanding battlefield. Pyres of cremated enemies lit the night sky with a dimly flickering, macabre glows.

Travis Hollingwood, a U.S. Marine of almost four years was blasting away at the enemies in a halo of gunfire next to Gerald. Travis was ruthless when it came to the sacred corps and defending the land of the free and abode of the brave. He was known to most for the most cold and callous acts among his division. Some of his own men watched the way they talked or responded to him, to be sure not to cross him in the wrong light. He once bashed in a bunk intruder's skull in and laughed about it as he bragged amongst the other men. Some of the soldiers even acquired a sick stomach just hearing the tone and sheer happiness he got from the retelling of the story. Each time he told what had happened, it was always with great enthusiasm; as if it were his first time explaining the deadly deed. Some recitals were accompanied with a grimly demonstrated and pantomimed reenactment. "I've already smoked about thirty of those bastards! More and more keep coming," he yelled to Ralph.

Alongside his brutality in defending his honor, Travis had always been a devout soldier that would gladly take a bullet to the face anytime for his beloved country. "Just aim for the knees and as they fall, blast them in the chest," Ralph told the men as they all continued firing at the waves of enemies.

Then, without warning, Travis began to violently convulse. "Hollingwood, what's wrong? *Hollingwood!*" Travis seemed as if he was mentally absent from the battle at hand. Ralph took out his radio. "Lieutenant! Come in! Come in! This is Peterson! Something is wrong with Hollingwood, sir!"

"Shit! What is it, is he injured? *Over,*" Lieutenant

Ledford responded through the fuzzy radio signal that was barely audible in the surrounding gunfire.

"I don't know, he just started to convulse..." Ralph eliminated his own words in dead silence and looked over at Travis, who was no longer convulsing. He looked directly into Ralph's eyes, stood up and walked directly into the line of fire. He held his arms out to his side and let out an unnatural growl before several bullets entered and exited his body.

"Jesus Christ, Hollingwood... What in the hell are you doing! Nooooo!" Ralph screamed in a shocking shriek of disbelief and terror. "Lieutenant Ledford!" Ralph called through the radio, "Hollingwood just pulled a fucking kamakaze!"

"What! Repeat that, Peterson! *Over!*" Lieutenant Ledford demanded.

"He just killed himself! It was suicide! He stood up and just took their bullets! *Over!*" Ralph screamed back to the Lieutenant and the men inside the bunker. Everyone around within earshot heard what he had witnessed. Several stood quiet with their mouths gaping in disbelief.

"I would take a million bullets for my stars and stripes. Always staying true to the red, white, and blue," had always been Travis' battle cry, but no one expected him to just give up to the opposition. He was proud to fight for what he stood for and solely believed in it with a fearless concrete solidity. He had died for his country by the hands of his enemies. Besides the fact that his action was a brave stand to follow through with, it still seemed very strange for him to act out this violent suicide in such a manner. He too, such as many others in his platoon, had a wife and children at home waiting for his safe return.

Ralph could not believe what he had just witnessed. He began to make his way back to the bunker with the Lieutenant and platoon. He felt something press firmly against his head. Ralph froze, like a deer in headlights, awaiting his execution. He was in a stooped position with his left foot in front of him and his sweaty palms above his head. He closed his eyes tightly with the heinous feeling of what would come next. He stood there and awaited a bullet blasting through the back of his skull... Nothing happened. Ralph was two steps from the safety of the bunker. He turned around to see who's hands and barrel was about to send him to his creator... and no one was there. Bullets kept whizzing by him, but he was the only one there. He opened the hatch to the bunker and put his boot on the top step of the ladder. He looked up one last time and then down to guide his way. Something slammed him in the face, knocking him all the way down onto the ground, flat on his back. Many of the soldiers came to his aid. He had been kicked in the face several times and knew just how it felt. He knew what had happened, but was well aware that it was only him at the top of the hatch. "What in the hell is going on up there," Private Brown asked as he rushed to Ralph with a canteen. He let Ralph drink from the canteen, but then Ralph snatched it from Private Brown's hands and started to pour the water all over him. He was trying to bring himself around. Ralph tried to speak, to piece together as many words into an explanation as he could. He tried to explain what happened to his Lieutenant and platoon, without fully understanding it himself.

"I... I don't... know who ... in the bloody hell... it was. Some- someone... kicked... me. They knocked... me down... the ladder," he explained in painful segments. He could barely breathe from the force of landing on his back. The wind was knocked out of him when he hit the ground. He remembered having the gun pressed to his head. It was still fresh on his mind, but he did not mention that part to anyone. Not only was he at a loss for words, he didn't know how to tell them because he knew for certain that

the entire platoon would think he had gone completely
nuts. He knew also that it could've been his mind playing
tricks on him. It happened all too often in the frenzied heat
of battle. It could have been the heat of the uniform and
helmet getting to him. It had to be something logical. It
didn't make sense to him and he knew the others would be
just as confused if he told them.

"Lieutenant! We need more man power up over
here. There aren't many of us left!... *Over!*" Major Carlson
wailed through the radio.

"Roberts, McDaniel, Louis, Nelson! Get up there...
now!" Lieutenant Ledford commanding voice gave the
order. Ray Nelson looked between his legs where he felt
something warm and wet ooze down his leg. It was his
released fear in urination form. He had just been drafted and
was not a fighter at heart. He was there to serve his country,
not to kill others in the process. His family was deeply
Baptist and he believed murder was a sin. He believed in
this very firmly, even in self-defense or protection. "Mr.
Ledford... I... I can't do this. I'm not supposed to be here. I
was drafted. I was supposed to go to college," Ray pleaded.

"For one, Nelson... It isn't Mr. Ledford, it's Lieutenant
Ledford. Do you see this, son!" Lieutenant Ledford pointed
to the patch on his jacket. "It says Lieutenant... *Ell Tee.
Ledford!* and you will do as I *command* or I'll be your fucking
worst nightmare! We don't build character in the corps, we
reveal it! Your only fear is *God*... and Lo and Behold Here...
I... am... Your *God in the flesh*! The saying in the corps is...
Core, God, country, family! Do you understand me?! You
are in the corps! I am your *God!* You will fight and die for
your *country*... and this... is... your... fucking *family!* Now
get up there and fight like a marine! Move, move, move,
move!"

Ray held in his tears with might and mustered the
courage he needed to climb the ladder with the other three

men. As he got out into the open air, he stomach lost the grip on his last meal. It splattered down the steps onto the two men following beneath him. He could feel the implanted bravery beginning to lose its grip. As the men reached ground level, they looked around at just how many dead platoon members laid before them. Michael Roberts had made good friends with Jeffrey Hillstorm. They'd bonded over many relations and common practices in the past. Jeffrey was now lying in the mud with the left side of his face missing. His jaw bone and skull were exposed, oozing liquid crimson life into the earth. As it seeped from his head and onto the ground, Michael shook his head in grief. He was going to miss his dear friend.

George McDaniel had always been a leader back home. He knew he could guide everyone to victory. "Nelson, get your ass on this side! Roberts, *you*, over here! Louis, you get beside me! We are going to form a wall and whatever happens, you keep firing!" He commanded the men as if he'd taken Mac Ledford's position in the platoon.

The three men did as they were ordered and began to fire. Ray could feel a flame of fearlessness slightly escalate as his fellow men surrounded him and fought against the opposition. He gained a sense of self-gratification with each and every kill he scored and each body he saw hit the ground. He looked down at his belt and grabbed a hand grenade. He stood, pulled the pin, and tossed it into the group that was charging with their guns blazing. Scattering body parts flew everywhere in instantaneous, simultaneous dismemberment.

Suddenly, something began to happen to Ray. Something that he could not feel and did not know he was experiencing. "Good shot, Sting Ray! You knocked out an entire... hey! What are you *doing*," George screamed in a gasp of terrified-laced breath.

"What in the... *everybody run*," Michael said as he

looked over at Ray intending to pat him on the back in congratulation. Ray had his last hand grenade placed in his mouth, with the pin sticking out and his hand ready to pull it. He looked back at the men with a blank and empty stare. There was no fear behind the mirrors to his soul. There was no courage... There was a deep pit of pure black nothingness behind his eyes. His finger curled around the pin and he pulled it as the men fled in all directions. The green metal scraped against his teeth as he retracted his steady hand. Ray's head exploded from his shoulders like a rotten watermelon being smashed between a sledge hammer and concrete. Michael got on his radio to report the bizarre incident to the rock hard Lieutenant. "Ledford!   Come in, Ledford! It's McDaniel! It's Ray Nelson, Lieutenant Ledford! He just offed himself with a hand grenade! He just put it in his mouth and pulled the God damn pin!... *Over!*"

"What did you say?! Come again!... *Over*," the Lieutenant blasted in a shroud of gargled fuzz. He was not sure that he'd heard the statement right, but thought he was correct in his assumption. The rest of the platoon below heard it as well. Ralph looked at Lieutenant Ledford in amazed discomfort. He had just witnessed the same phenomenon, but by a different self-mutilating method of operation. *What in the...* Lieutenant Ledford thought, but did not say. He knew the battle was going to be trying and some would not be able to take it and would take the easy way out. *Two of my men in a row*, he thought. He did not train them to destroy themselves, but to kill the opposition.

The remaining three men of the deployed group returned to their guns and continued to fire. The headless body of Ray lay beside them as they fought through the night.

After a few hours, the gun fire became few and far between. This had a calming effect on the soldiers as their tension levels collectively descended to relief. They dodged the occasional bullet and returned a little fire here and there.

At times a lonesome jet or helicopter would fly overhead in intervals of a few hours. Most of the enemy squad had been victoriously depleted, diminished and destroyed. The surviving men even found time to hold the occasional conversation, but all of them had their former battle buddy on their minds. The image of what he had done to himself would be burned in their brains forever, if they happened to live through the night.

"He was a good man. I don't see how he could've done that to himself. Did you see the look in his eyes? It was just... hollow. It was creepy," Michael said as he stared at former soldier and friend Ray Nelson's shoulder topped carcass. His spinal column could be seen protruding from where his neck used to be and his head once mounted. "I can't believe I was subjected to something like that. I could never tell my wife I saw that shit. It would kill her just hearing I had to go through it," Michael said as he bowed his head for a moment of silence. He knew it was right to honor Ray's time by his side, even if it was far from a proper burial. The other two men followed his lead standing in a dead silent flat line of shared sorrow. Other troops came and stood behind them to show their support for the fallen soldier.

"I remember when he first got here. He was such a nice, friendly guy," Fred Quakes announced as he knelt down in the midst of deceased air.

"Butcher... the weak" an anonymous and unfamiliar strange voice announced. The men looked around in disrespected confusion and repressed anger that was ready to be unleashed upon one of their own for the uncalled for comment. George could not resist his inner frustration any longer.

"Which one of you bastards said that?" He lashed out as he stood up, taking a fighting stance. He was ready to challenge one of his own.

"Said what?" Fred asked as he looked around and back at George with a hint of mutual disorder.

"You know what! Who in the hell said it? This one of *our* men we're talking about here, *not* theirs... *ours!* That's the most *dis*respectful load of verbal garbage that I've ever heard," he barked at the group of men standing around him and his headless former platoon pal.

The night crawlers of the ground and air were beginning to circle and swarm the inanimate corpse.

"I... I didn't hear anything," Craig Wilcox said in a cracking but steadily rising tone.

Fred could feel his blood beginning to boil with animosity for the group he was supposed to protect, the group that was required to protect him as well. "Listen... I know one of you disrespected him! I heard it with my own two fucking ears! Now be a man and stand up to your faults... Like a soldier should!" He spat in fire breathing fury and intolerance.

"Sir, I have no idea what you're talking..." Michael said as was quickly knocked to the ground with brutal force.

"Did you see that? What in the shit?" Craig said as Michael stood up and looked at the men like he had never seen them before in his life.

"Are you okay? What happened? It looked like someone punched you square in the face, but your neck didn't budge. I saw it... I mean, Fred seemed like he wanted to hit you... but... but he didn't. He didn't touch you, man. Are you hurt? That was fu..." Before he could spurt another word of condolence, Michael smiled, drew his rifle, and shot Craig directly in the face at point blank range. The other men stood in fear of what he would do next. Fred felt his bodily waste beginning to seep down his pant leg. He was once the leader, and had turned one hundred and eighty degrees in less than a few hours.

Everyone took a few steps back from Michael in fear of what he would do next.

Michael looked down at Craig. "Oh my God! What happened to Roberts? Someone shot him! Radio the Lieutenant! Hurry, someone call the medics!" The rest of the men were silent, as Craig was no longer with them. They were once again speechless, along with turmoil of other emotions, judgments and theories... but not a single pair of cracked lips could speak a solitary word in light of what had just happened. The options that swam around their craniums were either to run like hell, reason with Michael, or open fire on one of their own just as he had done to his own fellow soldier. "If someone isn't going to radio him, I will," Michael said as he pulled out his radio. "Lieutenant! Lieutenant! Come in! It's Wilcox! Someone shot Wilcox! There's barely anyone out here! No one saw who did it! His face is gone! I'm pretty sure it was at close range! *Over!*" Michael announced all this in disorientated oblivion. The rest of the men stood in silence around him and listened as Michael reported his own callous and cold blooded murder in a third person point of view.

For once, Lieutenant Mac Ledford was at a loss of words. He couldn't respond as he tried to grip onto shreds of dangling lucidness. He sat below his troop of men with his head between his hands. Ralph overheard every word from the dark corner in which he was huddled. He had seen similar occurrences in his men first hand before and had a front row seat to the destruction. He'd been subjected to manhandling by something that he could not see, even though he knew something was there.

"There is hardly anyone left. One of you had to have seen who did this," Michael shouted at the men around him.

"Are... are... you... sure that you're... in your right mind right now... Roberts?" Fred asked timidly as he took another step back and away from Michael.

"What in the hell do you mean? Why are you asking a question like that? Look at him! He's as dead as a fucking coffin nail! Do you not see him lying there, Quakes?"

Fred and the other men subtly eyeballed one another and tried to keep their attention directed anywhere but on Michael. They had a feeling that at any time one of them could be next.

***

"MORE OF YOU WILL die," an unknown voice invisibly blew through the wind from an unknown set of vocal chords and landed upon very short fused ears.

"*You're* going to die if you don't stop acting like this!" Fred blurted with as much control over his words as he had over his bowel movements.

"What in the hell did I do? Where does this *hostility* come from?!" Michael asked in a wondrous absence of clarity.

"You shot him, Roberts. You fell back, hit on the ground, got up and blew his fucking face to smithereens! Do you not recall that? You defiled Nelson's name and disrespected his honor... and now you just said more of us will die! Whose side are you on, anyway?" Fred blared these words in passionate anger. Then in the middle of Fred's rant, Jeremy Louis drew a pistol from his belt and slid the barrel under his protective head gear and pulled the trigger. Fred's helmet cracked in half as the bullet pierced it and he fell flat on his face.

"What in the fucking shit?!" Michael screamed in terror as he drew his gun and pointed it at Jeremy. "It was *you*! You sick son of a bitch! You're killing off the only men we have left! *We*... don't you get it? You... are one... of *us!*" Michael shouted as the rest ran like scattered fire ants on a burning hill back to the bunker. They were gripped by the fear of losing their lives to either of the two men.

As they reached the bunker entrance, their heads suddenly slammed together, knocking them senseless for a few moments. They felt an uneasy tension in their necks as it happened, but could not remember a thing when they came back into the real world. Then they noticed blood on each other's foreheads. The two stared at each other as Jeremy came walking towards them. They hurried into the bunker and quickly threw the metal latch closed, locking the only way to safety for the other men left above ground. "Lieutenant! They've all gone ape shit up there! They're killing each other off... Our own men! What in God's green Hell is going on around here!"

The hatch above started to shake as someone tried with relentless might to get in where the brain scrambled platoon once felt secure. Their security was abandoning them little by little.

Lieutenant Ledford watched with half attention as the others reached ground level. The hatch above the ladder continued to jerk up and down rapidly. A fuzzy frequency began to occupy Mac's radio. A scratchy voice spoke through the radio on his side. It was a malicious articulation that they had never encountered. The strange message cracked and faded in and out as if it were transmitted from a great distance. "The end... is... upon... you all. Everyone... will... be... wiped... out."

The soldiers could feel one another's bones beginning to give out around them as well as their own. An equal amount of fear consumed the cave of what use to be filled with strong men. "Who in the hell is this? Whose radio did you acquire? This is the Lieutenant! Answer me!... *over!*"

Lieutenant Ledford hissed in obscured fear. Caution and hesitation were blanketed under his solid demeanor. He knew deep within himself that his courage was beginning to crack and crumble like a sand castle being washed away by the rising tide. "

"All... of you... shall... parish... one... by... one," multiple voices announced on each of the soldier's radios, followed by loud and deep cackles. The ear scorching, simultaneous snickers sounded like that of ten thousand damned and condemned entities. They were surely inhuman and armed with inhumane intent in store for the survivors of the platoon. The men collectively turned pale as if they were already postmortem piles of flesh, walking in a daze to their summoning tombstones.

Just when the entire platoon was about to stain their camouflage apparel, a subtle knock began to clang at the wooden door above the ladder. It was the only way out and the only way in and someone was trying to reach them. "It's probably Louis. Let him stay out there, maybe one of them will get him before dawn," Private Brown said as he looked at the rest of the men. Another subtle blow wrapped upon the wood as the men looked at one another in confusion. "Someone help... me! I've lost... my baby! I'm wounded! Help... me!" It was an Asian woman's voice shouting through the slits in the small square entrance way.

***

"SHOULD WE FALL FOR that none-sense?" Private Brown asked the Lieutenant. Mac raised his head and shrugged his shoulders. His sharp wit and fire fueled determination was beginning to dwindle with every curve ball thrown his way. "You heard what was said over the radios! Don't answer it! I don't know what they have over there, but she's the bait, it's all a trap... and it's set for *us!*" Private

Brown snarled.

"No... I... I saw her earlier when I was helping first aid with some of the fallen. She did have a baby. Even though she's on their side, she's harmless and innocent. We need to help her," Gerald replied in a sympathetic cradle of reason.

"I have something for her," Private Brown added.

"Well, I'm letting her in. She needs us and she's absolutely harmless, besides the fact that she's carrying a child." Gerald said.

"She just said that she lost her child. Let her go find it," Private Brown replied.

"I'm letting her in, so shut the fuck up," Gerald said as he made his way for the ladder. He climbed to the top, amidst protests, and opened it. There was no woman, but a face that was very recognizable. It was Jeremy. He had Michael's severed head in one hand, a large machete in the other and a sinister grin stretched from ear to ear.

"No!" Gerald screamed as the blade went straight down his throat and through the back of his neck. He fell backwards to the ground without touching a single step. The ground bloomed a red tinged flower around his head. Jeremy began to crawl down into the bunker. All of the men felt as if they had suddenly transformed into scared little girls. They didn't know what to do about the situation. Jeremy got to the bottom of the stairs and looked at the soldiers in a baffled state.

"What are you all doing? I'm one of you! No... don't!" He pleaded as his entire former squad opened fire on him without thinking twice or giving him a verbal warning. They knew exactly who they were killing, but had the foggiest clue who they were actually shooting. They only knew that he could have taken their lives before they had a chance to protect themselves. Private Brown used Jeremy and Gerald's stacked and motionless bodies as a stepladder to get to the wooden steps, and shut the entrance. He peeked his eyes through the door and found no signs of an Asian woman. A few feet away, Michael's headless body was lying in the dirt.

"Damn," Private Brown mumbled as he closed the door and made his way back down the ladder.

"I don't know what is going on here, but there's none of them left and we're killing ourselves off as if we are the enemy." Lieutenant Ledford proclaimed. He couldn't believe what was unfolding before him and between his own platoon. He began to piece together the unimaginable in his scattered mind. *We've killed most, if not all of them... and they are coming back for us... in spirit.* He thought this, but could never vocalize this theory to the soldiers. It sounded too unreal, too fantastic, even to him, but he had no other explanation as to what could be happening. He did not want his own men to think he had flown the coo-coo's nest and went bat shit crazy from years of overlapping mental scars.

With this denial in mind, he knew a haunting could very well be possible, because everyone was experiencing the same strange occurrences. Just as the once fearless leader was gathering his thoughts and the rest of his men were losing their minds, they received another simultaneous broadcast over their radios. "Most... of... you... are... dead. The... rest... of you... will be dying... soon." The voice said as it multiplied into many. "Mark... our... words. Your time... is coming."

The men gazed at one another in hysteria and paranoia as the message ended with: "These... are... our... grounds."

"We're fucking shredded dog meat, every last one of us. They're silently leading us... or making us lead ourselves, blindly to the slaughter. *Look* at us... What's *left* of us. We need to get the hell *out* of here," Private Brown proclaimed this with a dreadful taste in his mouth. He knew what he was saying was against the code of honor and sounded cowardly, but he didn't care.

"I agree, Brown. We'll wait here until first light. At the hour of dawn, we're loading up and moving out, got it all of you?" Lieutenant Ledford said as he shifted his eyes across the small group of men.

"There's only a handful of us left and frankly, I don't know who in the hell I can trust among you," Private Brown said as he looked around the bunker.

"Well, we'll just have to see what happens. Until then, everyone shut off their radios. We don't necessarily need them due to the fact that this is all of us... Isn't it?" Lieutenant Ledford asked as he reached down and powered down his own. The rest of the men complied and followed his lead.

Most of the crew tried to get some sleep as soon as they possibly could so the hours would rush by and they could leave out at dawn. Lieutenant Ledford and Private Brown stayed up talking a little while after the rest of the men were sound asleep. "Private, tell me in your honest opinion what in the hell you think is happening here. I mean, this is fucked up beyond all recognition. In the years I've been in the service, I've never seen anything like this... Never."

"I don't know, Sir. I didn't think I could trust Ralph over there. Then it started happening to the others as well. I don't get what it could be," Private Brown replied in a watered down tone. He wanted to make sure not to wake the others. "I have my theories, but I don't want to be committed after leaving this hellhole. I'm never telling anyone about what we've experience down here if we get out of this alive."

"I don't blame you, Sir. I don't think I will either. My family would disown me, especially my wife's side.

They would think I'm loony as shit. I mean, yeah... Mental delusions and flashbacks are a well- known reaction from war. A lot have been through it... but nothing like this. This seems to be happening right before everyone's very eyes. We can't all be going mental, ya know. It's just too damn freaky. I wouldn't know how to explain it to anyone."

"Ten – four that, Private... Ten – four that. I feel the same way. As far as I'm concerned, this is staying between me and you men. Not a soul is going to know about this. I wouldn't even know where to begin."

Ralph rolled around in his sleep as Lieutenant Ledford and Private Brown conversed through most of the night. Then, he let out subtle moans of discomfort from his not so peaceful slumber. *They're going to kill us all. We can't escape them. There is nowhere for us to run or hide. We're all going to die down here... or up there.* The words drifting from Ralph's hallucinating mind as he journeyed through the land of Nod where of the morbid visions he'd witnessed above the soiled surface replayed themselves through his mind, over and over again. "None... of you... will... escape. The... time... of suffering... is among... you all." Ralph awoke a few hours before the sun was supposed to rise. He knew for certain that the voice in his head was not the voice of his own reasoning. It was surely someone else's and it did not come in peace, nor share the gift of any kind of hope whatsoever. "You... will all... join us!" Fuzzy voices of a malevolent tone announced. Every soldier in the bunker heard the same voice, at the same time all the men were jolted out of their sleep. "Our radios... We turned them off and they are powered up!"

Ralph screamed as he jumped up from his sleeping bag. The rest of the men looked down at their power knobs. All of them were set to the *off* position, but were still transmitting as if they were at full volume. "What in the hell is going on here?" Private Brown wailed as he looked down at his own radio.

"We... are... waiting... and you all... will join... us... in the place... in which... you... have accommodated... for us. We... are not... dead... as you... will be... This... is our... home. You... are... invited," the simultaneous voices announced through the radios.

"The batteries! Take out the God damn batteries!" Private Brown demanded as the men followed his given order of a possible solution. All of the batteries spilled onto the floor. "You... cannot... escape... your doom." several voices continued to announce. Private Brown jumped up, threw his radio to the ground and began smashing it to pieces under his boot. The rest of the men followed his lead once more. Scattered parts of dismembered radio units decorated the bunker. Each of the men were all silently expecting something else to happen. They stayed awake with their ears opened and their eyes peeled until the sun's morning beams seeped through the cracks of the wooden door. Until then, the voices of retribution remained silent.

The exhausted and starved platoon started loading up their belongings and gearing up for the trip out of the hole and hopefully to a station of safety miles from the occupied territory. What they didn't need to take, they agreed on leaving behind. There were no phones to call their families for miles. The only collective hope was to make it home alive, in one piece, and with a sane head still screwed on their shoulders.

"Alright, men... Let's get the rest of our supplies and surplus and get the hell out of here!" Lieutenant Ledford said with a new morning wind of self-confidence. He knew that once they were far away from the battle site, that everything would be okay and they would be able to go on living their lives. At least until another war.

On the bright side, Mac Ledford had a feeling that he and his men... his platoon... his "soldiers," would still be alive to fight at least one more battle, if need be.

The group of green attired men mounted everything onto their backs and made their way to the ladder. Private Brown and Ralph took it upon themselves to move the bodies of Jeremy and Gerald so they could make it up the ladder safely. Ralph closed his eyes tightly and removed the machete from Gerald's pie hole (as he lovingly called it) with a quick jerk. He may need the morbid, blood stained keepsake for future hassles. A trail of blood slithered behind their former platoon mates' bodies as they were dragged out of range. One by one, the men began to climb the ladder to the outside world and out of the dark earth. Lieutenant Ledford bravely guided the way up to the hatch as he unlocked it and crawled out onto the body and blood scattered sand. There was not a copter, tank, or jet in sight. The morning sun gave a radiant glow to the skies above. Private Brown took a deep inhale of the fresh air outside, laced with the wretched stench of decay and putrid rot. That did not bother him; they were all used to it.

In the distance, an Asian woman was on her belly, lying lifeless in the sand. They were all just happy to be out of the ground where they'd spent their last two weeks. The men looked around at the dirt beneath them. There were several bodies, limbs, and military accessories scattered about. Not a walking enemy was in sight as far as their relieved eyes could wander.

"Well, men... We're going home... We're fucking going home," Private Brown said as he looked around with a relaxed grin of confirmation. Ralph looked down into the pit in which he thought he would never have a chance to leave safe or alive. He exhaled and kicked the wooden door closed. "We're going to make it, men. We're going to get out of here and back home to our loved ones after all," Private Brown gleefully announced as a tear rolled down his cheek. He gave Lieutenant a high five, along with the rest of the survivors around him. Each man slapped hands with the other and gave a small brotherly hug and pat on the back. They had worked together as a team. "Over... and ... out," a voice whispered through the still air. "What did you say?" Private Brown asked Lieutenant Ledford.

"I was about to say let's get the hell out of here and blow this snow-cone stand, hahaha! Yeah!" Lieutenant Ledford said as he jumped in the air with boyish joy.

"No, I mean..."

Private Brown turned around to see Ralph staring him straight in the eyes. "Die," Ralph said in a voice that was clearly not his own. He shoved the machete straight into Private Brown's stomach, pulled it upward and shoved the blade completely through his back with a jerking twist. Blood poured from the Private's mouth in a streaming fountain of red as he slid off of the blade and backwards, onto the ground with the others. "No, Ralph, you son of a bitch! The Lieutenant screamed with an emotional cocktail of fear, confusion and anger swirling in his bloodshot eyes. Ralph let out a growling cackle as he tilted his head back and looked into the sky. The other men could not move, blink, or believe what they had just witnessed. Lieutenant Ledford drew his pistol, raised it and blasted Ralph's Adam's apple from his throat. He proceeded to scream maniacally as he relentlessly kicked Ralph's motionless, bleeding body where it rested in the dirt. The other men ran over to the Lieutenant and tried to stop him. They knew he had gone completely insane at this point. The usually nonvocal soldier in the platoon, Mills Bradley, tried to restrain the once sane Lieutenant Mac Ledford.

"Lieutenant, you have to stop this! You're going crazy! Stop, please! Let's just get the hell out of here, *now!* That was the mission at hand, right?" Mills asked in a forceful attempt of reasoning.

"You... are not... going... anywhere... maggot," the

Lieutenant proclaimed in a foreign tongue of deep scold. Lieutenant Ledford slowly turned to Mills and pressed his pistol firmly under his chin, clamping his bottom jaw to a shut position. "Please... no," Mills whimpered through his teeth as it became his final murmur of his few ever spoken words and Mill's fearless leader squeezed off two quick rounds. Sending the bullets through his chin and into his head.

All of his men had become one with the earth. The souls of those the platoon had executed were not done just yet. They were still roaming the land and had one last score to settle. Lieutenant Mac Alan Ledford, grade 0-2, of Platoon six, raised his pistol to his face, he clenched the cold metal barrel between his grinding teeth, almost to the point of cracking them... and pulled the trigger. The empty shell relieved of its bullet hit the ground a few seconds prior to the fallen soldier as the diabolic entity fled his once incarnate carcass.

"Now... we are even," words whispered throughout the air from an unseen tongue, but clearly presented resonance.

The Lieutenant joined the rest of his fearless platoon as they were left to mummify in the hot sun, which still had another fourteen hours to pulsate down upon their mangled remains. A subtle echo of sinister laughter continued to carry through the blazing winds. The countless enemies in which they had defended against and mercilessly slaughtered, for their own protection and honor of their country, had the last lingering machination among the unburied men of what use to be Platoon six. The ominous eyes of the seer of wandering souls observed among the dead as their spirits continued to swarm the land. The vengeful apparitions that lingered throughout the perimeter would always refer to this torment coated territory... as their eternal dwelling domain.

Thadd Presley Presents

Poisoned Meat
Jonathan Moon

EVERYTHING HAPPENED SO FAST.

Bobby blinks the blood out of his eyes and tries to catch his breath. He can't feel his legs and for that he is thankful. He lays his rifle across his lap and uses his hands to crawl to a tree behind him. Agony flares in his back as he drags his smashed legs away from the carnage of the clearing. His ears are ringing from all the sudden screams and close range gunfire. The high buzzing sound makes understanding what just happened to him near impossible. His mind flashes back to this morning with more vivid clarity than his gory current situation.

***

HE WOKE WITH THE sun, excited about his first day as a "hunter." Bobby splashed cold water on his face from the pan next to his bed and bound from his tent into the dawn. He bent down and zipped his tent closed quickly before putting on his gloves. He was in a hurry but he allowed himself a minute to soak in the beauty around the camp. He breathed the cold mountain air into his lungs and he rushed off through the rows of tents to the make-shift garage.

206

Bobby was born and raised in the city but the cities belonged to the dead now. The camp was called "Resurrection" and it was located high on a mountain ridge; far above the shambling dead. Tall evergreens surrounded the camp and the 400 campers had built a few tall look out/ defense towers that rose even further into the sky. Bobby loved the view from the towers and unlike others that had tower watch duty he never complained. From the top he could see down into the venison cages below or clear to the once lush valley floor at the foot of their mountain. Others complained about the smell of deer shit and the freezing wind. He knew once he turned eighteen he would be able bodied enough to become a "hunter" and that day had finally arrived.

David was standing right outside the door to the garage smoking a cigarette when Bobby approached. The older man nodded and stepped to one side allowing Bobby into the garage where the hunters gathered. David crumbled out his smoke and followed Bobby inside. Bobby walked into the room and everyone turned to look at him. He stared back at the men and women he admired and smiled nervously. Blake and Todd both nodded to him and Shannon smiled but no one else said anything. Their eyes were all cold and Bobby had shivered slightly as they bore into him.

"Our new hunter," David growled at them, "Say 'Hello'."

A meek chorus of greetings and uttered introductions made Bobby blush and David nodded at his flushed cheeks with a small grin. David strode to the wall and waited for everyone to surround him.

"This should be a nice easy run today folks," he told them with the confidence of a born leader.

"We haven't had any sighting of any "black-bloods", human or beast, in at least three days," he told them over his shoulder while tapping on the map tacked to the wall.

"That doesn't make me excited," Buck grumbled, "It makes me nervous."

Buck was one of the largest men in the camp and he was noticeably the biggest hunter. His size afforded him great attitude and he often shared it. He had been a bully before the dead started rising and that hadn't changed any when they ate everyone he ever knew. He had been one of the first to camp and he had been a steadfast defender of the camp but he really was an intolerable prick most of the time. David smiled at Buck as if he expected Buck to grumble.

"What are you smiling about?" Buck asked, anger twitching at his lips.

"I know why you're nervous, Big Man," David said shaking his head slowly; "you are thinking that something is scaring everything else away, aren't ya?"

Surprise sparkled in Buck's eyes and he nodded suspiciously at David.

"Noted. You, Blake, and Carol are on the four wheelers. Load up the big guns if it makes you feel safer…"

Buck interrupted him with a growl, "I'm not that worried about me, Little Man, I'm worried for the camp…"

David waved his hand and interrupted Buck back, "I didn't mean to hurt your feelings or make you feel challenged. Let me rephrase, I think you should load up the big guns, I'd sure feel safer."

Bobby swallowed hard as the mood in the cold room bristled with Buck's anger. David knew Buck to be a bully but he wasn't afraid as he'd dealt with bigger, badder men; dead and alive. David could fight the dead (or black-bloods as they were referred to in camp) and he knew how to track them. Not that human black-bloods needed much tracking but their undead animal counterparts still had their base instincts and that was a very dangerous thing for the band of survivors.

Shannon spoke quickly before anyone else could, "The camp would feel safer if we were out checkin' traps and laying new ones instead of sittin' in here primin' your testosterone to hunt dead things."

David and Buck exchanged looks but any argument was stopped dead in its tracks. David broke the hunters into their four member teams and the twelve living humans set out for the wall that surrounded the camp to face the death all around them.

***

THE RINGING IN BOBBY'S ears has tuned down to a loud hum and he can hear someone nearby gagging and taking deep ragged breathes. He pulled himself alongside the trunk of an ancient evergreen so he doesn't have to look at the small clearing and the crimson and black splattered and pooling there. He wipes blood off his face but his hands are numb inside his gloves and blood smears into his eyes. He winces while pulling his gloves off and dropping them next to his broken form. Every movement hurts. His hands are shaking and pale, but they wipe the blood from his eyes.

Bobby leans back against the tree trunk and tries to take deep breaths. He knows he has to calm down; there is no point in freaking out now. But every time he inhales a sharp fiery pain flares up and down his left side. He chokes on his breath and spits a mouthful of bright red blood all over himself. With the blood comes a release of pressure in his chest and he seizes the chance to lean forward. He looks from his broken and twisted legs, where each foot is pointed too far in odd directions, to the bloody trail he left dragging himself to shelter. The small swath of pine needles and gore ends abruptly at the corpse of the half rotted black blood elk.

***

BOBBY CHECKED THE STOCK in his semi-auto rifle twice while the group waited for the wall to be raised. The only opening in the entire wall was one ten foot wide section where the wall would slide up through a system of jerry-rigged pulleys. The entrance was built near the bottom of a steep rock outcropping to prevent any wandering black blood from finding the one weak spot in the tall log wall. Built high above and on either side of the gate were two guard planks each occupied by one heavily armed man. Neither sentry looked down on the group as they gate rose slowly. As soon as the gate allowed enough room Buck roared his four-wheeler out and up the rocks. The two other four wheelers, driven by Blake and Carol, followed. The remaining nine filed two by two out the opening and up the rocks on foot.

Bobby allowed everyone past until he was the last. A wide smiling Todd settled in next to him. As they walked through the gate Todd asked, "How long you been inside, Bobby?"

Bobby didn't look back at Todd; just focused on the steep path cut up the wall. He barely remembered entering the camp. Even walking up the same path he walked down at some point couldn't bring back his blacked out memories.

After a moment of going unanswered Todd said, "That long, huh?"

Bobby flushed and turned to the ever smiling man, "I'm sorry, sir, I don't remember much about before I got here."

Todd smiled and pulled a floppy fisherman hat from his vest and pulled it over his shiny bald head. He chuckled, a warm friendly sound that calmed Bobby's nervousness, and told Bobby, "First thing, easy with that "Sir" shit. Nobody out here likes to be called "Sir'. Well, maybe Buck but he's an asshole." Todd chuckled again and then said, "Second, feel lucky you can block it out."

"Yeah," Bobby sighed, "I hear them at night. You know, people that remember."

Todd smiled his good natured grin and nodded. They climbed the rest of the rocky path in silence. Once at the top Bobby stood and stared out in near disbelief. The camp sat high atop a ridge and the survivors burnt the valley around them to ash. The mountain side had been furiously logged for the wall but otherwise left untouched as the hard terrain and thick trees offered seclusion and natural defense. As he stared out thru the trees to the blackened valley below, memories flooded back to Bobby and they overwhelmed him. He knelt on the ground and tears warmed his eyes. Only Todd was standing close enough to notice and he helped Bobby back to his feet before anyone else saw his momentary breakdown.

Bobby wiped his eyes and managed a small smile, "I *was* lucky."

"Yeah, well, now you can move on," Todd told him quiet enough no one else heard.

David turned from the larger group to face Bobby and Todd. "Just my luck," he said to them, "I get the funny guy and the new guy."

Todd bowed and snickered, "Your lucky day, Dave, our shit luck, but your lucky day."

"Hey, you can switch with Shannon and go hang out with Buck if ya want," David smirked back.
"Easy, asshole," Todd warned through his wide grin.

Bobby laughed out loud and David's smile matched Todd's.

"You ever been hunting, Bobby?" David asked as they walked to Carol and her camouflaged four-wheeler.

"Once, when I was just a boy," Bobby answered honestly.

"I think a better question would be "You killed a mess of dead things yet, Bobby?"" Todd interjected with a grin.

"Good point and I was working towards it," David answered before walking over to Carol.

Carol and David talked and pointed downhill while Bobby checked his stock for the fifth and sixth time. Todd just chuckled softly and shook his head at the nervous kid. Carol fired her ATV to life and drove the direction she and David had been pointing. David nodded after her and all three started walking down the hill.

"We're checking traps today, Bobby, as I said before should be easy, but with black bloods you never know. Our cages are strong but they can't hold everything. Undead animals are fiercer and way more reckless than their living counterparts. Same rules apply, shoot them in their fucking heads," David told Bobby.

Bobby nodded his understanding and David continued, "Make no mistake, Bobby, we are hunters and we are hunting. We are hunting poisoned meat and it fights back."

***

THE BLACK BLOOD ELK is lying in a puddle of gore in the middle of the small clearing. Even though Bobby blew its decayed brains out of its rotted skull, it still looks to be staring him down with one hungry dead eye. Half its face and head are missing, and broken chunks of elk teeth are scattered around. One gray antler points to the sky with blood slowly dripping down it. Bobby clinches and unclenches his fists while he stares at the massive twice dead beast. His body is getting cold from blood loss and he stops clenching in favor of shaking.

To the left of the elk Bobby can see what's left of David

and it almost makes him sick. He gags and then chokes on the gag. Pain flares from his side and chest as he turns back away from David. Bobby sees Carol next; she is broken and bent in a bloody heap. Her corpse is near the pines where her four-wheeler was tossed by the rampaging black blood elk. On the other side of the elk Bobby spots Todd; gagging and choking on his own blood. He rolls weakly in the dirt with his hands held tight but useless at the massive wound on his throat. Bobby watches wordlessly as Todd's gags turn to gurgles and his hands flop away from his torn out throat. Bobby sobs and looks behind the elk corpse at the destroyed cage covered in both fresh and black blood.

***

DAVID AND TODD LEAD Bobby up and down the steep paths with the pace of men eager to either kill something or get the hell home. The hunters had placed traps ranging in size from small enough for rodents to large enough for bears. Dozens of traps were scattered across the forest floor and Bobby got his first chance to catch his breath when they came upon a cage containing a yowling and hissing undead bobcat. Fury darkened its dead eyes as it saw them and it crouched and drew its claws from skinless paws. David blew its brains out and trembled noticeably.

"Not good fellas, not good at all," David told them, all humor gone from his tone, "a predator like this could infect an ungodly amount of smaller creatures. The smaller the black blood creature is the harder they are to stop spreading. Birds, easy prey for this fella, can fly over the wall. An infected rodent will gnaw through our wall and the camp will be chaos and death before we have any chance to stop it."

They used a long barbed hook Todd carried to pull the thing out of the trap before David dug into his pack and pulled out a small slab of fresh meat to re-bait it. As they started for their last stop, a small clearing with a big cage, David finished, "Black bloods can still hunt. It is part of their instinct when they are hungry. They are always ravenous and vicious. I swear to god above, dead things are stronger than living things, animals and humans. That is what makes an undead natural predator so god damned dangerous."

He was going to say more but just then they entered the clearing. Both David and Todd raised their guns the instant they saw the mangled cage. David grabbed his walkie-talkie and made a frantic cry to Carol while Bobby raised his gun and stepped closer to David to allow him some cover.

"Let's hope to god that bobcat was in this cage first," Todd said in a vain attempt to ease the fear they all felt.

"Yeah, I don't think so," David said while scanning the tree line through his scope, "I don't know what happened but there is fresh blood and black blood. We could be looking at two of them."

They sat in nervous silence, guns at the ready, until the roar of the ATV cut thru the surrounding forest. Carol pulled into the clearing and turned off the ATV. She looked at the men and then at the smashed cage. The sweet smell of decay reeked around them and the air seemed to stir. She looked nervously at them and while she was reaching for her gun the black blood elk thundered out of the tree line and charged her.

***

BOBBY CAN HEAR THE sound of people and ATVs approaching. He has lost so much blood he can hardly sit up. His torso feels heavy and it tries to pull him to the ground. He almost lets it but then Todd twitches. Bobby gasps and strains to stay sitting up. Todd's fingers curl and uncurl. Bobby grabs his gun but drops it when it seems hundreds of pounds heavier than it did before. He grunts and pulls it on to his lap.

Todd's eyes blink and he starts to roll back and forth, spilling blood out of his wounds.

Bobby checks his clip, finds it empty, and he begins searching his pockets for a new clip.

Todd rolls awkwardly into a sitting position and he stares at Bobby with black eyes and black blood flowing from his throat.

Bobby attempts to slam the clip in the gun but he doesn't have the strength to make it lock.

Todd snarls and stumbles to his feet never taking his eyes off of Bobby.

Bobby strains and tries to slam the clip home but fails.

Todd takes a few slow steps forward as if he relearning how to walk.

Bobby screams in pain and frustration as he slams the clip one last time. It clicks loudly into place.

Todd growls and stumbles for Bobby.

Bobby raises his rifle but gets distracted by a shadow moving in the trees behind Todd.

Todd slaps the rifle away from Bobby and falls on him. He howls and blood splatters Bobby's face. At the same moment Todd snaps forward his head explodes with the crack of high powered rifle fire. His corpse falls next to Bobby's. Bobby's ears are ringing again. Buck and all the others rush into the small carnage filled clearing. Blake stands over Carol's now twitching corpse and fires a round into her skull. Buck walks over to Bobby and points his rifle at Bobby's forehead.

Bobby pushes the barrel away weakly and tries to talk but blood is bubbling in his throat. He wants to warn them. Buck kicks his arm away from the gun and points the gun back at Bobby's head. Bobby rolls to the side so he doesn't have to see it coming. In the split second before the bullet slams through his head he sees the black blood cougar crouched in the tree line behind Buck.

Author Page

Thadd Presley lives in Lancing, Tennessee and has written three books. He writes poetry and plays bass guitar. His second short story book is coming out in 2012 entitled "A Band of Black." You can find many of his stories and poems at his website www.thaddpresley.com Currenly he is an editor and works with writers from all over the world.

Michael Dortmundt is a modern horror writer in the style of Lovecraft, Machen and Poe. He is currently residing in Florida and attending med school and engaged to be married.

Todd Martin grew up in a small town in Kentucky where he spent his time watching 80's slasher flicks, reading comic books, and writing short stories about characters from The Masters of the Universe, Transformers, and other cartoons. He has been a huge horror fan his entire life and had a collection of short stories called "Nightmare Tales" published in 2006. Since then he has had many other short stories published in several collections and had "The Gardener," a novel he co-wrote with his wife Trish published. In addition to writing short stories and novels he also enjoys writing screenplays as well. He currently lives in Kentucky with Trish, their cat Buffy, and their wiener dog Cujo.

S. Wayne Roberts is currently writing his debut novel, Two Weeks Notice; as well as a short story collection, Foibles

& Follies. He's been published over 50 times in various magazines, anthologies and collections; both print and e-book form, prose and poetry, comedies and tragedies. He also, as Steve Roberts, writes nonfiction, mostly comedy, for Cracked Magazine, Comstock Greeting Cards, as well as various works to be found here and there. S. Wayne Roberts, Steve to most, resides in the Baltimore area of his beloved Maryland, with his supportive family, where he enjoys taking life by the Bay one day at a time.

Charlotte Emma Gledson currently resides in the south-coastal town of Gosport , UK . Her heart however yearns to return to her roots in the Northwest of England, specifically Cumbria . With over 30 stories and poems published in Anthologies and Magazines, including 'The Serial Killer Magazine', Charlotte is also penning a supernatural novel entitled 'Bluebells for my Baby'. Her collection of 'unsettling' stories, 'The Lonely Tree and Other Twisted Tales of Torment' is available at all good book retailers.

Married with four gregarious children and a collection of ventriloquist dummies and porcelain dolls, she finds time relaxing sipping wine, singing Karaoke and going on paranormal investigations.

Charlotte has reviewed a few novels and is happy for authors to submit their work to her. Send to charlotte@gledson.co.uk
For all updates visit www.charlottemmagledson.com

JD Stone is the pen name for Daniel Fabiani, a native New Yorker with a bullet mouth and sharp opinion. His stories have been featured in Sins & Tragedies, Pill Hill Press, Library of Horror Press and more. He's writer currently disguised in scrubs at his day job, but is breaking out as a journalist. You can contact him at: SolitarySpiral@gmail.com

Nate Burleigh lives in Vancouver, Washington with his wife and three children. He has published short horror stories in multiple anthologies, magazines and ezines. Some of his most recent work can be found in the anthologies "Bleed and They Will Come", and "Soup of Souls". His debut novel "Sustenance" is currently published by *Panic Press* and available at lulu.com. Please stop by his Facebook page or his blog natedburleigh.blogspot.com and let him know how you liked the story.

Jason Hughes grew up in Texas. He has been a lifelong fan of the Horror genre for thirty - five years and counting. He graduated *The Tom Savini's Special Effects Make- Up Program* in 2004 and still does Special Effects today. He is the Editor the anthology, *Moral Horror*. He is a contributing Writer for *The Houston [Horror] Examiner* and *ScreamTV*, and Film, Book and Magazine Reviewer for *Horrornews.net*. His writings can be found in such anthologies as *Nocturnal Illumination, Ladies and Gentlemen of Horror 2010, Soup of Souls, The Nine Circles of Hell,* and *House of Horror Magazine, Beyond the Dark Horizon Magazine* and *Twisted Dreams Magazine* among many others. He is a multi-published (and transferred to audio) Poet. Jason was chosen as one of the top ten best new Horror Authors of 2009 - 2011. He has written screenplays for Rebellious Cinema, Sick Flick Productions & American – International Pictures (released *The Amityville Horror* and much more). He is also a Drummer, t-shirt Printer, Sky Diver and avid fifteen year Supporter of *The West Memphis Three* (www.wm3.org).

Stacy Bolli is a busy single mother of three beautiful children. She hails from the sun soaked state of Florida. She has several published pieces in anthologies, including Sins and Tragedies, DOA: Stories of Extreme Horror, and Ollie, published by Dopamalovi Books to name a few.